Long-Term Care

Cover Photographs

In the bottom left photo Doris Martini, Betsy's mother-in-law and Betsy's husband John Martini pose with Milo, Betsy and John's golden doodle.

The other three pictures are from 123RF.com with the following photo credits: Top left: Wang Tom, Top right: Fabio Formaggio, Bottom right: Cathy Yeulet.

Long-Term Care

for
Activity Professionals, Social Services Professionals, and Recreational Therapists
Seventh Edition

Elizabeth (Betsy) Best-Martini, MS, CTRS
Mary Anne Weeks, MPH, SSC
Priscilla Wirth, MS, RHIA

Published and distributed by

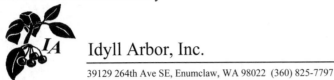

Idyll Arbor, Inc.

39129 264th Ave SE, Enumclaw, WA 98022 (360) 825-7797

Idyll Arbor Editor: Thomas M. Blaschko

Apple Valley Post-Acute Rehab calendar provided by Calendars USA.
AgeSong University assisted living calendar provided by AgeSong.

ISBN 9781611580617

Contents

Table of Forms

Index of Activities

Acknowledgments

This book was created from the many years of combined direct clinical experiences, teaching, and consulting expertise of the three authors. It was not only these experiences that melded together in the philosophy of the work, but, much more important, the people whom we each have worked with who inspired us and taught us about what one needs in order to live a life with meaning and purpose.

There are many familiar faces of friends and family throughout these years who have left an imprint on my life and work and I wish to acknowledge them in this book: Thanks and love to my treasured husband John who believes not only in me but also in the importance of my work, Aunt Barbara who encouraged and taught me how to venture into this business, my grandmother who taught me appreciation of the elderly, my mom and dad, and each of my family members for all their love, thanks to Mary Anne and Priscilla for their expertise, all of the activity professionals and recreational therapists I have had the honor of teaching and working with, and joan and Tom (our editors) for seeing the potential of this book.

— Betsy Best-Martini, MS, CTRS

I've always considered myself to be lucky; and now, with the opportunity to write this book, I once again need to say, "Thank you." All of my life experiences have led me up to this point and I hope that I have done justice to the world full of people who have inspired me along the way. Some have left their vision with me, some only a word in passing. I am the sum of all that.

Thank you to all the residents and their families who have taught me my job and given a special meaning to my life; thank you to Betsy and Priscilla: it's been fun; thank you to joan and Tom for having faith in us and thank you always to my family — from the beginning in Holley, New York, to the present in Sonoma, California. Thanks, Mom and Dad; thanks Nick, Nick, and Lucia.

— Mary Anne Weeks, MPH, SSC

I have been most influenced by the countless staff members in many nursing facilities who constantly remind me that health records reflect peoples' lives and that documentation is much more than recording vital signs. I wish to acknowledge Brenda Huntsinger, ART, who first introduced me to long-term care consulting; Sharon Carrier, RN, ART, who made it real and fun; my parents who encourage me always; my husband Tom; and all of the medical records directors who teach me new ways of looking at things every day. My thanks to Elizabeth Best-Martini for envisioning this book and asking me to contribute and to joan burlingame and Tom Blaschko for pulling it all together.

— Priscilla Wirth, MS, RHIA

We would also like to recognize the authors who contributed to the various sections in this book.

Chapter 2: People We Serve

- Theories on Aging by joan burlingame
- Mobility Losses and Multiple Medical Issues by Mary Kathleen Lockett, RPT
- Demographics of the People We Serve by Jane Martin, BS, ACC and joan burlingame
- Myths and Realities of Aging by the National Council on Aging

Chapter 3: The Work We Do

- Recreational Therapist by joan burlingame

Chapter 4: Resident and Family Environment

- Cultural Competency by Tameka Battle
- Survey Form 19: Signage, Figure 3: Wheelchair Turning Space, Figure 38: Storage Shelves and Closets and Figure 45: Minimum Clearances for Seating and Tables from the United States Government

Chapter 6: Meaningful Person-Centered Activities

- Leisure Room by Pat Hubbard, AC, SSD and Elizabeth Best-Martini, MS, CTRS
- Mountain Theme by Ann Argé Nathan and Elizabeth Best-Martini, MS, CTRS
- Theme Weeks by Mary Anne Clagett, CTRS, ACC
- Intergenerational Programs by Marcia Weldon

Chapter 7: Specific Programs for Dementia and NCDs

- Sensory Awareness Ideas: Shadow Design, Hair Dryer Bubble Blow, Free Form Ball Toss, Free Form Pillow Toss, Powder and Facial Scrubber Time and Tactile Finger Walk by Lois Herman Friedlander, RMT, MFCC

Chapter 8: Programs for Individuals with Mild to Moderate Cognitive Impairments and Dementia

- Let's Talk: Fifty Topics Guaranteed to Get Discussion Started by Harriet Berliner, RN-C, MSN, ARNP
- Men in a Women's World — Discussion by Michael Watters, CTRS

Chapter 9: Short-Term Stay: Rehabilitation-Oriented

- Short-Term Rehab Activities by Lauren Newman, OTR
- When the Participant Is in Need of Recreational Therapy Services by joan burlingame
- Recreational Therapy Services in Community Integration Programming by joan burlingame

Chapter 11: Assessments

- Recreational Therapy Assessment, Standardized Scales, and Assessment Tools by joan burlingame

Chapter 17: Quality Assurance, Infection Control, and Risk Management

- Infection Control, Risk Management, and Immediate Jeopardy by joan burlingame

Chapter 18: Management

- Behavior Management by Kay Garrick, LCSW
- OBRA '87 Regulations by Centers for Medicare and Medicaid Services, State Operations Manual

Purpose

Long-Term Care is a programming and documentation manual for professionals in long-term care settings. The book is designed to be a "how to" guide which will review the people we serve; the environment we are working in; programs that we can provide; work descriptions for activity professionals, recreational therapists, and social services professionals as members of the health care team; documentation of our programs; and management issues for the positions, including federal regulations and interpretive guidelines.

All of the authors have been working in the field of aging and long-term care since the late 1970s. It has been a time of great change and progress in the provision of services and the types of places we work. One of the greatest changes of all has been the expansion of the types of services provided and where these services are provided. No longer is health care provided only by nursing. Now the focus is much more holistic. In order for an individual to progress, to heal, or to accept a new lifestyle with limitations, all services must work together as a team and blend their perspectives and treatment goals. The individuals we serve benefit from the diversity of outlooks and develop new strategies for coping both within and outside the facility.

Because of this focus, professionals need to have a greater understanding of diagnosis, assessment, and team approach. In order to be a vital part of the interdisciplinary team, they need to be both articulate and assertive along with being skilled in documentation and federal and state regulations. They also need to be versed in the varied levels of programming required by the people they serve, from the individual who is very alert and independent to the person who is profoundly regressed.

This book is the joint effort of a Certified Therapeutic Recreation Specialist, a Social Services Coordinator with a Masters in Public Health, and a Health Information Consultant who is a Registered Health Information Administrator.

We dedicate this book to the many individuals who have inspired us with their resilience and wisdom. We also dedicate it to you, the reader, in the hopes of bringing continued inspiration so that your work improves the quality of life for others.

Publisher's Note:

We have promoted the development and publishing of the seventh edition of this book because we feel that the people we serve deserve the best of care. This book was written for activity professionals, social services professionals, recreational therapists, occupational therapists, occupational therapy assistants, and gerontologists.

To the best of our knowledge, the procedures and recommendations of this book reflect currently accepted practice. Nevertheless, they cannot be considered absolute and universal. For individual application, recommendations for therapy for a particular individual must be considered in light of the individual's needs and condition. The authors and publisher disclaim responsibility for any adverse effects resulting directly or indirectly from the suggested procedures, from any undetected errors, or from the reader's misunderstanding of the text.

1. Introduction

The professional opportunities to care for the growing number of people who will use the supportive assistance offered in day treatment, assisted living, and long-term care settings are expanding faster than professionals can be trained. These positions can be rewarding, challenging, and fulfilling — if the individual feels that s/he is competent because of his/her training and is able to feel like an accepted member of the health care team. The purpose of this book is to provide you with the knowledge and skills you need. There are increasing options for people who need assistance with daily living — from help a few hours a day to 24-hour care. Some of the main choices are home health care, home health aids, adult day programs, assisted living communities, long-term care, and specialty units.

This book covers both parts of providing care successfully. It looks at what the people you serve need based on what they can do. It also looks at what the regulations and rules (laws and standards) require you to do. We'll start with a look at the ever-changing requirements of health care practice.

What Has Changed

With every new edition of *Long Term Care*, there is information on regulatory updates pertaining to the jobs of Activity Professionals, Social Services Professionals, and Recreational Therapists. All of the previous editions have been based on the CMS Federal Regulations, OBRA '87. The sixth edition referred to some of the changes to these regulations that were made in 1993. These federal regulations are at the base of our work in long-term care settings and change all of the time. Here is a list of some of the changes made in 2017. In 2017, the OBRA '87 regulations did not change but their interpretations and expectations increased. Some examples are

- The F-Tag numbers have all changed. You will find reference to both the old numbers and the new numbers throughout the book.
- A greater focus on abuse and mandated reporting requirements. Every person who works with the elderly is a mandated reporter by federal and most state regulations. You have a great responsibility in protecting and advocating for each resident to assure they are free from all types of abuse
- Emergency preparedness and implementation. Keep up with all required in-services pertaining to emergency preparedness. Your department should have a plan for all "what ifs." If you are in a room leading a group and need to secure that room due to an earthquake, flood, or active police activity, be prepared to become the leader and keep everyone safe and secure. Write a policy and procedure for the activity department and review this with staff and volunteers. Also update it with all new regulations.
- Consider getting CPR/First Aid Certification
- End-of-life decisions: Do you know the advanced directives of residents? If you take residents on an outing and they have a health emergency, do you know their wishes?
- Immunizations: Check to see what tests your volunteers are required to have. Do they have TB screening and flu shots?
- Infection control-universal precautions: Do you know what types of cleaning and disinfectants are used for different types of issues such as NoroVirus, C-Diff, MRSA, etc.? Are the supplies that you use to clean equipment

and sensory items the same as the environmental services department is using? Be sure they are.

- LGBTQ (lesbian, gay, bi-sexual, transgender and queer): There is a greater federal outreach to assure protection and implementation of rights and benefits of this population and an emphasis on cultural sensitivity, inclusive legal provisions, and civil rights of all. Be sure you address this in your policies and procedures.
- Privacy and confidentiality: These are all protected by HIPAA regulations. All information, both verbal and written, is to be kept confidential to protect residents and staff. Assure that there are no breaches including breaches of electronic records.

The following websites have information that will keep you up to date on changes that impact our work.

- www.cms.gov/Regulations-and-Guidance/Regulations-and-Guidance.html
- www.cms.gov/Medicare/Quality-Initiatives-Patient-Assessment-Instruments/NursingHomeQualityInits/MDS30RAIManual.html
- www.pioneernetwork.net
- www.cms.gov/Medicare/Provider-Enrollment-and-Certification/SurveyCertEmergPrep/Emergency-Prep-Rule.html

Special Thanks to Carol Bartolo Loeffler, MA, OTR/L, Occupational Therapy Consultant with California Department of Public Health, Licensing and Certification, Sacramento, California Office for these updates and websites.

Culture Change in Long-Term Care

> 'Culture change' is the common name given to the national movement for the transformation of older adult services, based on person-directed values and practices where the voices of elders and those working most closely with them are solicited, respected, and honored. Core person-directed values are relationship, choice, dignity, respect, self-determination, and purposeful living.
>
> — *Pioneer Network*

This quote reflects the personalization of services in the model that we refer to as long-term care. The settings are as unique as the people who live in them and work in them. Federal regulations overseeing nursing facilities were developed to assure the same standards of care throughout the United States. Unfortunately, the attention to regulatory compliance has many times taken the focus away from the residents' ability to make personal choices and have more control over their lives on a day-to-day basis.

The first mention of culture change occurred in the late 1970s with a group in California called The Live Oak Institute. Betsy Best-Martini was fortunate to be a member of this culture change team in the 99-bed facility in which she worked at the time. The team was very innovative and interested in providing professional and progressive personalized services for their elderly residents. Live Oak was founded by Barry Barkan who continues to pioneer culture change through workshops, training manuals and resources, and website access. In 1994, William H. Thomas, M.D. wrote *The Eden Alternative* with the same desire to empower nursing home residents and staff, to create a life worth living by addressing what he considers to be the greatest "plagues" of nursing homes: loneliness, helplessness, and boredom. In 1997, nursing home change leaders formed the Pioneer Network. The vision of this network is a culture of aging that is life affirming, satisfying, humane, and meaningful (Fagan, 2003). This focus was one that moved away from the medical model and more towards a home-like environment and family culture model.

HCFA (Health Care Finance Committee — now called CMS, Centers for Medicare and Medicaid Services) called for a study of quality of life issues in nursing homes after the 10th Circuit Court ordered a plan of action to make changes in long-term care settings and the survey process. The report of these findings, *Improving the Quality of Care in Nursing Homes*, was published in 1986. This became the basis for the Nursing Home Reform law of OBRA '87. Now there were specific regulations, a clearly stated and standardized assessment form, the MDS, a standardized survey process, resident's rights, and, most of all, accountability for the highest-level quality of care and life.

This federal law and survey process have changed the face of long-term care in many positive ways. With the changing laws and the culture change movement occurring at the same time, in 2002 CMS created a Satellite Broadcast called *Innovations in Quality of Life — The Pioneer Network*. Karen Schoeneman, CMS Project Officer, and Carmen S. Bowman of Edu-Catering, LLP, co-authored *Artifacts of Culture Change Tool*. This is a CMS tool made available for public use. For review and information, contact Karen Schoeneman at Karen.schoeneman@cms.hhs.gov or Carmen@edu-catering.com. You can also get more information and great resources at www.calculturechange.org or www.pioneernetwork.net.

On March 10, 2006, CMS released the new surveyor guidelines for federal tags (F-Tags) F248 and F249. The F-Tags for activities are now F679 and F680. These regulations pertain to the activity service in skilled nursing settings. The regulations have not changed, but the intent of the guidelines and the surveyor guidance has been modified significantly. These can be found in the State Operators Manual (SOM). Check with your administrator for a copy of this manual. Quality of life is at the core of these new guidelines.

One of the important terms used is "person-centered" or "person-directed." This term is derived from the Pioneer Network definition, Person-Centered Culture. It reflects the philosophy shift from staff-directed and staff-centered to person-centered and person-directed. More information can be found at www.pioneernetwork.net.

CMS has embraced the philosophy of culture change as a modality of change that directly enhances quality of life. Culture change is improving life for residents living in long-term care settings today as well as preparing for the baby-boomer generation. This generation will be the largest population of elders to come into retirement in our history. It has been coined the silver tsunami.

This CMS endorsement has created a stamp of approval along with a federal expectation that all long-term care settings begin to make these changes, which will all be reviewed in the yearly survey process.

An important component of culture change is the language that we use in staff, family, and resident-to-resident communication. The Pioneer Network has posted on their website an excellent article, *The Language of Culture Change*, by Karen Schoeneman. Karen has created a chart with old words and new suggested words for staff to use. An example of some of these would be the change from "Patient" to "Resident," "Feeders" to "People who need assistance with eating," "trays are here" to "dinner is served," etc.[1]

Quality of Life/Quality of Care

The responsibilities of professionals are based on the need for quality of life and quality of care for each of the people we serve. The federal regulations called OBRA '87 define the quality of life component as including the services of recreational therapists, activity professionals, and social services professionals and also address the emotional and physical environment in which the resident lives.

[1] www.pioneernetwork.net/Culture/Language 2/2/10

The people we serve have more power in making decisions concerning various types of activities, treatment, and schedules. They or their representatives must be part of the team in care conferences, resident council, the survey process, and much more. Documents such as the Resident Bill of Rights (in assisted living communities and nursing homes) will be at the forefront of quality of life.

The Ombudsman is a federal program established in nursing homes to review resident complaints and assure quality of life issues. Each state has an Ombudsman program in individual county governments. The role of the Ombudsman has grown in importance into an integral part of the survey process.

With the implementation of the Final Rule of OBRA '87, the Department of Health, Licensing, and Certification has the option to invite the Ombudsman to participate in the survey process and the final exit interview with staff. The Ombudsman can also inform the survey team about any complaints or concerns registered with and/or by the Ombudsman office. It is very important for the professional to develop a good line of communication with the Ombudsman.

The Settings in Which We Work

Living situations of older adults and people with disabilities have changed a great deal over the last twenty years. They used to have just two choices: living at home (or with a relative) or living in a nursing home. Now the people we serve have many choices including home health care, hospice, adult day programs, assisted living, and nursing homes. As professionals our services can be provided in any of these settings.

The types of services you provide for the people you serve should remain pretty much the same, regardless of where you provide the services, because you are providing what they need. However, the manner in which you provide the services (e.g., based on formal assessment, care plans, etc.) and how you record the services (and the person's responses) can vary significantly. What drives the differences in the manner services are provided is based on regulations (laws) and standards (peer-set expectations of performance). Regulations and standards vary depending on the type of setting where the services are provided and the state in which the facility is located.

Below is a quick overview of each type of setting where you may be providing services.

Home Health Care

Home health care is a program in which the patient receives health care services in his or her own home. The type of services may vary from a one-time visit to make sure that the necessary adaptive equipment (e.g., raised toilet seat, shower chair) has been correctly placed to regular, long-term visitation for therapy and/or nursing services. Patients may have IVs placed, receive chemotherapy, or receive help with range of motion, activities of daily living, wound care, respiratory treatment, and many other types of care. There are federal regulations and accreditation standards from the Joint Commission that set minimum levels of quality of care for home health care. The Centers for Medicare and Medicaid Services (CMS) require that all home health care agencies provide skilled nursing services and at least one of the following other therapeutic services: physical, speech, or occupational therapy; medical social services; or home health aide services. The federal law specifically excludes home-based services whose primary function is to provide for the care and treatment of mental illness. Hospice care is often classified as a specialty of home health care.

Hospice

Hospice is as much a way of thinking as a type of service. The goal is to provide comfort and support to a patient and the patient's support system of family and friends when the patient is no longer responding to cure-oriented treatments. The primary goal of hospice is to provide quality of life during an individual's last days while neither prolonging nor hastening death. Pain management and other medical treatments are provided to enhance comfort and dignity. Hospice workers, usually a team of health care professionals, volunteers, and the patient's support system, try to address the patient's emotional, social, and spiritual needs while minimizing pain and discomfort.

Dr. Cicely Saunders is credited with starting the first modern hospice program in Great Britain in the 1960s. The first hospice program in the United States was established in 1974 in New Haven, Connecticut. People living at home can participate in the hospice program. In addition, residents of assisted living and skilled nursing facilities can be under contract with hospice for services. In these settings, the hospice team becomes an integral part of the interdisciplinary team on site. According to the National Hospice and Palliative Care Organization's 2010 findings, almost 1.56 million people in the United States received hospice services in 2009. That is almost 42% of all the people who died in the U.S. in 2009.

The Centers for Medicare and Medicaid Services (CMS) list specific core services that must be part of a hospice program. They include nursing care; medical social services under the direction of a physician; physician's services; counseling (including dietary and bereavement counseling); physical, occupational, and speech therapy; home health aide services; and homemaker services.

Adult Day Care Programs

Adult day care programs offer daytime assistance for individuals who need the structure and support offered through a formal program. There are two different types of adult day programs: social programs and medical programs. These programs may be freestanding (not part of a larger health care system) or be just one part of a larger continuum of care. Adult day care centers may be located in a shopping mall, church, community center, assisted living center, or other type of building. Adult day programs do not provide overnight lodging for their participants but may be affiliated with a hospital, assisted care living facility, or other respite care type facilities where overnight lodging for short-term stays may be arranged when the participant's condition deteriorates.

Socially based adult day programs provide services for seniors who benefit from a structured program and from the opportunity to reduce time spent in isolation. Social adult day programs have fewer regulations so they tend to be more informal than medically based adult day programs. Due to the lack of regulations and standards, there are no specific staffing requirements, documentation requirements, or program/activity requirements.

Medically based adult day programs tend to be a low-cost (about $50 per day per participant), organized day program consisting of health, social, and recreational services for adults with physical and mental disabilities. Under the direct supervision of professional staff these programs assist in maintaining or restoring, to the fullest extent possible, an individual's capacity for self-care. These programs usually provide assistance in activities of daily living, cognitive stimulation, leisure activities, and at least one meal each day.

While regulations vary slightly from state to state, they frequently require the medical adult day program to provide many services, such as transportation to and from the facility, medical monitoring, group activities, and medication administration. The types of individuals who use adult day programs have similar medical needs to individuals who are in assisted living facilities or nursing homes. The primary difference between these populations is that adults in adult day programs tend to have very supportive family networks that are committed to keeping their family member at home. Some states have different names for adult day care. For example, in California it is called California Community-Based Adult Services (CBAS). Be sure to check your state website for more information.

Assisted Living Resident Profile (from National Center for Assisted Living)[2]

Category	Statistic
Age	In 2006 the average age of an assisted living resident was 86.9 years.
Sex	Nearly 3/4 of assisted living residents are female; 1/4 are male.
Typical Resident	The typical assisted living resident is an 86-year-old woman who is mobile, but needs assistance with two activities of daily living.
Number of Residents	Approximately one million people nationwide live in assisted living settings.
Receive Help with Housework	A full 91% of assisted living residents need or accept help with housework.
Medication Assistance	Eighty-six percent need or accept help with their daily medication.
Average Length of Stay	The typical resident stays 27 months. Thirty-four percent will move into a nursing facility. Thirty percent will pass away. The remaining will move home or to another location.
Activities of Daily Living	The following percentages of assisted living residents need help with these activities of daily living: Bathing 68% Dressing 47% Toileting 34% Transferring 25% Eating 22%

One of the biggest problems facing adult day programs is the provision of safe and reliable transportation to and from the program. Some of the individuals in the program may be able to retain some independence by using public transportation. If this option is to be part of the treatment plan, a therapist may want to assess the individual's level of independence by using both the Environmental Safety and the City Bus assessments found in the *Community Integration Program* by Armstrong and Lauzen (1994) or the *Bus Utilization Skills Assessment* (BUS) by burlingame.

Assisted Living

According to the National Center for Assisted Living, almost one million Americans reside in assisted living facilities. Assisted living refers to residential care, personal care, adult congregate care, or board and care. According to the US Department of Health and Human Services, there are approximately 36,000 assisted-living facilities in the United States. The average size is 58 units but the size and type vary greatly.

Assisted living communities have regulations (governmental laws) and standards (peer-set performance standards) that outline the minimum level and quality of services expected. Assisted living communities must provide basic housing and meals, help the individual coordinate his/her personal needs, offer 24-hour supervision and assistance, and offer an activities program and health-related services. The staff must design and offer services that allow each individual to remain as independent as possible, for as long as possible, while providing an atmosphere of respect, dignity, and autonomy. Supporting and encouraging the involvement of the individual's significant others is an important component of the assisted living community. The level of assistance provided can be minimal to comprehensive. The types of services offered are custom-tailored while also providing routine activities. This allows individuals to avoid paying for more care than they need, while

[2] This information is from the National Center for Assisted Living's web site on June 18, 2010. http://www.ncal.org/about/resident.htm

enjoying all the advantages of a caring environment.

Skilled Nursing Settings

In years past, the skilled nursing (convalescent, nursing home) setting was almost always a facility that provided services to frail, elderly people in need of 24-hour nursing attention. This was what defined a skilled nursing facility/long-term care facility. Today, this setting is referred to as a long-term care facility or a Nursing Facility (NF) according to the OBRA '87 regulations. The people or residents of a nursing setting today vary in age from teenagers to people over 100. There is no "typical" resident.

The need to be admitted is identified not according to age, but according to acuity level (how sick or disabled someone is) in relationship to how much assistance the individual needs. Some of the people we serve can be placed within the general nursing home population on units with residents who have a wide variety of needs. Many facilities also have "special care units" which function as an individual unit providing specialized services and programs to residents with disorders such as Alzheimer's disease and related dementias (neurocognitive disorders). These have separate activity and treatment programs designed to meet special needs. Because they have become so common, the Joint Commission on Accreditation of Healthcare Organizations (JCAHO) has created standards for special care units and criteria for accreditation of these units.

The nursing facility can also be a special unit within the framework of an acute care hospital. This may be called a Transitional Care Unit, Subacute Unit, Medicare Unit, or Extended Care Unit. In an acute care hospital, a patient can be transferred from the acute to subacute unit while remaining in the same hospital. The subacute care unit provides the patient with continued coverage of services until s/he is discharged. Medicare coverage continues, so this unit benefits the hospital financially. It benefits patients because they do not have to go through another transfer or the trauma associated with moving while trying to recuperate. Because of these factors, many acute care hospitals are reorganizing their beds to create a nursing facility unit.

This unit is under the same licensure as a nursing facility. It must comply with both governmental regulations and voluntary accreditation. The activity programs are required as a service within the bed rate. The uniqueness of the setting and the high level of acuity of these residents create quite a challenge, especially within the context of regulations that were created before the setting was! Most of the residents — who prefer to be called patients as they are focused on short-term stays — are too ill and frail to be out of bed and in groups. In a unit such as this the person we serve may also be dependent on machines and equipment that the professional from a more traditional nursing home may be unfamiliar with. The majority of therapeutic activities are provided on a very specialized, one-on-one basis. The greater the acuity level, the more specialized the activity.

As health care reform continues to affect each of us individually in terms of coverage and special services, it will also play a role in determining which professional services will be provided and covered within a managed care system. The long-term care facility is required by law to provide an activity program. Because of this, activity programs in this setting, whether a separate long-term care facility or a transitional care setting, are protected and will become more important both as a service and as a marketing tool. Professionals need to be vocal, goal oriented, and clear as to how they play a significant role in the interdisciplinary approach to health care.

Subacute Care

Subacute care is a level of medical or rehabilitation care that is less intense than what would be provided in a hospital unit but more than what would normally be provided for a resident admitted to a nursing home for long-term placement. "Transitional care" is another term used in place of subacute care. The individual transitions from requiring many hours a day of specialized medical or rehabilitation care to needing only about two to five hours of specialized care a day. Much of the emphasis on treatment will be to help the individual improve his/her ability to take care of himself/herself so that discharge to a less restrictive environment is possible.

The American Health Care Association (AHCA), the Joint Commission on Accreditation of Healthcare Organizations (JCAHO), and the Association of Hospital-Based Skilled Nursing Facilities have developed a definition of subacute care:[3]

> Subacute care is comprehensive inpatient care designed for someone who has an acute illness, injury, or exacerbation of a disease process. It is goal-oriented treatment rendered immediately after, or instead of, acute hospitalization to treat one or more specific active complex medical conditions or to administer one or more technically complex treatments, in the context of a person's underlying long-term conditions and overall situation.
>
> Generally, the individual's condition is such that the care does not depend heavily on high-technology monitoring or complex diagnostic procedures. Subacute care requires the coordinated services of an interdisciplinary team including physicians, nurses, and other relevant professional disciplines, who are trained and knowledgeable to assess and manage these specific conditions and perform the necessary procedures. Subacute care is given as part of a specifically defined program, regardless of the site.
>
> Subacute care is generally more intensive than traditional nursing facility care and less than acute care. It requires frequent (daily to weekly) recurrent patient assessment and review of the clinical course and treatment plan for a limited (several days to several months) time period, until the condition is stabilized or a predetermined treatment course is completed.

What's in this Book

This book is intended to help you meet the challenges of your profession in many different types of settings. It will explain how to:

- Assess and work with people at their current level of functioning
- See how you fit into the larger health care picture
- Deal with federal and state regulations
- Provide a safe and stimulating environment for the people you serve
- Deal with all of the details of your work (surveys, laws, budgets, quality assurance, time management, diversity of client needs)

This book is about each of us on our journey of aging. It is important that we accept ourselves and respect and honor those who are our elders. We soon shall be them. Treat each person for his or her uniqueness, life experiences, and cultural richness. Treat each as you would your own parents and family members.

The book is divided into chapters that focus on the various aspects of your work:

Chapter 2. The People We Serve describes the people we serve. Understanding the variety of residents with their range of skills is an important aspect of understanding how to help them lead the best possible lives. Diagnoses that affect people in long-term care are included in this chapter.

Chapter 3. The Work We Do describes the work involved with being an activity professional, a social services professional, or a recrea-

---

[3] American Health Care Association. (1996) "Nursing facility subacute care: The quality and cost-effective alternative to hospital care." www.rai.to/subacute.htm

tional therapist. This is an overview of these positions. Many of the details of the work are described in later chapters.

Chapter 4. Resident and Facility Environment describes the environment that exists for the people we serve, their families, and the health care team.

Chapter 5. Meaningful and Person-Centered Activity Programs has information about taking your participants' personal interests and requirements for care and quality of life issues and devising a program for your facility that meets all of the residents' needs along with satisfying regulations.

Chapter 6. Meaningful Person-Centered Activities gives you the foundation you need to run groups and activity programs. Leisure, therapy programs, using themes, and thoughts about participation are all covered in this chapter.

Chapter 7. Specific Programs for Dementia and NCDs provides you with information about how to design and implement programs for residents dealing with varying levels of dementia and neurocognitive disorders. The key is to find personal strengths and enhance these through meaningful programs.

Chapter 8. Programs for Individuals with Mild to Moderate Cognitive Impairments and Dementia talks about the people you serve will who still be able to assist in their care and want to engage in meaningful activities that bring them happiness and purpose. This chapter provides you with ideas of how to work with these individuals and options for activities.

Chapter 9. Short-Term Stay: Rehabilitation-Oriented helps you understand the differences inherent in people who have a true opportunity to work their way to a less restrictive environment versus people who are appropriately placed and are interested in maintaining the skills they have. This chapter has extensive information on cognitive stimulation and retraining. These cognitive strengthening activities may also be used with participants who are moderately impaired or who are at a lower functioning level.

Chapter 10. Documentation discusses the legal requirements for documenting the care you are providing. It includes information about assessments, care plans, and monitoring care plans.

Chapter 11. Assessments covers the discipline-specific assessment process, including setting discharge goals as part of the participant's admission to the program.

Chapter 12. Resident Assessment Instrument: MDS + CAAs talks about the required assessment and care planning process for nursing homes. We will cover specific information on filling out your part of the interdisciplinary Resident Assessment Instrument.

Chapter 13. Care Planning takes you beyond the assessment and helps you create a care plan. writing a care plan from the assessment information, updating the care plan at appropriate (and legally required) intervals, and planning a program based on residents' needs.

Chapter 14. Monitoring the Treatment Plan provide information to help you understand the types of tools you will need to monitor your participant's progress (or regression) on the objectives in the care plan. Specific types of progress notes and updates are discussed at the end of the chapter.

Chapter 15. Councils discusses the OBRA '87 requirement that you give residents (or their guardians) control over their lives, in general and through the specific use of resident and family councils.

Chapter 16. Volunteers talks about using volunteers in your programs.

Chapter 17. Quality Assurance and Performance Improvement, Infection Control, Risk Management, and Emergency Preparedness deals with being part of the quality assurance program at your facility, being sure that your environment and your activities meet infection control guidelines, and understanding the basic elements of risk management and emergency preparedness.

Chapter 18. Management gives you help understanding resident rights (especially the right to be free of restraints), writing policies and procedures, complying with laws, dealing constructively with surveys, developing a budget, and other topics.

Appendix A. Abbreviations provides you with a short list of the most commonly used health care abbreviations.

Appendix B. Minimum Data Set and the Resident Assessment System shows you examples of the Minimum Data Set (MDS 3.0).

Appendix C. Care Area Assessment (CAA) provides sample CAAs for Activities and Social Services

References and Further Reading gives you places to learn more about long-term care.

Terminology

According to the Federal OBRA '87 guidelines, there are five different types of training or professional certifications that qualify an individual to work as an activity professional, as shown below.

The new OBRA '87 interpretive guidelines for F-Tag F249, which is now F680, have an addition that is very important to understand in regards to who is qualified to be an activity professional. The new guidelines state, "F680 is a tag that is absolute, which means the facility must have a qualified activities professional to direct the provision of activities to the residents. Thus, it is cited if the facility is non-compliant with the regulation, whether or not there have been any negative outcomes to residents." Simply stated, this means that during the survey process, a surveyor does not need to find a deficient practice in order to find non-compliance. It is non-compliance if a non-qualified individual is hired as the activity professional.

The activity professional is a person who is responsible for designing and running activity programs for the people we serve. Most of the book is appropriate for all of you who are responsible for programs. In the particular cases where we discuss the activity professional who is responsible for the administration of the activity department, we are referring to an individual who meets the requirements in F680

A recreational therapist is a person who is responsible for designing and implementing rehabilitation-oriented treatment that is prescribed by a physician. This type of treatment is outside the typical services offered by the activity professional. Most of the accreditation standards require the recreational therapist to be nationally credentialed as a Certified Therapeutic Recreation Specialist or hold the equivalent state credential after completing a bachelor's degree program from an accredited university. The recreational therapist who is working in a long-term care setting may be providing the general recreation program along with leisure education services and physician-ordered recreational therapy.

Skilled Nursing Facilities: Regulation F680:

(2) The activities program must be directed by a qualified professional who —
- (i) Is a qualified therapeutic recreation specialist or an activities professional who
  - (A) Is licensed or registered, if applicable, by the State in which practicing: and
  - (B) Is eligible for certification as a therapeutic recreation specialist or as an activities professional by a recognized accrediting body on or after October 1, 1990; or
- (ii) Has 2 years of experience in a social or recreational program within the last five years, one of which was full-time in a patient activities program in a health care setting, or
- (iii) Is a qualified occupational therapist or occupational therapy assistant; or
- (iv) Has completed a training course approved by the State.

In earlier editions we generally used the term "resident" when we referred to the people we serve. This term is not always appropriate when we are talking about issues that may also impact the delivery of services in adult day programs, home health care, subacute, and rehab-oriented facilities. Generally, when we do use the term "resident" in this book, we are talking about issues related to long-term care facilities.

We will use the term "patient" for people in subacute settings whose focus is on leaving the facility and going back into the community. In general we will not try to label particular segments of people who receive health care, calling them, instead, the "people we serve."

2. The People We Serve

The long-term care and assisted living settings have no typical resident or client. The types of individuals who find themselves living either for a short time or a long time in these settings span the categories of age, disability, socioeconomic status, cultural background and diagnosis. An 82-year-old man with a fractured hip may share a room with a 19-year-old man suffering from a head injury sustained in a motorcycle accident. In the next room, a 17-year-old woman who is comatose from a drug overdose may have as her roommate a 74-year-old woman who is incontinent, suffers from short-term memory loss, and is blind.

Many people over 65 will spend some time in a long-term care facility. Some will live out the rest of their lives there. A much larger percentage of the residents will be admitted for a short period to deal with an acute problem. After their stay they will return to a lesser level of care.

It is important to address the diversity and its consequent impact on programming needs.

This chapter will talk about the people we serve and some of their important issues. We will look at the expectations of these individuals and their families, the kinds of physical and cognitive disabilities that they may have, and opportunities for continuing a meaningful lifestyle in a long-term care or assisted living setting.

Theories on Aging

A theory is a speculation on why and how something happens. Over the years, biologists, psychologists, and anthropologists have all speculated on why and how people react and adjust to growing older. The belief is: if we can understand why common problems and strengths have developed, then we can know what to do to improve the quality of life for the community as a whole. This section will introduce you to the most common theories of aging including biological and psychological theories of aging. We hope that this will help you better understand the people you serve and that you can improve the overall quality of life for the individual and for the larger community.

For thousands of years people have been curious about the aging process, striving to find everlasting youthfulness or immortality. Our history is full of stories such as the one about the Spanish explorer Ponce de León, and his search for the Fountain of Youth in Florida in the late 1400s. There are many relics from ancient Egyptian and Chinese towns that show interest in potions and ceremonies to prolong life or to achieve immortality.

While the use of extracts made from tiger testicles and other rituals may seem laughable now, look at our everyday advertising to see all of the products offered. We have products to make wrinkles fade, megavitamins to prolong life, and the increased use of cosmetic surgery. People study the aging process to help us better understand the body as it ages, to improve our abilities to cope, and to improve our interpersonal relationships through the life cycle.

Because there is no single action or event that can cause or prevent aging, the complex aging process cannot be described by just one or two theories. Additionally, over the last century there has been a change in how we look at theories that add to the complexity of speculations on the whys and hows of aging. During the early and middle 1900s, the people who studied development and aging focused on descriptions of milestones at each phase of life, asking "what happens?" and "when does it happen?" At the end of the twentieth century, researchers started focusing on the explanations of how the changes occurred by asking "why?" and "how?" This led to theories based on both descriptive and explanation-based ideas.

Biological Theories of Aging

Biological theories on aging focus on anticipated changes in the organs of the human body. The aging process is called senescence, from the Latin word *senescere* meaning to grow old. The aging process usually involves a decline of the body's ability to function in almost all biological systems including respiratory, cardiovascular, endocrine, immune, and genitourinary. However, the myth that people experience significant cognitive and physical capacity losses as they age has been shown to generally be false. Many people retain a significant portion of their cognitive and physical abilities as they age.

Three of the more common biological theories on aging are the Genetic Factors Theory on Aging, the Nutrition Theory on Aging, and the Environment Theory on Aging.

The Genetic Factors Theory on Aging states that one's DNA plays the primary role in how well one will age and how long one can anticipate living. Both the person's genetic ability to continue normally dividing cells (thus, prolonging life) and the person's genetic ability to reduce the amount of organ decline through avoiding mutations of DNA determine how long the person will live.

The Nutrition Theory on Aging stresses the importance of good nutrition (an adequate amount of vitamins and other nutrients and a limited amount of refined carbohydrates, cholesterols, and fats). This is one of the older theories on aging and prolonging life, although the sophistication of this theory has increased as more research has gone into it. The relationship between eating in a healthy way and living longer has been documented for thousands of years. Even though we do not understand many of the specifics of nutrition and aging, enough is known to lead to the belief that a good diet may minimize or even eliminate some of the negative effects of aging on the body.

The Environmental Theory on Aging focuses on the elements of our environment — toxins in the environment, viruses, density of population, smoking, the effects of the sun, and other factors — that are thought to influence how we age. In his book *The Stress of Life*, Dr. Hans Selye lists elements of the climate and environment that cause the biology of the body (due to stress reactions) to suffer trauma and reduce longevity. They are air and water pollution, social and cultural stressors, crowding, sensory deprivation and boredom, isolation and loneliness, captivity, relocation and travel, urbanization, catastrophes, meteorological factors, and neuropsychological stressors. As an example of one of the stressors, Selye says of relocation and travel

> For the aged, the stress of being transferred into "old folks' homes" is exacerbated by the feeling of being useless burdens on their families and of having no further purpose in life. (p. 390)

The biological factors that impact the body and aging process are complex. All of the theories of aging discussed above are part of the "what, when, why, and how" of aging.

Psychological Theories on Aging

There are three main psychological theories on aging: the Personality Theory, the Activity Theory, and the Disengagement Theory.

The *Personality Theory*, often referred to as the Developmental Theory or Continuity Theory on Aging, is based on the belief that the personality, coping skills, and behavior patterns that one used during his/her earlier stages of life will remain basically the same as one ages. This theory recognizes that individuals may choose to react to changes and challenges in the environment and community based on how they chose to react to similar events in their past, bringing in things learned as they move through the change(s). Theorists feel that healthy developmental aging happens when an individual is able to successfully fulfill the developmental tasks of aging, making the necessary changes to be ready for the next developmental challenge. The developmental tasks of aging are adjusting to one's losses (both physical and interpersonal losses), developing a sense of satisfaction with one's accomplishments in life, and preparing for death.

Erik Erikson listed eight stages of human development, the last being old age. Erikson felt that the challenge of getting older was to accept and find meaning in one's life. Finding such acceptance would give the individual "ego integrity," allowing coping skills and the ability to adjust to the reality of aging and death. Erik H. Erickson, Joan M. Erickson, and Helen Q. Kivnick continued to explore development in old age and addressed the importance of creativity in old age. They found that it is important to participate in life review while continuing to be involved in each day's work and play. Their book *Vital Involvement in Old Age* was published in 1994. This is an excellent resource for activity professionals. Aging is a complex process and, of all the psychological theories on aging, the personality theory considers these dynamics more than others.

The *Activity Theory of Aging* was developed during the 1960s by Robert J. Havighurst. The basic premise of the activity theory is that as individuals age, they make a choice not to turn inward and be self-absorbed, but instead keep about the work of their lives and remain an active participant in all that brings importance to them. Activity theory includes the use of activity (and adapted activity) to help someone through the multiple losses associated with aging. One of the adaptations associated with this theory is the elder's use of "brain instead of brawn" to solve problems.

The activity theory suggests that the older individual continues to try to live a middle-age lifestyle as long as possible, unlike the continuity theory that emphasizes a continual passage to the next developmental task. The activity theory suggests that just because people age, it does not mean that they change in terms of their emotional and social needs.

A third theory of aging, which is highly controversial and now generally considered to be discredited, is the *Disengagement Theory of Aging*. This theory suggested that as people got older they slowly withdrew from society and society slowly withdrew from them. A mutual satisfaction with this separation as one prepared for death encouraged health care professionals and family members to allow the elder to isolate himself/herself from activity, social interaction, and societal roles. While individual elders may go down the path of increased isolation, this action is considered to be pathological and health care workers these days work to prevent it from happening.

Demographics of the People We Serve

There are many changes in our lives that affect how (and how long) we live. Some of these changes, such as the computer and information revolution, are currently causing major changes in our lives. One of the greatest changes is the length of time people live. Life expectancy is the term used to describe how long the average newborn infant can be expected to live. During the time of the Roman Empire the life expectancy of the average newborn was only 28 years. From the time Christ was born until 1900, life expectancy increased three days a year. Such dramatic changes have taken place since the turn of the last century that we are now seeing an increase in life expectancy of 110 days a year. Much of this change is due to better medications, surgery, personal exercise, better eating habits, and general prosperity.

As we move further into the twenty-first century, we are finding that global migration of cultural groups is changing the dynamics of our communities. Combining this with our increasingly greater life expectancy, we must ask ourselves, "Who is this group of seniors that we serve?" Are we just increasing the number of older people who are sick and in need of care or are we increasing our number of healthier and more active seniors? And how does the blending of cultures impact those we serve? Row and Kahn (1999) state:

> When you compare 65 to 75-year-old individuals in 1960 with those similarly aged in 1990, you find a dramatic reduction in the prevalence of three important precursors to chronic disease: high blood pressure, high cholesterol levels, and smoking. We also know that between 1982 and 1989, there were significant reductions in the prevalence of arthritis, arteriosclerosis (hardening of the arteries), dementia [now also called NCD], hypertension, stroke, and emphysema (chronic lung disease), as well as a dramatic decrease in the average number of diseases an older person has. And dental health has improved as well; the proportion of older individuals with dental disease so severe as to result in their having no teeth has dropped from 55 percent in 1957 to 34 percent in 1980, and is currently approaching 20 percent.
>
> But what really matters is not the number or type of disease one has, but how those problems impact on one's ability to function. For example, if you are told that a white male is 75, your ability to predict his functional status is limited. Even if you are given details of his medical history…a history of hypertension [and] diabetes, and has had a heart attack in the past, you still couldn't say whether he is sitting on the Supreme Court of the United States or in a nursing home![4]

This section will cover what we know about the people we serve by looking at statistics such as the number of individuals who experience specific illnesses or other major events at specific ages. We will also look at the numbers of individuals based on cultural and other backgrounds. Next, we will look at a health initiative sponsored by the US government (and other groups) called Healthy People 2020. This initiative is aimed at improving health and quality of life.

Profile of Older Americans[5]

It is always helpful to have access to current statistics on aging. These statistics give us a basis for our work and help explain how public policy is created. Some highlights from the *Administration Agency on Aging Report: 2015* include:

- The older population (65+) numbered 46.2 million in 2014, an increase of 10 million or 28% since 2004.
- Between 2004 and 2014, the population age 60 and over increased 32.5% from 48.9 million to 64.8 million.
- Over one in every 7, or 14.5%, of the population is an older American.
- Persons reaching age 65 have an average life expectancy of an additional 19.3 years (20.5 years for females and 18 years for males).
- Older women outnumber older men at 25.9 million older women to 20.4 million older men.
- In 2014, 22% of persons 65+ were members of racial or ethnic minority populations: 9% African American (not Hispanic), 4% were Asian or Pacific Islander (not Hispanic), 0.5% were Native American (not Hispanic), 0.1% were Native Hawaiian/Pacific Islander

[4] Rowe, J and Kahn, R. (1999). "The future of aging." In *Contemporary Long-Term Care, 22* (2), 38.

[5] The information from this section comes from the *Profile of Older Americans: 2015 report*, United States Administration on Aging, www.aoa.dhhs.gov/aoa/stats/profile/default.htm, 5/02/17

(not Hispanic), and 0.7% of persons 65+ identified themselves as being of two or more races. Persons of Hispanic origin (who may be of any race) represented 8% of the older population.

- Older men were much more likely to be married than older women — 70% of men vs. 45% of women. In 2015, 34% of older women were widows.
- About 29% (13.3 million) of non-institutionalized older persons live alone (9.2 million women, 4.1 million men).
- Almost half of older women — 46% of those ages 75+ — live alone.
- In 2014, about 554,579 grandparents aged 65 or more had the primary responsibility for their grandchildren who lived with them.
- The population 65 and over has increased from 36.2 million in 2004 to 46.2 million in 2014 (a 28% increase) and is projected to more than double to 98 million by 2060.
- The 85+ population is projected to triple from 6.2 million in 2014 to 14.6 million in 2040.
- Racial and ethnic minority populations have increased from 6.5 million in 2004 (18% of the elderly population) to 10 million in 2014 (22% of the elderly) and will increase to 21.1 million in 2030 (28% of the elderly).
- The median income of older persons in 2014 was $31,169 for males and $17,375 for females.
- Median money income (after adjusting for inflation) of all households headed by older people declined by 2.7% (which was not statistically significant) between 2013 and 2014. Households containing families headed by persons 65+ reported a median income in 2014 of $54,838.
- Major sources of income for older people in 2013 were Social Security (reported by 84% of older persons), income from assets (reported by 51%), private pensions (reported by 27%), government employee pensions (reported by 14%), and earnings (reported by 28%).
- Social Security constituted 90% or more of the income received by 35% of all Social Security beneficiaries (21% of married couples and 46% of non-married beneficiaries).
- About 4.5 million elderly persons (10%) were below the poverty level in 2014 which is not statistically different from the poverty rate in 2013 (10.2%).

Diseases of the People We Serve

As people get older, their health status tends to change, not as fast as they expected when they were young, but the trend is still there. In 1996, 27% of older people reported that their health was only fair to poor. In the population as a whole, only 9.2% said that they were experiencing only fair to poor health. If we look at cultural and ethnic difference, we see a different story. While 27% of people who were over 65 years of age reported that their health was only fair to poor, a far greater percentage of minorities reported their health to be only fair to poor. Among African-Americans, 41.6% said their health was only fair to poor. Of people of Hispanic origin, 35.1% reported poor to fair health. Poor health does not just mean more visits to the doctor. Over one third (36.3%) of people over 65 reported that they had limitations on their activities because of chronic conditions. A full 10.5% said that the limitations were significant enough to make them unable to complete a major activity. For individuals under the age of 65, only 3.5% reported such a significant limitation.

In 1997 the Health Care Financing Administration (now called the Centers for Medicare and Medicaid Services) reported that there were a total of 14,852 nursing homes in the United States, which had a total of 684,656 beds. In the previous year 1,325,993 people were admitted to a nursing home with 1,423,224 discharged in the same year. The larger number of people being discharged than admitted reflects a national trend to shorten the length of stay in a nursing home.

Individuals from different cultural groups are also less likely to be admitted to nursing homes. Wallace et al. (1998)[6] found that individuals of African-American backgrounds were less likely to be admitted to a nursing home than if they were white. African-American elderly were more likely to use paid home care, unpaid home care, or no care at all. Forty-five percent of blacks and 32 percent of whites used unpaid community care. The study determined that older blacks had a higher need for long-term care than whites when measured by inability of complete ADLs and/or by the severity of symptoms from strokes, diabetes, and hearing difficulties. Fifty-three percent of older whites who required help with three to five ADLs lived in a nursing home while only 34% of older blacks with similar functional limitations lived in a nursing home.

While cultural background plays a part in whether someone is admitted to a nursing home, so does loneliness. Over 3,000 individuals over the age of 65 years were interviewed in rural Iowa to determine their degree of loneliness and lack of peer companionship. Four years later, 42% of the individuals who were severely lonely had been admitted to a nursing home, while only 10% of those who scored lowest on the loneliness scale had been admitted to a nursing home.[7]

Healthy People 2020

As professionals we need to have an understanding of the population we serve. What we do can help increase the quality and length of life for this population. To do this we must understand the diverse nature of the people we serve. There are health inequalities among this diverse population. *Healthy People 2020* is a "broad-based collaborative effort among government, private, public, and non-profit organizations." It has set national disease prevention and health promotion objectives to improve the health of all Americans, eliminate disparities in health, and improve years and quality of life.

Healthy People 2020 reflects the scientific advances that have taken place over the past twenty years in preventive medicine, disease surveillance, vaccine and therapeutic development, and information technology. The changing demographics of our country, the changes that have taken place in health care, and the growing impact on our national health status are areas that need in-depth analysis. There are twenty-six Leading Health Indicators (LHI) that have been chosen as focus areas to improve the health and well-being of the residents of the United States[8]. They are organized under the following 12 topics:

1. Access to health services
2. Clinical preventive services
3. Environmental quality
4. Injury and violence
5. Maternal, infant, and child health
6. Mental health and mental disorders
7. Nutrition, physical activity, and obesity
8. Oral health
9. Reproductive and sexual health
10. Social determinants
11. Substance abuse
12. Tobacco

Myths and Realities of Aging 2000[9]

March 28, 2000: The National Council on the Aging (NCOA) launched its fiftieth anniversary conference by unveiling the results of *Myths and Realities of Aging 2000*, a wide-ranging survey on Americans' attitudes about aging. For the second time in twenty-five years, a major NCOA study has overturned stereotypes about aging in America. Conducted with the International Longevity Center and supported by Oppenheimer Funds and Pfizer Inc., *Myths and*

[6] Wallace, S., Levy-Storms, L, Kington, R., and Andersen, R. (1998). "The persistence of race and ethnicity in the use of long-term care." *Journal of Gerontology: Social Sciences 53B*(2), S104-S112.

[7] Newsfronts. *Contemporary Long-term Care 21*(5), 13.

[8] For more information about Healthy People 2020 or to access Healthy People 2020 documents online, visit: http://www.health.gov/healthypeople/ or call 1-800-367-4725

[9] Used with permission from The National Council on the Aging. (www.ncoa.org)

Realities of Aging 2000 showed that most Americans would be happy if they lived to be 90. Nearly half of the respondents age 65 and over (44 percent) described the present as the best years of their lives — a 32 percent increase over 1974 results.

The survey of more than 3,000 U.S. adults produced a number of surprises, besides the percentages of elders who considered their current years to be their best. The survey demolished the myth of intergenerational conflict, showing that most Americans favor spending more — not less — on older people. Older people are less worried about their health, their finances, and the threat of crime than they were twenty-five years ago. *Myths and Realities of Aging 2000* showed that in the minds of many, old age begins with a decline in physical or mental ability, rather than with the arrival of a specific birthday. The survey also indicated that younger people tend to overstate the financial and social isolation problems of older people.

Myths and Realities of Aging 2000 has far-reaching implications, according to a panel of experts who spoke at the March 28 announcement event. Money and health, said survey research director Neal Cutler, PhD, are more likely than chronological age to determine retirement decisions. Only 24 percent of survey respondents cited "reaching a certain age" as a key potential factor in deciding to retire. The relationship of age, work, and retirement, said Cutler, is undergoing profound change.

Survey results suggest the need to respond with optimism, but not over-confidence, to the present challenges of aging, according to Robert Butler, MD, president of the International Longevity Center in New York City. Although science has dramatically altered aging-related declines in health, stubborn problems remain. Alzheimer's disease remains a formidable challenge that may affect millions of baby boomers as they age.

Although Americans know what they should do to protect their health, they often fail to take steps that could promote their own longevity. The epidemic of obesity in our society, for example, reflects our failure to act on growing knowledge about predictors of longevity. Also, said Butler, we have failed to include long-term care in our Medicare system, or to educate people on the need to plan how to finance their own long-term care.

For the serious health problems that complicate late life, the medical profession and corporate America are actively seeking solutions, said Tom McRae, MD, of Pfizer, Inc. Physicians now aggressively treat conditions that they used to accept as inevitable complications of old age. Pharmaceutical companies are working on treatments for heart disease, hypertension, cancer, arthritis, osteoporosis, and other conditions that affect older people. He stressed the importance of educating people with chronic conditions about the need to take their medication and to assume responsibility for staying healthy.

Wealth, as well as health, greatly determines happiness in old age. Although 60 percent of respondents took responsibility for key financial decisions, many Americans lack the knowledge and confidence such decisions require. Oppenheimer Funds president and CEO Bridget A. Macaskill noted that as longevity increases, the need for careful planning and extensive discussion increases. Yet 44 percent of married respondents had never discussed with their spouse when they would retire; 40 percent had never discussed where they will live; and 45 percent had never talked about how much money they would need. To guide long-term financial planning, Macaskill recommended professional guidance for individuals and a higher savings rate for Americans.

Policy makers, like individuals, must plan for the future of retirement. Yet the survey reveals a chasm between individuals' expectations about government programs and current political priorities, according to Humphrey A. Taylor, chairman of Harris Interactive, Inc. The current stress on cutting government programs threatens the benefits people expect to receive from Social Security and Medicare. Few new proposals address the need to alter working conditions for those who must work well beyond "retirement" age to make ends meet. Such tough challenges will intensify as the number of elders increases in future years.

Myths and Realities of Aging 2000 presented grounds for optimism and careful thought. NCOA's goal, said president and CEO James Firman, is to ensure that within the next decades, all elders can live the "best years of their lives" in old age. To transform the "twilight years" into the "highlight years," added Bridget Macaskill, NCOA's landmark survey should begin to lead the way.

Older Americans Act

The Older Americans Act (OAA) Reauthorization Act, S. 192, was signed into law by President Barack Obama on April 19, 2016. This bipartisan legislation reauthorized the OAA for three years and made improvements to benefit older Americans and their families. Three important provisions are

- Improving access to benefit programs through the creation of a National Center on Senior Benefits Outreach and Enrollment.
- Providing broader opportunities for seniors' civic engagement and enabling seniors to make important contributions to their communities.
- Expanding evidence-based health promotion and disease prevention programs.

Imagine Yourself at 84

One of the best ways to sensitize yourself to the aging process is to personalize the experience. So many times there is an imaginary divide between older people and those not quite there. We are all aging and need to get in touch with any stereotypes or personal issues related to getting older.

A good experiential lesson is to imagine yourself at 84. Describe yourself, how you look and feel both physically and emotionally. Include family, hobbies, and activities. Now look back and write a short life review as if you were sitting in the living room, reviewing your life and all of its experiences. Are you satisfied and content? Are there more things you wish to accomplish? Would you do anything differently? What have you left for the world around you?

Complete the following page. Add to it with photographs, collages, and any other creative or expressive ideas that enhance the experience. It can be very powerful.

Psychosocial and Behavioral Health Issues

The people we serve often have psychosocial and behavioral health issues that are as significant as their health issues. Some are part of aging. Some happen because of physical health issues. Others reflect changes in friends and family. This section looks at some of the important ones for activity professionals to consider in their care.

Dealing with Now

People change as they go through their lives. When adults begin to require help for their basic needs, they are different in some way than they were before. They may have slowly become less capable of taking care of themselves as a result of disease or impairment or disability. These changes may have come about slowly, as with Alzheimer's disease, or there may have been a sudden event that drastically changed their lives, such as a motorcycle accident. We need to understand that *how* they came to need care is a significant aspect of their future expectations. We also need to understand that other people who knew the person before s/he came to the facility may react very strongly to the change they see in the person.

Imagine Yourself at 84

How do you see yourself looking physically?

How do you see yourself feeling emotionally?

What is an average day like for you at 84?

Look back on your life and tell your story as a Life History

Often a family member or friend cannot relate to their loved one because s/he has changed so much from what s/he was before. But for us, whenever we meet an individual, that is how we will know that person.

As a staff member, you meet the people we serve as the person s/he is today. You may not have a complete understanding of who s/he was, but you can form a realistic vision of what his/her needs are now. You can see the individual without his/her past, which allows you to see a different present and future.

The difference in expectations is not always obvious, but there are some general trends. Typically a sudden event leaves the family and friends with strong memories of the person before the event. Consequently, they often unrealistically hope for a complete recovery. You will need to deal with the reality of the situation and develop a program that takes the changes into account.

In a gradual process, the family and friends may see the move into supported living or into a long-term care facility as a final step after which they have no further expectations for the person. In those cases you may expect more from the person, when those who knew them before harbor fewer expectations and hopes.

Helen is a good example. She was a regal woman of 82 years. Married twice, both times to high-ranking navy officers, she had lived in exotic lands and treasured her possessions that reminded her of adventures and interesting people from those trips. As a widow, Helen had decided to rent out rooms in her spacious home to artists and musicians so that she could enjoy their company and talents and continue entertaining as she always had.

As Helen became less able to continue this lifestyle with all of its responsibilities, she found herself depending on family more. Her only family was a niece who lived close by. The niece encouraged Helen to seek the care that she felt was needed and to enter a long-term care facility. Helen was still fiercely independent, accustomed to attention, good conversation, good books, and three shots of whiskey daily. Within a short time at the facility, Helen was experiencing frustration, anger, and depression. Her physical strength began to diminish and her memory began to fade. The books that had brought her such joy sat unopened by her bed.

Helen and I still recited her favorite poems and verses during our frequent visits. She shared with me many intimacies, one of which was her unhappiness with her present life. Helen was a frail woman now, but still with the capacity for relationships and friendship.

When Helen died, her niece invited me to attend her memorial service. I found myself alone in a church full of friends and some distant family members, all of whom were wondering how I fit into Helen's life. No one could understand how Helen, in her "obvious state," could have developed a friendship with someone. This is understandable, because she was not the woman whom they had known. But I had never known that Helen, and I never established expectations of what she could or could not accomplish. Still, I was her friend.

We share this story because of the lesson learned. No one is to blame. The lesson is that at any age and at any specific time in our lives, we may encounter someone whom we do not completely understand. At these times we need to pay close attention to what is happening now. We should expect as much as we can, anticipate change, and look for miracles — because one person can make a difference.

The individuals we are working with are who they are in the present because of the sum total of many rich and varied experiences. We need to help them get in touch with the good feelings associated with pleasurable experiences, sensory experiences, companionship, exercise, and success in doing and being alive. At the same time, we need to be sensitive to the fact that they have limits on what they can do and we should not push them beyond those limits. We need to work with the people who are with us as they are now.

Reactions to Illness

People react in different ways to their illnesses and disabilities. And depending on events in their lives, the way they react may change. It may help to be able to identify the manner in which the person is reacting to the illness or disability before determining a treatment plan. (If the person you serve is denying that s/he will need to live in a long-term care facility the rest of his/her life, having a goal of adjusting to living in the long-term care facility will probably not be very well received.) You will usually see one of these five identifiable responses:

1. The "I Can Live with It" attitude. These people accept their illness or disability and are in the process of going on with their lives in the best way possible. Chances are they will cooperate with therapy as long as it has a meaningful, positive impact on their well-being.

2. The "How Do I Get out of Here?" attitude. These people are being limited in their ability to express who they are and to do what they have enjoyed in the past because of their illness or disability (e.g., multiple sclerosis which limits mobility, chronic obstructive pulmonary disease which limits activity level, and early dementia which limits the choice of behavior). These individuals may have unrealistic goals for improvement, waver between anger and depression (about the situation) and bargaining and ability (over hoped changes). This makes consistent performance during therapy difficult.

3. The "I'm Not Really That Sick" attitude. These people are not able to accept their illness or disability and are therefore denying the severity of their limitations. Engaging these individuals in therapy may be difficult, as they may not recognize that they need to work to improve function.

4. The "Is There Really Any Other Way to Be?" attitude. These individuals define their role in life as being "sick" and must have others take care of them and feel sorry for them. Some people define themselves by this role for their entire lives, while others ease into it. In either case, it's the assumption that one has the *right* to be and act ill. These individuals tend to want treatment to be done *to* them, not to initiate and be self-guided in treatment.

5. "Unable to Comprehend." The last category is not associated with an attitude, but the reality that due to the severity of the illness or disability the person is not able to engage in meaningful thought about his/her problems. This is especially true for residents with advanced dementia, severe head injuries, or other significant insults to the brain. These individuals will tend to be guided by the stimulation (noxious or pleasant) in the environment and by internally felt impulses.

When we set goals for the people we serve, we need to take into account how each person is reacting to being in the facility.

Along with the reaction to his/her illness or disability, there is one reaction that we see in almost every person: the need to be in control. The need to control one's life is one of our greatest needs. From the robust to the frail, feeling like we are in control of what happens to us is important.

The Patient or Resident Bill of Rights goes a long way toward guaranteeing this control. However, we must use good judgment when we offer choices to the people we serve. We must take into account previous lifestyle, current abilities, and the person's health status when deciding how to offer the choices.

The People We Serve and Their Families

One of the most common myths of long-term care — spread far and wide — is that the typical long-term care facility resident is dumped into an institution by society or by an uncaring family. In truth, it is the rare resident who has *no one* to care for him/her. This fact actually extends whom we serve and requires that we consider not only the needs of the resident but also the needs of his/her family. To a lesser extent, the same considerations apply when someone starts receiving home health care services or is placed in an adult day program.

As a response to loss of function or declining health with the need for assistance and placement in a program, we find some very complicated, yet common, responses by both the person we serve and the family. Reactions to placement and the progression of feelings are actually the same as we see in any situation where loss is involved:

1. Denial that the loss of independence has occurred and that the need for placement really exists.
2. Anger and hostility about or toward the placement.
3. Searching for alternatives and bargaining to try to change the situation.
4. Sadness and depression in response to the loss.
5. Acceptance of the loss of independence and the need for placement.

The question is "What do we do with all of these feelings and the actions and interactions that result from them?" They will all be there and we need to deal with them effectively.

Any satisfactory placement depends on appropriate staff interventions related to these feelings, actions, and interactions. We will analyze them to help you prepare to interpret them and work through them when you see them in your facility.

At any given moment, any of these responses may be occurring between one or another resident and family because the facility is dynamic, with new admissions, new adjustments, and continuing attempts to cope with the circumstances of placement.

From your side, you will see the same set of problems played out many times. Remember, though, this may be the first time for the person you serve and the family. Even though you have seen the situation many times, each situation will be different. There will be a difference in the intensity of each reaction depending on what has come before. For example, the family that has had previous admissions to a transitional care unit in a hospital resulting in discharge to a lesser level of care will have had the opportunity to think about this (re)placement and will come in with a different set of emotions and reactions based on already having worked through the progression of reactions to loss. Others will need every opportunity to interpret this new set of life circumstances and will then progress naturally from one through five.

What to do? We suggest that you trust your basic instincts. Ask yourself the questions: "What might I need if I were in this (these) situation(s)? How might I wish to be treated if this were my family?"

We do not pretend to know all of the answers, but there are a few things that all of us can do to bring some comfort and reassurance. No matter what else you say or do, be sincere. Your words may not be remembered but your reactions, the way you act, have the potential of forming a lasting impression and may set the tone for further helpful interactions.

Listen to anger and hostility without reacting defensively; offer to seek answers to questions and concerns and then follow up. In any case, genuine warmth and compassion mean the world at times of loss and transition.

In the next five sections, we will identify expected feelings and suggest interventions that will help the person you serve and his/her family progress toward acceptance of the situation.

Denial

There's no place like home. Who hasn't felt the comfort of returning home after being away for any length of time? How can home, that place where we most belong in the world, become one day a place that is no longer physically or emotionally nurturing? In fact, how can it represent potential harm for us?

The loss of home, warmth, and comfort underlie the person's denial, especially for people who have been admitted to a long-term care facility for the first time. It is unimaginable to most to give up the place where one not only belongs, but is also independent and safe.

Typical timing. Admission to two months

Feelings and thoughts

Person we serve: "I'm really not as ill or needy as everyone is saying; if you let me go home, I will be able to take care of myself."

Family: "This is really only a temporary placement; soon, Mom/Dad will be out of bed doing just what s/he has always been able to."

Interactions

Person we serve: "My home is so well organized for me; I have a routine there which allows me to function." "Everyone is counting on my leaving, so I have to."

Family: "I wonder if this might be a permanent placement. I hate to bring the subject up because I don't want to discourage Mom/Dad from making progress so I will continue to speak about his/her discharge as a given."

Intervention

False hope is worse than the truth and only postpones facing the facts. But arriving at the truth is an evolutionary process. For example, first ask both the person you serve and the family to describe actual functioning level and then ask them to describe what level of function is necessary, especially related to the return to the previous environment (usually taking care of themselves). This process takes time; the two steps we recommend are not easily or truthfully answered upon admission. We find, in fact, that an individual admitted to a long-term care facility is not usually ready to admit that placement may be long-term for at least two months from the time of admission. By that time, a sense of security may have set in and, with support from staff and family, the realization that care is required. (We are, of course, speaking only of those needing long-term placement.)

We feel that involving the person we serve, continually asking him/her to assess and reassess the reality of his/her level of function will remove the pressure from the family. It is a tremendous burden for the family to feel they are making this decision against someone's will. The decision is seldom crystal clear. All available resources, including the physician and staff, should be called upon to paint the picture of what is and what isn't possible, what can and what can't be.

Anger

We will preface this section by saying that this is often the most difficult reaction to deal with because of its intensity. Most of us shrink from anger in ourselves or in others and are frightened by it. As a result, we tend to deny its existence or negate its necessity. But it is necessary to let us know when something is wrong. By becoming aware of the usefulness of anger, you can be more compassionate, looking beyond the words and actions to find the motivating pain.

Typical Timing. Two weeks to two months

Feelings and Thoughts

Person we serve: "You've put me here; you're dumping me and leaving me to die. I hate this place and I hate these people. I am not like them." "I am terribly disappointed in what you have done to me." "You're treating me like a child. I can still take care of myself most of the time."

Family: "Everything is topsy-turvy in my life now; not only has my parent been taken from me, but you don't know how to take care of him/her the way I do. The food doesn't suit him/her; no one comes when s/he calls."

Interactions

Person we serve: (to staff) "Everything I eat tastes the same! Why?" "Last night instead of helping me, the aide turned my light off. That's no way to treat me!" (to family) "When will you take me out of here?" "You don't love me any more and are glad that you got rid of me!" "You've rested enough. How can you leave me here?"

Family: "I know I come early in the morning, but I like to see that Mom/Dad eats breakfast, has his/her dentures cleaned properly, and is dressed warmly. That's the way we did it at home and I want to continue doing it that way."

Intervention

The family's frustrations often are seen as anger toward the staff. They need our help to understand what has happened and where they need to go from here.

Think about what makes a family angry. It may be caused by a lack of control over what is happening to both the individual and the family. It may be guilt about making the placement, the inconvenience of visiting during perceived visiting hours, driving mom or dad to the center, or the stress of needing to deal with others who have different cultural values. It may be that at home everything was always neatly in place and easy to find while now the person can't even be sure that his/her socks will get back from the laundry. We need to look at the possibility that the anger is justified and deal as best we can with concrete and correctable complaints.

In addition to problems that can be fixed, we also need to consider whether the role reversal — parent to child, child to parent — doesn't somehow produce a tremendous sense of responsibility, which shows up as an increase in anger related to expected levels of care. That is, the idea of becoming the parent to our parent may be so threatening emotionally that we feel fear or grief that manifests itself as anger. How can we ever adequately parent the person who gave us life? How can we ever do enough? And will we ever be old enough to outgrow the need for being parented ourselves?

These are all issues we must learn to deal with. They are important because those of us who work in facilities often greet the mad or angry face. If we return anger, it is a significant deterrent to warm relationships between family and staff. If we can wade through some of this emotion, interpret it to the staff, and help the family see ways of getting beyond their fears and anger, we will be further along in meeting resident and family needs.

Allow for healing time so that trust can be developed. Time is needed for both the person we serve and the family. We are entrusted with a great responsibility and it is appropriate that the way we work is closely scrutinized. Do your best to not return anger by realizing that the anger of the family and the person we serve is an attack against the situation, not an attack against *you*.

Advise and inform all concerned about what can be expected of the facility. Guide them in the choice and style of visiting and encourage families to trust the facility resources and to pursue their own, sometimes abandoned, lives.

Establishing trust in communication is most effective in dissipating anger. Become a familiar, reliable source of information and comfort.

Searching for Alternatives

As a result of recognizing and acting on the anger surrounding the placement, the person we serve may prevail upon the family to get him/her "out of here." Likewise, the family may respond to their own feelings by shopping around in hope of finding a program or facility that will be more suitable. Sometimes there is a clear need to change programs or facilities to find one that is more compatible with their needs. Other times simply altering the location of the placement (even if there are only subtle differences in care) will allow the person we serve and the family to regain some of their lost control. Most of the time, the search for alternatives does not result in the person we serve leaving, but it is still necessary for both the family and the person we serve to know that they have done their best to make the situation as ideal as it possibly can be. When they are sure that the situation can't be improved, they can move on toward accepting the situation.

Typical timing. 6 weeks to 3 months

Feelings and thoughts

Person we serve: "I feel abandoned and isolated. I just don't think this is the best place." "If I could just go home, I know it would be so much better." "There must be a better place."

Family: "I heard of a place that really is good about getting people back on their feet. I want to check it out." "There must be some way we can take care of him/her at home." "There must be a better place."

Interactions

Person we serve: "I think I can walk as well as I did before. You won't have to lift me at home." "I'll work very hard in therapy so I get well enough to go home." "Please, please, find someplace else. I just don't fit in here."

Family: (to person we serve) "We're looking for a better place. They are not that easy to find, though." (to staff) "We're trying to find a way to take care of Mom/Dad at home. Do you know of any resources that can help?"

Intervention

Some families never reach the point where they feel they have found the best alternative and this can be hard on everyone. For many, the weight of responsibility is tremendous; spouses especially may feel guilty whenever they are enjoying themselves and the person we serve can't share it. We find this to be especially true for spouses of people we serve who have Alzheimer's. The spouses have to watch the person slowly dying and feel in limbo — neither married nor widowed — and guilty for thinking of fun or normalcy in life. If you really feel that the current situation is appropriate, help the person and family to accept the situation, too.

Support groups help both the person and family to resolve many of the issues of searching for alternatives. It helps to see how others have dealt with feelings and restructured their lives. Individuals may need to redefine their lives within the confines of a smaller community (the care facility) and family members must re-enter the community at large with a different identity. Advise individuals and their significant others about support groups and use your experience to assist in reshaping roles and responsibilities.

Remember that there is a chance (even a good chance) that the family and the person we serve will find a better alternative. Support them in their search, especially by helping them find resources in the community that will make it possible for the person we serve to return home or to a lesser care setting. Try to remain open to, and applaud, the possibility that the person we serve would be better suited somewhere else and is actively pursuing this goal.

Sadness and Depression

Sadness and depression are very individual responses. The depth and length of this period depend on the person's philosophy of life, the support available from family and staff, and the medical problems the person is experiencing. (Some medical problems, such as a stroke, may cause an organically induced depression lasting months.)

Typical timing. 6 weeks to 1 year

Feelings and thoughts

Person we serve: "There is nothing, absolutely nothing that appeals to me here." "I really don't feel like getting up and I certainly don't want to do anything as silly as having my hair done."

Family: "I miss him/her. It just isn't the same at home any more." "I hate to visit — it makes me feel badly when I come in feeling happy with news from home."

Interactions

Person we serve: Sitting, doing nothing, not interacting with staff or others. "I'm sorry. I really don't feel like doing that now." "I suppose we can talk, but this whole thing just makes me want to cry."

Family: "I cry a lot when I'm home; the only time I'm happy is when I'm here with you." "I just can't visit. It makes me too sad." "It's always good to talk with you about how I feel. It just makes me feel better."

Intervention

Once again, time, opportunity to experience control, and security of placement will contribute to a change in mood away from sadness. It is essential, however, to acknowledge the feelings, never trying to negate or "soft pedal" sorrow or grieving.

In order to encourage ongoing family visiting and to make it a positive experience for everyone involved, you might give some of your favorite ideas for visiting:

- Come during a meal when you will be assured of having something to focus on; use the meal's beginning (or end) as the beginning (or end) of your visit, a natural breaking point.
- Come just before the person's normal bedtime to offer pleasant good night wishes.
- Bring in a special treat — a milkshake, a spring bouquet from your garden, or some homemade soup.
- Bring in a special friend or a new great-grandchild; encourage friends to visit, even for a moment.
- Personalize the room with a picture from home, family pictures, a favorite vase. Not only will this trigger happy memories, but these objects will also be icebreakers for conservation when facility staff are in the room.
- If the person is enrolled in an adult day program, develop a special routine that is enjoyable to the person either before or after each time s/he attends the program.

The important thing is to work toward accepting the sadness at the loss of independence and to start looking for the good things that are still possible in the new situation.

Acceptance

There are those who appear to acknowledge the need for placement from the time of admission — immediate acceptance! But don't be fooled! Almost everyone who starts out seeming to accept the placement will still go through the previously described reactions. Even a person who is being readmitted is back again because something has changed (and probably something has been lost).

We have seen almost everyone work his/her way through all four of the previous stages. Once those stages have been experienced, you can look for true acceptance.

Typical timing. May start at 2 months

Feelings and thoughts

Person we serve: "I am enjoying the activities here, especially cards and travel presentations. I have chosen Saturday for one of my shower days so that I can feel good about myself for church on Sunday. My room looks so comfy with my TV and chair and all those family photos. Best of all, my son goes to the bank and tends to all of my affairs for me."

Family: "I enjoy visiting a lot more now. It's so nice to see Mom/Dad smiling again. It's fun to bring in flowers from the garden for the room and for the staff. It's nice to have Mom/Dad in a place where s/he feels comfortable. It's nice to be able to get out of the house and do things without worrying all the time if Mom/Dad is all right."

Interactions

Person we serve: You will observe relaxed body language and warm relationships with others. "I've made so many friends here, residents and staff. I trust that they do care about me, maybe not as much as my family, but I can still complain and express my true feelings without worrying about what will happen. I know you can't really make me get a lot better, but I certainly appreciate your help making me comfortable."

Family: You will see an easygoing relationship with staff and a warm and friendly attitude. They will freely seek to resolve grievances as they occur. "Everyone is friendly here. You are always willing to listen when I have a concern and you usually take care of it right away."

Intervention

Acceptance comes after much hard work and usually some emotional stress. It is welcome as a time for appreciating relationships and enjoying the time left. At this point, everyone involved (the person we serve, family, and staff) is visibly satisfied with the quality and quantity of interactions. An easy camaraderie exists between individual and family and the feeling generates goodwill with the staff. There is usually free give and take and consistent involvement in all aspects of care. During this period, you may find individuals and families needing more encouragement to attend resident care conferences because they will say, "We're here so often." "We speak with you regularly." "I trust you to phone if there is a new problem." "I know you take good care of me."

A final note. The five reactions we have described here are a continuum and people generally go through them step by step. However, residents and families will often seem to drop back several levels. When this happens, look for some additional loss that has occurred. We go through the stages with each loss and there is no guarantee that it gets any easier with time. But our struggles and our eventual acceptance show the lifelong potential for growth and change that all of us carry within ourselves.

Diagnoses and Chronic Disorders

Diagnosis refers to "the process of identifying a medical condition or disease by its signs, symptoms, and from the results of various diagnostic procedures."

A diagnosis is important to you for many reasons. It helps identify known risk factors during activities (what you can expect of the person now). It gives you some indication of prognosis (what you can expect of the person in the future). There are other factors that interact with the diagnosed condition to affect what the person is capable of doing. The two most significant factors are the acuity of the condition and the excess disability resulting from the person's environment.

Acuity refers to the severity or the level of intensity of the diagnosed illness or condition at the present time. Perhaps this condition represents a crisis or acute situation as opposed to a chronic condition that is more stable and long lasting. People on an intensive care unit represent a higher level of acuity than an individual who is recuperating from a broken leg. The acuity of the condition can have a significant influence on the types of activity that the person can successfully participate in. Knowing the level of acuity also helps professionals know how quickly they can expect a change.

Excess disability refers to a "decline of functional abilities, alertness, cognitive status, orientation, communication, physical status, and socialization attributed to the environment and not specifically attributable to a disease process."[10] This decline is greater than, or in excess of, the decline expected from the illness or disability. Something besides the illness or disability is making the person worse than expected. One of the jobs of the professional is to help identify what this "something" is.

Excess disability refers to all potential factors that can impact an individual's cognitive and functional level more profoundly than their diagnosis. One set of reasons for this excess disability comes from the environment: the physical environment, social issues, and attitudes exhibited by staff and family. Other reasons for excess disability are found in individual beliefs and attitudes including problem solving skills, life skills, and the ability to be resilient during stressful experiences. Many of these factors causing excess disability can be improved through changes in the facility environment, group activities, and one-on-one interactions between the professional and the individual or family. One other contributing factor is medication, which may increase memory loss, depression, lethargy, and balance problems. You can often provide information to the health care team about effects of medication that may not be obvious in other settings.

You are often the member of the interdisciplinary team who assesses how a person's diagnosis, acuity, and excess disability influence his/her leisure needs, interests, and quality of life. Goals need to specifically correlate to the individual's present functional level. Federal law (OBRA '87) mandates that the nursing home facility provide quality of life experiences to all individuals residing in a long-term care setting. (When the quality of life component is out of compliance, the facility is deemed to be in

---

[10] Katsinas, René, 1995, *Excess disability: Recognizing the hidden problem in long-term care*, presented at the American Therapeutic Recreation Association Conference, October, 1995.

substandard compliance.) As with other determinants, you should understand all of the limitations a person is experiencing related to his/her diagnosis and use that knowledge to find and focus on abilities, rather than disabilities, a holistic rather than medical model approach for planning the activity program.

MDS List of Active Diagnoses

The following list of diagnoses shows the categorization in the MDS Version 3.0, Section I: Active Diagnoses. We will be referring to these categories in the material that follows.

Cancer

- I0100, cancer (with or without metastasis)

Heart/Circulation

- I0200, anemia (e.g., aplastic, iron deficiency, pernicious, sickle cell)
- I0300, atrial fibrillation or other dysrhythmias (e.g., bradycardias, tachycardias)
- I0400, coronary artery disease (CAD) (e.g., angina, myocardial infarction, atherosclerotic heart disease [ASHD])
- I0500, deep venous thrombosis (DVT), pulmonary embolus (PE), or pulmonary thromboembolism (PTE)
- I0600, heart failure (e.g., congestive heart failure [CHF], pulmonary edema)
- I0700, hypertension
- I0800, orthostatic hypotension
- I0900, peripheral vascular disease or peripheral arterial disease

Gastrointestinal

- I1100, cirrhosis
- I1200, gastroesophageal reflux disease (GERD) or ulcer (e.g., esophageal, gastric, and peptic ulcers)
- I1300, ulcerative colitis or Crohn's disease or inflammatory bowel disease

Genitourinary

- I1400, benign prostatic hyperplasia (BPH)
- I1500, renal insufficiency, renal failure, or end-stage renal disease (ESRD)
- I1550, neurogenic bladder
- I1650, obstructive uropathy

Infections

- I1700, multidrug resistant organism (MDRO)
- I2000, pneumonia
- I2100, septicemia
- I2200, tuberculosis
- I2300, urinary tract infection (UTI) (last 30 days)
- I2400, viral hepatitis (e.g., hepatitis A, B, C, D, and E)
- I2500, wound infection (other than in foot)

Metabolic

- I2900, diabetes mellitus (DM) (e.g., diabetic retinopathy, nephropathy, neuropathy)
- I3100, hyponatremia
- I3200, hyperkalemia
- I3300, hyperlipidemia (e.g., hypercholesterolemia)
- I3400, thyroid disorder (e.g., hypothyroidism, hyperthyroidism, Hashimoto's thyroiditis)

Musculoskeletal

- I3700, arthritis (e.g., degenerative joint disease [DJD], osteoarthritis, rheumatoid arthritis [RA])
- I3800, osteoporosis
- I3900, hip fracture (any hip fracture that has a relationship to current status, treatments, monitoring (e.g., subcapital fractures and fractures of the trochanter and femoral neck))
- I4000, other fracture

Neurological

- I4200, Alzheimer's disease

- I4300, aphasia
- I4400, cerebral palsy
- I4500, cerebrovascular accident (CVA), transient ischemic attack (TIA), or stroke
- I4800, dementia[11] (e.g., non-Alzheimer's dementia, including vascular or multi-infarct dementia; mixed dementia; frontotemporal dementia, such as Pick's disease; and dementia related to stroke, Parkinson's disease, or Creutzfeldt-Jakob diseases)
- I4900, hemiplegia or hemiparesis
- I5000, paraplegia
- I5100, quadriplegia
- I5200, multiple sclerosis (MS)
- I5250, Huntington's disease
- I5300, Parkinson's disease
- I5350, Tourette's syndrome
- I5400, seizure disorder or epilepsy
- I5500, traumatic brain injury (TBI)

Nutritional

- I5600, malnutrition (protein or calorie) or at risk for malnutrition

Psychiatric/Mood Disorder

- I5700, anxiety disorder
- I5800, depression (other than bipolar)
- I5900, manic depression (bipolar disorder)
- I5950, psychotic disorder (other than schizophrenia)
- I6000, schizophrenia (e.g., schizoaffective and schizophreniform disorders)
- I6100, post-traumatic stress disorder (PTSD)

Pulmonary

- I6200, asthma, chronic obstructive pulmonary disease (COPD), or chronic lung disease (e.g., chronic bronchitis and restrictive lung diseases, such as asbestosis)
- I6300, respiratory failure

Vision

- I6500, cataracts, glaucoma, or macular degeneration

None of Above

- I7900, none of the above active diagnoses within the past 7 days

Other

- I8000, additional active diagnoses

The Diagnostic Intervention Grid

This Diagnostic Intervention Grid was designed to provide professionals with a quick overview of specific disorders that may affect the people they serve. It also summarizes what the individual may be experiencing and the consequent implications for programming and communications for those individuals.

The Diagnostic Intervention Grid is a quick reference to diagnostic groups and corresponding therapeutic programming needs and psychosocial needs. You need to work with the rest of the health care team to coordinate the specific guidelines and treatment plans. In addition, you have much to offer in terms of continued training and understanding of the people we serve.

This form cannot cover all the people we serve or all situations, but it will help explain some of the diagnoses seen. It is also useful as a training tool and can be successfully shared with staff and volunteers alike who work with you. After becoming acquainted with this chart and its underlying ideas, they will better understand how and why specific activities are designed to meet specific needs.

Using the Diagnostic Intervention Grid

The grid is designed to give you important information about specific disorders and what this individual may be experiencing. After you have met and begun your assessment of the person, use this grid as a reference to determine

[11] The MDS 3.0 Manual came out in 2012, the year before the DSM-5 came out and changed the diagnosis of dementia to neurocognitive disorder (NCD). Both terms are currently used in settings with older adults.

what type of person-centered programming may be both appropriate and therapeutic.

There is an important change to one term that is used in the diagnostic grid. When the *Diagnostic and Statistical Manual of Mental Disorders, Fifth Ed.* came out in 2013, the psychological community changed the term dementia to neurocognitive disorder (NCD). In long-term care the most widely accepted term is still dementia. In this book we will continue to primarily use the term dementia until the Centers for Medicare and Medicaid Services change their terminology.

Diagnostic Group (Column 1)

This column defines some of the diagnostic categories that may be found in the populations we serve.

Implications and Symptoms (Column 2)

This column describes some of the implications and symptoms of the diagnosis found in column one. A review of these issues will help you understand the disorder more clearly by observing common signs, symptoms, and issues.

Psychosocial Impact (Column 3)

This column deals with the psychosocial aspects that may be related to the health issue. Some of these may be perceptions of an individual's condition that his/her family members and other visitors may also experience. In order to better understand the diagnosis and current needs of the individual, you must be sensitive to all of the emotional and psychological aspects that affect not only the individual but also his/her significant others' ability to cope with the diagnosis or illness and the interventions.

Programming Ideas (Column 4)

This column suggests a variety of therapeutic programming ideas specific to the health issues in column one. Which activities are appropriate depends primarily on the needs, interests, and abilities of the individual. Many of these ideas can be found in the program chapters of the book. Take into account current levels of cognitive function.

Diagnostic Intervention Grid

Diagnostic Group	Implications and Symptoms	Psychosocial Impact	Programming Ideas
Diabetes Type 1: Diabetes Mellitus (insulin dependent) Type 2: Non-Insulin Dependent Diabetes Mellitus (NIDDM)	Low tolerance to heat and cold	May avoid groups in crowded spaces or outdoor activities in the heat or cold May feel anxious	Activities should not tax physical ability Be sure to remind individuals to eat complex carbohydrates and keep snacks with them as recommended by the physician
	Poor circulation in legs and feet with potential for sores that do not heal	Poor safety awareness due to lack of sensation	Staff need to be aware of positioning and placement especially at tables and in group settings
	Possible visual deficits	May feel insecure due to vision loss	Avoid activities that require good vision for success Avoid exercises that can increase blood pressure because this can harm the retinal blood vessels
	Potential for hypoglycemia (insulin reaction)	Concern about risks	Staff need to be aware of symptoms (such as faintness, sweating, dizziness, hunger, loss of motor coordination, rapid pulse, and/or confusion) and respond immediately so that the individual feels safe
	Limited endurance	May need reminders to take breaks and hydrate	Teach energy conservation techniques Encourage physical activity to increase endurance and strength, but discourage exercise that may be too strenuous
	Potential for dehydration	Feeling thirsty and potentially anxious	Remind person to drink water frequently during activities and at other times
Sensory Deficits vision hearing touch taste smell	Partial to total loss of one or more of the senses Great potential for isolation Potential pain Stiff and swollen joints Limited dexterity and coordination Blurred vision and/or lack of color discrimination Loss of sensation and sense of touch Lack of sufficient stimulation Need glasses and/or hearing aids	Perceived as mentally impaired or incapable of conversation and/or normal activity Socially isolated related to sensory impairment Depression related to losses Potential for injury in environment	Sensory stimulation Weaving Theme activities Exercise/movement Visual cues Auditory cues Activities to learn strategies to compensate for losses Focus on senses that remain intact Social interaction Provide adaptations for sensory losses

Diagnostic Intervention Grid

Diagnostic Group	Implications and Symptoms	Psychosocial Impact	Programming Ideas
Osteoporosis	Potential for falls and fractures	Fear and anxiety about physical activity and leisure activities that may be too difficult	Avoid activities that require lifting or carrying heavy objects
	Possible balance and posture problems	Insecure about participating due to pain and possible injury	Encourage exercises that improve posture and/or balance to build confidence in movement
	Kyphosis (severe spinal deformity)	Lack of motivation to participate due to pain and fear of injury	Encourage postural exercises that bring the shoulders back and enhance the ability to stand and sit straighter Avoid overloading the back Avoid exercises that increase spinal flexion (bending forward at the waist)
	Chronic back pain and stiffness	Uncomfortable to sit for an extended amount of time due to back pain	Stretching exercises and slow, pain-free range-of-motion exercises Provide seated exercise classes Provide activities that can be done in segments so that individual can change position or return later to complete
	Fatigue	A stooped posture can impair pulmonary function and thus limit endurance and create fatigue	Small amounts of exercise or activity at a time Remind individual to change positions and take a rest as needed Adapt activities to the functional level of the individual
Language Barriers	Inability to make needs known and to communicate in primary language	Perceived as mentally impaired or incapable of conversation and/or normal activity Loss of familiar language, customs, and music	Communication cards in primary language Visual cues Communication board Tapes in primary language, music, and foreign newspapers

Diagnostic Intervention Grid

Diagnostic Group	Implications and Symptoms	Psychosocial Impact	Programming Ideas
Dementia/Neurocognitive Disorder (NCD) Dementia due to Alzheimer's Disease Vascular Dementia Dementia with Lewy Bodies Dementia due to Parkinson's Disease Frontotemporal Dementia Dementia due to Traumatic Brain Injury Dementia due to HIV Infection Substance/Medication-Induced Dementia Dementia due to Huntington's Disease Dementia due to Prion Disease Mild Cognitive Impairment (MCI) Delirium (see section on cognitive impairments for more information)	Short-term memory loss and/or long-term memory loss Short attention span Loss of executive functions Decline in decision making skills (moderately impaired to severely impaired) Disorientation and confusion Possible agitation, aggression, anxiety, apathy Pacing Psychosis Catastrophic responses, possible combativeness Possible decrease in activity levels and physical fitness Communication deficits Difficulty with directions (e.g. path finding) Depression Decrease in ability to learn new things Sleep disturbance Possible aphasia, apraxia, agnosia Impulsivity	Depression based on realization of loss No longer treated as an intelligent person by others due to loss of ability to communicate well in conversation The need for structure increases with disease progression Loss of previous lifestyle, life roles Feelings of helplessness and hopelessness Personal awareness of cognitive losses during more alert periods Decreased safety awareness Inability to perceive physical threats within the environment Catastrophic responses to environment and interactions caused by inability to interpret multiple stimulating events	Tap into the abilities that remain Reality awareness Validation therapy Sensory stimulation Music activities Outdoor activities Object identification, sorting Reading Breathing exercises Body awareness Physical activity, physical games Flash cards, Etch-A-Sketch Velcro activities Compensatory skills training Provide activities that access long-term memory Decrease the stress and fear the individual may be experiencing by using structured, safe, and relaxing activities Create activities that encourage socialization Provide fun experiences that are age-appropriate

Diagnostic Intervention Grid

Diagnostic Group	Implications and Symptoms	Psychosocial Impact	Programming Ideas
Comatose (persistent vegetative state with no discernible consciousness)	Non-responsive Limited or no vision Communication deficit Potential for skin integrity problems Possible nasogastric tube or other feeding tube Possible tracheotomy Possible respirator	Isolation Family and friends feel helpless or hopeless about visiting unless able to assist in the rehabilitative process Potential sensory deprivation Unknown outcome Loss of previous relationships and income	Music Eye tracking experiences (mobiles and/or, posters if eyes are open) Soft range of motion exercises Hand over hand activities Tactile stimulation Auditory stimulation Reading out loud Pet therapy Fresh air
Head Injury	Need for compensatory skills Impaired memory and judgment Impulsivity Weak problem solving Catastrophic reaction to stress Irritability due to limited cognitive, motor, and language abilities Slow processing of information and learning and remembering new information Poor safety skills	If the injury is not visible, expectations are often greater than potential, resulting in frustration for the person and caregivers Lack of initiative Decreased ability to structure or manage time Change in social relationships and behavior Decreased ability to perform in work, academic, and leisure activities	Sequencing activities Sensory integration Sorting games Word games Body awareness and movement Word search activities Hangman Crossword puzzles Large sectional puzzles Attention to task building activities Theme activities Links to community resources Focus on abilities that remain
Chemotherapy **Dialysis**	Limited mobility Low level of energy Need for close proximity to equipment	Loss of control based on limited mobility Feelings of vulnerability Exhaustion due to condition and therapy Fear of the future and unknown outcome	Mild exercise and movement Talking books Oral history visits Reinforcement of therapy goals Environmental and relaxation CDs, music Art interventions Memory book

Diagnostic Intervention Grid

Diagnostic Group	Implications and Symptoms	Psychosocial Impact	Programming Ideas
CVA (stroke) **Left Brain Damage (right side paralyzed)**	Right hemiparesis/hemiplegia Language/reading/writing problems Aphasia (word-finding problems) Perseveration (repeating same word or phrase) Possible dysphagia Attention deficits Difficulty distinguishing left and right Visuospatial neglect Memory deficits Lability (mood swings) Low frustration tolerance Sleep disturbances Difficulty naming objects, but can use them Impaired verbal and math skills Loss of ability to plan movements (apraxia)	Isolation depending on location of CVA and degree of impairment Depression — both physiological and related to loss(es) and/or expectations beyond current potential Impatience and frustration with new functional status and lack of speedy recovery Self-conscious about appearance and language difficulties Loss of function and frustration from inactivity Frustration with group experiences Lack of inhibition Behavior is slow, cautious, anxious Underestimates ability	Involving in appropriate exercises as soon as possible after stroke Activities which stimulate cognitive functioning Body image activities Retraining cognitive and perceptual abilities Repetitive tasks and movements to achieve mastery and therefore transfer skills to other activities Sensory integration activities Sequencing activities Communication group experiences Working with significant others to identify leisure interests and opportunities Exercise activities Opportunities for community reintegration as part of rehabilitation Life skills training Memory enhancement exercises Word and trivia games
CVA (stroke) **Right Brain Damage (left side paralyzed)**	Left hemiparesis/hemiplegia Perceptual problems Poor spatial orientation and concepts of direction Gets lost easily Decrease or increase in sensation Change in vision Seizures Decreased eye-hand coordination Impaired concrete thinking Sleep disturbances Left-side neglect Short attention span Speech usually not affected Possible dysphagia	Isolation depending on location of CVA and degree of impairment Depression — both physiological and related to loss(es) or expectations beyond potential Impatience, frustration with new functional status and lack of speedy recovery Self-conscious about appearance and language difficulties Loss of function and frustration from inactivity Behavior is fast, impulsive, with lack of inhibition and verbal outbursts Overestimates ability Emotional lability, apathy	Focus on using intact strengths and abilities to help overcome limitations

Diagnostic Intervention Grid

Diagnostic Group	Implications and Symptoms	Psychosocial Impact	Programming Ideas
Hip Fractures, Joint Replacements	Limited energy and endurance Easily fatigued Pain Temporary loss of mobility and previous level of function At risk for falls	Relationships may be strained due to pain and due to the resident needing to adjust to new (usually lower) ability Impatience with the current situation Primary focus on therapy goals Fantasies about home and about the ability to care for him/herself Lack of information about home health care and unreasonable expectations can cause anxiety for individual and family	Reading Relaxation CDs Exercise/movement Bird watching Outdoor social activities Work/service oriented activities Community integration Reinforcing therapy goals Resident council Volunteering Memory book
Huntington's Chorea	Severe mood swings Involuntary movements Twitching Nervous behavior Depression Communication problems Aggression Hallucinations Difficulty swallowing	Hopelessness, isolation, and feelings of anger and abandonment Guilt based on the genetic component of this disease Inability to feel independent due to tremors Difficulty communicating related to slurred speech Intoxicated appearance which can overwhelm people nearby	Exercise Expressive opportunities Weaving Music for relaxation Ceramics Homemaking activities Adaptive switches Verbal word games Communication groups Theme activities
Parkinson's Disease	Resting tremors Rigidity Bradykinesia (slow movement) Has difficulty with more than two movements at one time Softness of voice Depression Need extra time to respond Unsteady gait Possible limb apraxia Poor coordination Possible dementia and hallucinations	Isolation as communication becomes more difficult Perceived as having dementia when this is not necessarily true Flat affect (disease related) may be perceived as disinterest or dementia	Exercise Expressive opportunities Weaving Music and relaxing Ceramics Homemaking activities Adaptive switches Verbal word games Communication groups Theme activities

Diagnostic Intervention Grid

Diagnostic Group	Implications and Symptoms	Psychosocial Impact	Programming Ideas
Multiple Sclerosis **Amyotrophic Lateral Sclerosis (ALS)**	Possible loss of fine and gross motor skills Possible speech and language disorders Possible vision impairments Fluctuation both physically and emotionally Possible fluid retention Gastrointestinal problems Depression Possible limb apraxia	Total loss of control is possible Anger Attempts to manipulate the environment in order to have needs met Fantasizing about home and the ability to care for oneself Lack of participation in activities Anxiety Impatience and frustration over situation Depression	Exercise and movement activities Need for energy conservation techniques Relaxation Creative outlets Opportunities to socialize with peers in age-appropriate activities Visualization Empowerment activities Adaptive switches Communication activities with yes/no responses Body awareness and posture exercises
Pulmonary Problems **COPD** **Asthma** **Heart Circulation /Cardiac** **Hypotension** **Hypertension**	Anxiety Coughing Light-headed depending on body positioning Inability to breathe deeply Decreased endurance Low tolerance to dust, odors, and crowded spaces Depression Activities requiring raising the arms over the head are too taxing Limited time up Added stress on heart	Attempts to manipulate the environment and personnel secondary to feelings of anxiety and claustrophobia Need to feel in control of personal environment as much as possible Need for stress management and coping mechanisms	Handwork Breathing exercises Relaxation Energy conservation techniques Need for balance of active and passive activities Slow-paced activities Activities which do not require lifting heavy objects Crossword puzzles Puzzles Body positioned leaning forward to reduce strain on respiratory system Reading Creative writing Theme activities
Critically Ill **Terminally Ill** **Hospice**	Limited energy and time awake Depression Potential for pain	Changing moods depending on state of anger, depression, and acceptance Existential issues of life and death May have unfinished business that needs to be completed including questions of religion and spirituality	Relaxation Being read to In room travel slides or environmental CDs One-on-one volunteers Memory book Companionship Visualization Opportunity to talk Light range-of-motion activities Interventions to manage pain

Diagnostic Intervention Grid

Diagnostic Group	Implications and Symptoms	Psychosocial Impact	Programming Ideas
Ventilator Dependent	Potential for sensory deprivation Lack of mobility or freedom of movement Potential for skin integrity issues Communication problems Lack of endurance Potential for significant hours a day in bed Pain related to injuries and condition Cardiopulmonary issues Partial to total loss of one or more senses May be non-responsive Potential for total care ADLs May have a tracheotomy May be fed by tube	Inability to move around without equipment causes loss of independence Depression related to condition Anxiety related to breathing ability Limited emotional outlets Potential for social isolation Short- or long-term need for ventilator Potential for embarrassment in groups related to equipment and equipment sounds	Visualization and relaxation CDs Mobiles Music Slide shows Activities related to body awareness and directionality games Opportunities to be outdoors Range of motion activities Pain management techniques Reading and being read to Intellectual activities Pets Theme-related decorations Volunteer visitors Small fish bowl in room within visual range Computer games Dot-to-dot puzzles Wristbands with bell to enhance movement and auditory stimulation Drinking straw with streamer attached to enhance breathing exercises
Spinal Cord Injury[12]	Loss of mobility Loss of motor strength Loss of sensory awareness Depression Change in self-image Change in physical fitness Loss of bowel and bladder control Susceptibility to pressure sores Potential for long-term pain	Change in vocational abilities Change in independence Change in self-image Change in social relationships	Assess physical and psychological dysfunction Increase functional abilities through the use of recreation and leisure-oriented programs Teach functional skills, recreational skills, and provide adaptive equipment Provide opportunities for creative self-expression Teach progressive relaxation techniques Teach stress management skills Build community resources and skills

[12].Spinal Cord Injury information from the American Therapeutic Recreation Association, 1992, *Therapeutic Recreation Services*, ATRA, Hattiesburg, MS.

Neurological Disorders and Psychiatric Disorders

Many of the people we serve have some form of cognitive impairment or psychiatric disorder. We need to understand the impairment to understand the possibilities for the individual. There are two ways to divide the impairments:

- whether the impairment is a neurological disorder or due to a psychiatric diagnosis
- whether the impairment is acute or chronic.

Neurological disorders are caused by a physical (usually known) impairment in the brain such as Alzheimer's, vascular disease, and other causes. Psychiatric impairments are disturbances related to personality and life experiences, which do not always appear to have an obvious organic cause. Examples include phobias and psychoses.

Acute cognitive impairments include any situation that changes quickly (within hours or days) and has a reasonable chance of returning to normal. Alcohol intoxication and overdoses of medication are usually acute impairments. Chronic impairments change slowly and usually do not allow the individual to return to normal functioning. Dementias and other damage to the brain such as that resulting from long-term alcohol abuse are chronic.

There are a few diagnoses that cover most of the impairments that we see. Before we look at the list, there is an important point to be made about some of these diagnoses — they don't always give us a clear-enough picture of what is happening with and for the person. For example, dementia is the most common cognitive

Classification of Cognitive Impairments

	Organic Impairments (Related to impairments in brain and brain tissue, reversibility depends on cause)	**Psychiatric Impairments** (Related to personality and life experience, may be organic in nature, frequently treatable)
Acute	Caused by trauma, infection, diabetes, chronic heart failure, drugs and alcohol, reversible to some degree Delirium Medication Overdose Alcohol Intoxication Stroke (acute phase) Traumatic Brain Injury (acute phase)	Caused by events in one's life, his/her perceptions of life, and may be organic in origin, can be treated with psychiatric and other mental health intervention, reversible although there may be recurrences Depression Anxiety Panic attacks Phobias
Chronic	Caused by physiological degeneration or damage to the brain, generally irreversible, some daily variation in skill level Dementia due to Alzheimer's Disease Vascular Dementia Dementia with Lewy Bodies Dementia due to Parkinson's Disease Frontotemporal Dementia Dementia due to Traumatic Brain Injury Dementia due to HIV Infection Substance/Medication-Induced Dementia Dementia due to Prion Disease Stroke (chronic phase, psychosis is a possible result)	Caused by events in one's life, has not been helped by mental health interventions, probably irreversible Depression Psychosis

impairment seen in individuals of long-term care facilities. Of the 1.3 million individuals, approximately 60% are estimated to have some form of dementia. (Dementia means that the individual has "a disorder in which the primary clinical deficit is in cognitive function, and that [is] acquired rather than developmental."[13])

If you are working with an individual who has "dementia," you need to know more. You need to know why the individual has been diagnosed as having a dementia:

- Is it because the doctor prescribing the pain medication didn't realize that the dentist also prescribed pain medication and thus the individual is getting overdosed on medications? (Speak up at team meetings about your medication concerns. Expect the "dementia" to improve if the medication dosages are more appropriate.)
- Is the individual simply not hearing what is said so s/he can't respond appropriately? (Work on alternate means of communication and expect an improvement.)

There are many more examples, of course, but the idea is to understand that a diagnosis is never the final answer when you are working with a particular individual. Everyone is unique and continues to have strengths and talents to share. In addition, all individuals deserve a life with meaning and respect regardless of limitations and diagnosis.

The chart on the previous page shows one method of classifying cognitive impairments. The cognitive impairments in the table can be divided into eight general categories:

Dementia is not a disease but rather a cluster of symptoms. These symptoms significantly limit a person's ability to perform normal, complex tasks associated with taking care of himself/herself. With dementia there has been a loss of cognitive function. The cognitive losses may be in the following domains:

- Complex attention. This includes difficulty in environments with multiple stimuli, being easily distracted, difficulty retaining information or remembering what was just said.
- Executive function. This is a significant impairment in the ability to think through problems, to work on complex projects, to initiate purposeful activity, to decide in what order actions should be done (as in dressing), to appreciate the significance of one's actions (understanding that picking up the unit's cat by the tail may make the cat angry), and to be able to stop what one is doing (to stop pouring milk when the glass is full).
- Memory and learning. Repeats self in conversations, can't keep track of a short list of items, and requires frequent reminders about the current task. Newly learned information is more likely to be lost than previously learned information.
- Language. This includes aphasia, the ability to recognize an object or a person but the inability to find the right word to describe the object or person resulting in the excessive use of words such as "thing" or "it." Apraxia, the inability to remember how to move your mouth and tongue to correctly pronounce words. Agnosia, the inability to recognize what an object is or who a person is.
- Perceptual-motor. Difficulties with familiar activities and finding familiar places, including more confusion at dusk.
- Social cognition. Behavior out of acceptable range, insensitivity to social standards, behaves without regard for other's feelings or personal safety, and has little insight into these changes.

Approximate 50–60 percent of dementia cases are irreversible. This means that anywhere from 650,000 to nearly one million people with dementias are being cared for with no hope of significant improvement. According to the

[13] American Psychiatric Association, 2013, *Diagnostic and statistical manual of mental disorders-5*.

Alzheimer's Association,[14] "More than 5 million Americans are living with Alzheimer's. By 2050 this number could rise as high as 16 million."

Dementias may be chronic or acute. They are organic.

The types of dementias are

- Dementia due to Alzheimer's Disease
- Vascular Dementia
- Dementia with Lewy Bodies
- Dementia due to Parkinson's Disease
- Frontotemporal Dementia
- Dementia due to Traumatic Brain Injury
- Dementia due to HIV Infection
- Dementia due to Huntington's Disease
- Substance/Medication-Induced Dementia
- Dementia due to Prion Disease
- Dementia due to another medical condition
- Dementia due to multiple etiologies (causes)
- Dementia due to Developmental Disorder Age-Associated Memory Impairment

Dementia due to Alzheimer's disease is the most common type of dementia. It is an incurable neurological disease in which changes in the nerve cells of the outer layer of the brain result in the death of a large number of cells. This disease is organic, chronic, and currently irreversible. Research suggests it may be caused by what is being called type-3 diabetes, which primarily affects the brain. If the research is correct, there may be ways to stop the progression of Alzheimer's.[15]

Delirium involves disorganized thinking and an inability to attend to external stimuli and appropriately shift to new external stimuli. It typically occurs suddenly and lasts a short time — it's acute. The causes are organic and include infection, fever, post-op conditions, drug-induced states, etc. Delirium is not dementia but the DSM-5 considers it to be a neurocognitive disorder.

Stroke refers to any damage to the brain resulting from lack of blood supply to the affected part. It usually results in the loss of particular functions that vary greatly depending on the part of the brain that is affected. It is organic and has both an acute phase and a chronic phase. Some recovery is usually seen.

Traumatic Brain Injury describes damage to the brain caused by physical injury to the brain including car accidents and gunshot wounds. The impairment is organic and has both an acute and chronic phase. Recovery may go on for ten or more years after the accident.

Depression is characterized by "being down in the dumps" or sad for most of the day for many weeks. Over a period of time, this sadness is present more days than not. An individual who is depressed may also experience a change in eating patterns (poor appetite or overeating), a change in sleeping patterns (insomnia or hypersomnia), a drop in energy (fatigue), a drop in self-esteem, a drop in the ability to concentrate long enough to make decisions or to respond to situations, and a decrease in the ability to be hopeful. Between 20% and 25% of individuals with major medical problems (e.g., stroke, heart disorders, cancer, diabetes) will experience a major depression disorder. Depression may be chronic or acute.

Anxiety is the most common psychiatric disorder experienced by the general population. There are twelve major psychiatric disorders grouped under the heading of Anxiety Disorders including Panic Disorder, Agoraphobia, and Social Anxiety Disorder. Anxiety impairs the individual's ability to respond to events and people in normally expected ways. Anxiety may be due to a variety of organic and other causes and may be either acute or chronic.

Trauma and Stress-Related Disorders occur when a trauma or stress is part of the diagnosis. Post-traumatic stress disorder is the most common one seen in the people we serve.

Psychotic Disorders are psychiatric disorders where the individual may experience hallucinations; manifest disorganized thoughts,

---

[14] Alzheimer's Association, 2017 Alzheimer's Disease Facts and Figures. www.alz.org/facts.

[15] de la Monte, Suzanne M. & Wands, Jack R. 2008. Alzheimer's Disease Is Type 3 Diabetes–Evidence Reviewed. *J Diabetes Sci Technol. 2008 Nov; 2*(6): 1101–1113.

speech, and actions; may be delusional (severe lack of normal insight); and/or even have catatonia. Psychotic disorders include schizophrenia, delusional disorders, paranoia, and other conditions.

Mild Dementia (Mild Neurocognitive Disorder) is a diagnostic term that refers to mild changes in cognitive function. Some of the criteria for this diagnosis are memory complaints from client, family, or physician; memory performance below age-appropriate mean; normal activities of living, clinical dementia rating 0.5 (Berg, 1988); normal global cognitive function (MMSE>26) and not demented (McPherson, 2005). These criteria identify an individual who is still living independently, but does present with mild cognitive losses. A Mayo Clinic study (Peterson, 2004) found that 80% of patients with mild dementia will convert to full dementia within six years.[16]

Dementia

Dementia is such a common diagnosis in long-term care facilities that it is important to understand the possible strengths and weaknesses of a person who is diagnosed with dementia. Creating a person-centered program requires truly understanding all aspects of the person.

Even when a dementia is present there are still many abilities and strengths that remain. These may include:

- Long-term memory — a trivia game can be successful for a person with dementia because it draws on long-term memory
- A sense of humor
- Many physical abilities
- Compensatory skills
- Crystallized intelligence (skills learned from living a long life)
- Ability to still experience enjoyment and happiness within a safe environment
- Ability to make some needs known nonverbally
- Recognition of familiar things such as pets, children, music, movement, friendship, religion, a handshake
- Awareness of respect and dignity given by family and caregivers
- Continuation of previous life roles through activities
- Past social skills and learned behaviors are still available to them
- Appreciation of the present moment in time

The following are communication issues related to dementias:

- **Agnosia**. The inability to interpret sensations and recognize familiar objects
- **Anomia**, The inability to find the right word to name an object or express an idea
- **Aphasia**, Difficulty understanding and or expressing language
- **Apraxia**. Difficulty translating thought into action
- **Paraphrasia**. Syllables, words, and phrases becoming jumbled and mixed up
- **Perseveration**. A persistent repetition of an activity, a phrase, or a movement such as tapping, wiping, picking

Wandering[17] or continuous walking can be major problems for people who have dementias. Different types to be aware of include tactile wandering, environmentally cued wandering, reminiscent wandering, recreational wandering, and agitated purposeful wandering. Understanding why the person is wandering is important in figuring out an intervention to reduce the risks to the resident.

There are several other possible "disturbing behaviors" that require behavioral interventions in the activity care plan. These include:

- Apathy
- Motor restlessness

---

[16] Best-Martini, E., 2007. "Cognitive stimulation, cognitive retraining and mental wellness interventions: Implications for recreational therapy practice." *ATRA Newsletter*, *23*(2). Part One.

[17] Buettner, L. & S. Fitzsimmons. 2003. *Dementia practice guidelines for recreational therapy: Treatment of disturbing behaviors*. ATRA. Alexandria: VA. p. 10

- Repetitive movements
- Rummaging
- Hoarding
- Repetitive verbalizations
- Picking
- Rubbing
- Biting
- Screaming
- Weeping
- Crying
- Moaning
- Argumentativeness
- Angry outbursts
- Paranoia
- Social isolation
- Disinhibition
- Pica (putting non-food items in mouth)
- Hair-pulling

Sensory Loss

Everyone who has read about Helen Keller has marveled at her ability to adapt to her sensory losses. Her compensatory skills were incredible; her will and her talent, monumental; her support system, constant. But what happens to everyday people like the individuals we serve when they suffer sensory losses? Do they have the skills and the talent to compensate adequately for their losses? How does loss influence one's adjustment and involvement in the long-term care facility?

Sadly, by the time older people come into supportive care, most have already experienced diminished visual or auditory capacity — or both. Vision and hearing can be a factor in the smooth and complete integration into facility life. Loss of one or the other can create a barrier to adjustment and, frequently, to the ability to socialize. As sensitive health care providers, we must be acutely aware of the potential for isolation inherent in this and make every effort to increase the opportunities for interaction.

Imagine how we become comfortable in new surroundings, such as a hotel. We use our vision to orient ourselves to the placement of doors and windows. We find the bathroom. We learn to identify, by sight if not by name, those who might be useful in assisting us with information or problem solving. If we can't see, we depend on our auditory sense to sharpen our awareness of traffic patterns, new or identifiable noises around us, and the daily rhythm of activities.

As we age, it is possible that, even if we do not lose total capacity, our senses may diminish enough to make most situations (especially new ones) awkward. In defense, compensatory skills are developed to mask the deprivation and to allow at least the illusion of normalcy. For example, people with a hearing loss may smile at everything they think they hear in every interaction or may answer yes to all questions. People are frequently embarrassed to ask us to repeat ourselves, and sometimes repeating doesn't help if the hearing loss is significant.

So what is the issue here? That this person may be labeled confused or senile and left to his/her own memories. With the additional loss of social stimulation, memory loss may become an actual problem — and we still haven't solved the original problems: a lack of social interaction and the possibility of an incorrect interpretation of the individual's condition.

So what do we do? Look for the underlying problem. If it's hearing loss, make sure that others know that the problem is hearing and not cognition. Speak clearly, face the person directly, repeat as necessary, use gestures, and use communication boards if possible. For a surprisingly small number of people, a hearing aid can help.

As for vision loss, if an individual has low vision but is alert, a vivid word picture can create a colorful image. Of course the individual with a visual impairment is more likely to need assistance to move around the facility and cueing at meals, but coupling this person with a peer as a volunteer can avoid a potential problem.

The really unfortunate thing is that sometimes nothing works well. As a result, we find that people engage in parallel existences. How often family members will say, "My mother has such a nice roommate; I wish they would talk to each other." In actuality, we have attempted on numerous occasions to introduce new roommates to each other only to be thwarted in our efforts by each one's inability to hear the other's voice. What happens? They only coexist, their lives never really touching in a meaningful way; two oriented, interesting, and social people unable to fully enjoy the company of the person they live with. This same problem will preclude involvement in many activities. But, all is not bleak as the truly interested individual will (if able) develop a level of involvement s/he is comfortable with and many times this means establishing a relationship with one or more staff members.

It is not uncommon for people to choose staff as kindred spirits. Part of this may be desire; part a refusal to identify with the other residents; but a large part of this may be because these individuals can hear the staff when they are educated to be patient and to repeat as necessary. Staff also have the ability to be heard by projecting their voices, whereas another resident may not have this ability.

Sensory losses pose terrible dilemmas and in many cases frustrate the person, the family, and even the staff. Staff should employ a great variety of creative skills and sensory tools to alleviate isolation and communication barriers. If all else proves to be unsuccessful, remember that the sense of touch is likely to remain intact until near death. A kind and gentle touch will almost always be well received. Be sure to review the sensory stimulation/integration section of the book for more therapeutic interventions.

Saying Goodbye: The Way We Grieve, the Way We Die

What act that we perform in our whole lives is more personal, more private, more self-centered than our death? Many authors have written eloquently about the stages leading up to death. Perhaps the best-known authority on the subject of death and dying is Elizabeth Kübler-Ross. Her five stages of death and dying are well recognized as guideposts in understanding this process for others and ourselves. These stages do not necessarily come in any set order. They are

Denial. At first we tend to deny the loss has taken place, and may withdraw from our usual social contacts. There is a feeling of disbelief that this could really be happening to us.

Anger. There is great anger in loss. This anger is based on our inability to control the circumstances of loss and death. There is a feeling of "If only…"

Bargaining. At this stage, we attempt to control the situation by bargaining. We may bargain with God, the doctor, or our loved ones. "If you give me three months so that I can go to my son's graduation…"

Depression. Reality sets in. We feel numb, although anger and sadness may remain hidden under the depression.

Acceptance. This is the stage when the anger and sadness taper off. We begin to accept the reality of the loss or impending death.

Each person's individual grief experience is different. And so each of us will experience this process in varying stages.

If you are working with an individual who is angry and unable to accept his/her situation, do not be quick to judge and do not assume that your role is to help him/her move through these stages. Instead, be a good listener, encourage sharing of feelings and fears, and lend emotional strength in any way possible.

If you are not informed about preparing for death, you should read one or more of the books listed below:

- Kübler-Ross, Elizabeth. *On Death and Dying*. Scribner, 2014.
- Stearns, Ann Kaiser. *Living Through Personal Crisis*. Idyll Arbor, 2010.

- Lewis, C. S. *A Grief Observed.* HarperOne, 2015.
- Staudacher, Carol. *Men and Grief.* New Harbinger, 1991.
- Caplan, Sandi. *Grief's Courageous Journey: A Workbook.* New Harbinger, 1995.

Death is inevitable and we know that it causes the least negative impact on the survivors when the person who is dying has reached an "acceptance" of his/her death. It means that the person understands the inevitability of death and feels prepared to die. We are often fortunate to have a chance to help the people we serve prepare for death and to be a witness to the hopefulness of impending death.

Let's draw a context here. Imagine having lived a full life, having created positive associations and memories. Imagine further having lost close family, then friends, then function, and, finally, a physical environment that was supportive of one's illness and disabilities. Having dealt with loss and change, step by step, problem by problem, people will usually arrive at the point of acceptance with a degree of relief. Ongoing love, support, and counseling will allow them to find peace in that emotional setting and, instead of mourning what life has been, there is pleasure in one's memories and hope for a peaceful end.

One does not have to have lived a life of comfort and joy to be able to arrive at such a state. In fact, one can still produce a positive face for the future, even without the pleasant memories that we hope will accompany each of us. It is no secret that the resident frequently accepts the inevitable placement in a long-term care facility before the family does. We sense that it relates to the comfort of letting go of all the unnecessary trappings in our lives, of already having made the hard choices and now being stripped to that part of self that is most vulnerable, most human. Without the distractions of the world, there is peace in having our needs met and peace in the assurance that we will be made comfortable to the end of our lives.

Of course, the need to control is still in evidence. In fact, that need is so ingrained in us that many people orchestrate their own dying. It is with pleasure that they cause families to rally round, to feel the power of being responded to, of being capable of living by choice until the end.

This is not true for everyone; but, among us, we often discuss — and believe — that people die the way they wish to. Some wish to die with family nearby; others prefer to be alone (to save family the possible pain of witnessing this final separation?). Most wish to die pain-free, which is often our only viable goal as caregivers — comfort for the individual who is dying.

Frequently there is a useful and wonderfully productive time to be lived as people proceed toward death. This can be a more open time, more emotional, more honest, with communication among family members at its best. Reminiscing is appropriate, especially if family members have never taken the time to explore the past with each other. (Amazingly, we find this is often true, as when we ask a resident for a social history and become aware that the family members are hearing life details for the first time, too. "Oh *that's* how your parents chose your name, Mom.") Sharing memories and stories revives lives led and provides the material for future reminiscing and for creating family legends and folklore.

Caregivers need to pay special attention to changes in health status that may be leading to the terminal state. At such times, it is imperative that you are even more available to the individual and family in order to address any terminal care needs:

- Do they wish clergy to be present?
- Do they wish a private meal with friends and family?
- Are there special arrangements that need to be made, such as an autopsy?

Sometimes your presence — sitting with the person and being with the family — is the best you can do. If appropriate, participate in the reminiscence. Help the family interact with the dying resident by modeling: speak to the resident; assure him/her that s/he is not alone and that his/her family is with him/her. Ask if the family wishes to be alone or if they are more comfortable having others in the room. The family may wish you to interpret physical changes. Encourage them to speak with nursing staff as they observe alteration in color, breathing patterns, and body temperature.

Finally, determine if anyone in the family wishes to view the resident after death and before the body is removed to the mortuary. Some people draw great comfort in this final good-bye, this private time. Most facilities are able to make accommodation for this.

When there is a death, be certain that the people most involved with the deceased have the opportunity to verbalize feelings of loss or fear. Include them in the dying process. If it seems feasible, allow them to sit with the dying person. Predictably, other residents seldom display any anxiety after a death. There is sadness, and a sense of loss and of missing a companion, but the pervasive feeling is of peace with the inevitable. We witness the ability of people to carry on when the natural has occurred.

It often seems to us that when we lose an individual, we lose twice, especially if the person had an active and interested family. The staff misses the spirit and energy of the resident and also the socializing and communicating with the family.

In order to allow all of us to make our final good-byes, — to the deceased and to the family and the routine that have become a part of us — we strongly recommend having a memorial service. We are not proposing that you conduct one after each death, but having one monthly or quarterly can be an emotional release. Be sure to invite the families and special friends of all the residents who have died. With or without a memorial service, it is highly recommended to send a condolence card to the family of a resident who has died. They have been a member of your community.

The service is simple with perhaps a prayer or a psalm reading led by a clergyman; this brings an appropriate solemnity to the occasion. These formalities are followed by spontaneous reminiscences, with staff and other individuals at the facility also making their contributions. When the formal service is concluded, there is time for refreshments and informal exchanges. For some, this is the only memorial service they will have. For others, it is their second, more private one. For everyone, it provides the opportunity for closure.

It never ceases to amaze us how truly uplifting it is to be with someone who is dying. We will qualify this by saying that this is especially true if the death is accepted, anticipated with joy as the natural ending to a life that has been well spent and is essentially pain free at the end. The emotional release is cathartic for all involved and opens our hearts to emotions that keep us most human: compassion, sympathy, and, in some cases, empathy.

It is always a privilege for caretakers who witness and ease the way to death; and no matter how one chooses to let go, it is always personal and private and special.

Hospice

Hospice care can be provided in the skilled nursing facility. It is a sort of ancillary service for the terminally ill — a provider is brought into the facility to minister to the resident and his/her family in a special way.

The hospice care provided must be coordinated between the facility and the hospice service. For that reason, it is very important to have ongoing contact with the team leader, the hospice social worker, and the hospice caregivers. A schedule must be shared so that the facility staff know when the hospice team will be coming in to give personal care so that no resident is left without essential care.

The social services professional, along with the activity professional, has a special role with hospice patients and their families. The care plan must focus on relief of psychosocial pain and the measures used need to be documented with appropriate, specific notes in the chart.

If a patient or family requests a hospice referral, or if the physician writes one, the patient and family must be given a choice of hospice providers. This is the same as giving a choice of home care agencies to follow discharged residents.

Once the patient has signed on for hospice, a note should include:

- Why was hospice considered as an intervention? What was the healthcare situation that pointed to the need for end of life care?
- Who (physician, patient, family) was involved in the decision?
- What is the diagnosis for hospice admission?

Next is the care plan entry. Nursing will always focus on relief from physical pain. In fact, that is a hospice specialty. Social services must focus on relief of psychosocial pain. These include the terminal care the resident wishes to have, private time with family, a liberalized diet, pet visits, clergy, phone calls, etc. Social services must meet frequently with the resident and the family to assess and address these needs.

To assure coordination, an initial care plan conference takes place as soon as possible after the patient is admitted to hospice. Of course, the hospice team is invited. Following this initial care conference, they are invited to all quarterly meetings.

At other times, social services communicates with the hospice team, especially the hospice social worker, to discuss any unmet or troubling psychosocial issues which they will then work together to resolve.

Finally, given that the patient is in a terminal state, charting should address the patient's end-of-life psychosocial issues and note that the facility and the hospice team are working together for the well-being of the patient.

3. The Work We Do

This chapter describes the history of our profession and the work done by the various professionals who work with the people we serve. For each of these professions we have included a description of the work that they do, an example of a typical day, and a formal position description.

These are rewarding professions, but they can be difficult at times. Significant complications will arise if you are disorganized. We have included some ideas for controlling the chaos of your setting so that human needs, professional needs, and bureaucratic needs can all be met without total loss of sanity. (Some loss of your sanity, some of the time, and the ability to regain it are part of the informal work description for all of these professions.)

Our History

The use of "leisure time" has changed dramatically over the last 6,000 years. "Emerson declared that all history is biography" (James, 1998, p. 7) so our history is really a retelling of the actions of many individuals. This section will provide you with a short history of leisure, social services, recreational therapy, and activity professionals through the actions of individuals.

Origins of Leisure, Activity, and Social Services

The concept that leisure time is separate from work time is a relatively new concept. Until about 6,000 years ago humankind wandered the countryside hunting and gathering food and foraging for other elements necessary for survival. This was the time of *preliterate society*. How people played or aged is something we can only speculate about. However, what we can extrapolate from archeological records is that early humans mixed work and leisure. Leisure appeared to be a key element of life involving music, chanting, art, and games. As today, it is thought that children played at being hunters or climbed and splashed, practicing skills that would aid survival when they became adults. Adults carried on traditions of music, dance, art, and games, often with spiritual overtones. Life expectancy was not very long, and elders who could no longer travel were likely left behind.

Eight thousand years ago in Mesopotamia and six thousand years ago in Central America humankind domesticated animals and tilled the soil. Thus the *agricultural era* started. This changed life to a more settled and stationary existence. Gathering and storing food, along with the building of more permanent residences allowed increased stability. Life and time became more seasonal with periods of less work. These periods of less work allowed society to pursue the arts, do scientific research, develop religions and governments, and start formal schooling of some of its citizens. A philosopher from Athens, Aristotle, spent many hours discussing the importance of both work and leisure, with leisure being preferable because it allowed the pursuit of intellectual inquiry. The Romans, coming from a society based on military strength, saw many of their leisure pursuits support excellence in military skills. Elders could now be taken care of at home even if they were no longer mobile.

Around the late 1700s in Great Britain (the mid-1800s in the United States) new inventions allowed the mass production of goods, introducing the *industrial era*. The mass production of goods increased the number of individuals who did not toil for work; they hired others to do the work for them. So society went from having leisure time for individuals to pursue artistic, intellectual, and religious pursuits to society having an actual leisure class of people. As the numbers in the leisure class grew, many now had more time and resources to follow intellectual pursuits. The invention of the printing press four hundred years previously allowed the mass dissemination of intellectual material. For the first time civilization had both the leisure time and the written material to begin educating large numbers of its citizens. A true middle class was being formed. With larger numbers of people educated and having both leisure time and money to conduct research, medical and other advances occurred faster than any previous time in history. In the 1900s life expectancy increased by three days each year.

During the industrial era the division between work and leisure became more sharply defined. For the individuals working in factories, life was hard. During the agricultural era, children worked alongside their parents and grandparents. But agriculture allowed for play as well as work. Playfulness and games occurred both in the fields and during the "off" seasons. Children were also required to work during the industrial age, but factory work did not allow leisurely breaks with parents and grandparents. In the lower classes all generations worked long, hard hours in factories just to make ends meet.

Around the same time that the industrial revolution helped emphasize the division between leisure and work, a shift was taking place in health care. In Great Britain, Florence Nightingale pushed for changes to the nursing profession. After she started making significant headway in modernizing the nursing profession, she expanded her vision to the reform of health care as a whole. The following passage by James (1998) in *Perspectives in Recreational Therapy* explains (pg. 8):

> Nightingale protested to all who would listen that the dreary conditions of the hospital were counterproductive and that the monotony endured by the patients adversely affected their recoveries.
>
> People say the effect [of a pleasing environment] is only on the mind. It is no such thing. The effect is on the body too. Little as we know about the way in which we are affected by form, by color and light, we do know this, that they have an actual physical effect. (Nightingale, 1859, p. 34)

Nightingale's observations also led her to conclude:

> It is a matter of painful wonder to the sick themselves how much painful ideas predominate over pleasurable ones in their impressions; they reason with themselves; they think themselves ungrateful; it is all of no use. The fact is that these painful impressions are far better dismissed by a real laugh, if you can excite one by books or conversation, than by any direct reasoning; or if the patient is too weak to laugh, some impression from nature is what he wants. (Nightingale, 1859, p. 34)
>
> Nightingale wrote of the benefits that accrued to patients from caring for pets, listening to and performing music, doing needlework and writing. She chastised health care administrators to be more inclusive in their provision of services to patients: 'Bearing in mind that you have all these varieties of employment which the sick cannot have, bear also in mind to obtain them all the varieties which they can enjoy.' (Nightingale, 1859, p. 36)

In Great Britain during the fall of 1855 a combination recreation room and coffee house, called the Inkerman Café, was created from a building on a hospital's grounds. While hobbies, arts and crafts, and other leisurely pursuits were offered to help the patients heal, Inkerman Café also offered the convalescing patients a place to pass the time instead of the taverns next to the hospital. Overall, it was a win-win situation. The patients stayed sober while benefiting from leisure activities during convalescing.

Similar changes were taking place in the United States under the guidance of physician Benjamin Rush and the Quakers. The concept of moral treatment," especially of patients with mental illness, was beginning to replace warehouse-like hospital facilities with homelike facilities surrounded by gardens. Progress was being made during the first half of the 1800s toward Moral Treatment of patients that included activities run by nurses and others. But this was soon to change. As the 1800s advanced, the United States became a country increasingly populated by interdependent urban dwellers instead of self-sufficient farmers. Work hours in factories were long and few recreation facilities were built in the urban areas. Combined with increased crowding because of immigration and more people in hospitals because of the Civil War, the country's resources were strained trying to accommodate all the unmet needs of the urban dwellers and of the people who over-filled the hospitals.

For the working masses, leisure had become a frivolous pastime. Adults were expected to be productive. At the same time, middle and upper class reformers pushed for changes in child labor laws. By the last quarter of the 1800s many children, no longer allowed to work, but having both parents still working the long factory hours, spent many idle hours in the streets of the cities. Between the rampant alcoholism of the adults and the mischief of the children, it became evident to many that further change was needed.

By the 1890s over sixty reform groups had formed, many with the belief that guided recreation experiences would help heal the moral and health problems of a society that were caused, in part, by an imbalance of work and healthy leisure activity. A relatively new field, social work, joined forces with teachers and government reform groups to try to address the problem.

The pendulum was swinging back again. Leisure activities moved away from being considered frivolous to being the modality of choice to create morally and physically strong citizens. Joseph Lee, a graduate of Harvard Law School, was so interested in the potential for leisure activities to help cure the social ills of society that he built sandpile play areas and, later, playgrounds in the Boston area. Lee hired and trained activity leaders to run groups and gather data for his research on the benefits of recreation. At the turn of the last century, physician Luther Gulick helped change the YMCA's direction from one of exercise to moral and physical health through recreation. Gulick also proposed that an association of playground professionals be formed. So, in 1906 the first national organization for recreation and activity professionals was formed, called the Playground Association of America (PAA).

That year, US President Theodore Roosevelt invited eighteen people from around the country to the White House to celebrate the formation of the PAA. Eight of the original eighteen founders of PAA were women. The second national conference was held in Chicago in 1907 with 200 delegates from 30 cities. One of the outcomes of that conference was the formation of an advisory committee on "play in institutions" aimed at furthering the work of Nightingale, Rush, Gulick, and others.

One of PAA's most influential and insightful members was Neva Leona Boyd. She was hired as a social worker at Hull House (a settlement house in Chicago) in 1908 to work with the immigrants who lived there. Her job description was to organize social clubs, play, and other small group activities to help Hull House's residents develop appropriate physical, social, and intellectual skills. Hull House, originally founded by Jane Addams, provided Neva Boyd with a lab and classroom space to train others. She would accept students who had already completed two years of college to enter her one-year social work/recreation leader program.

> Besides offering extensive technical training in group games, gymnastics, dancing and dramatic arts, the school provided course work in the theory and psychology of play, social behavior problems, and 'preventive and remedial social efforts' (Simon, 1971, p. 14).[18]

Ms. Boyd called her school the Chicago Training School for Playground Workers and termed the work "recreational therapy." In 1927 the school became part of Northwestern University. Similar programs developed at other universities including a Department of Recreation Leadership at the Teachers College, Columbia University.

The United States entered World War I in 1917. The American Red Cross built 52 recreation centers, all using the same design, at military hospitals across the country. The Red Cross hired the Department of Recreation Leadership at Columbia University to help train and staff these centers with professionals who used recreational activities as part of the patient's medical and therapy program.

> The program drew from activity areas consistent with those used by group work services at the time. Among those were music, dance, gardening, community trips, drama, games, and social recreation. The military was assigned supervision of physical education. Following the precedents established by the terms social work and group work, the Red Cross titled this new service 'Hospital Recreation Work.' (Program of Recreation, 1919)[19]

By the 1930s the use of recreational therapy in mental health hospitals was well established. Not only had Boyd promoted the use of recreational therapy in psychiatric hospitals since the early 1900s, but so did the Drs. Menninger (father C. F., brothers Karl and William). The Menningers formed the Menninger Clinic in Topeka, Kansas, and used recreational therapy as one of the core treatment specialties at their facility.

The use of activities and recreation as a therapeutic intervention continued to gain recognition. However, the last 70 years of the twentieth century would prove volatile for the professionals who used recreation and activities as a means to improve people's health and well-being. Political struggles based on philosophy along with different views on scope and content of professional preparation caused numerous factions to split off, forming new national organizations. At their 1935 National Conference of Social Work, the national organization broke with Boyd's previous group work using recreation so social work and recreational therapy became distinctly different fields. It was almost forty years later, in 1977, when President Gary Robb of the National Therapeutic Recreation Society, directed a study that lead to the registration of therapeutic recreation specialists (recreational therapists), and a clear split between recreational therapy and activity professionals took place.

Professional Organizations

There are currently four national organizations who represent people working in nursing homes in activities and social services; the American Therapeutic Recreation Association,

[18] Simon, P. (1971). *Play and game theory in group work: A collection of papers by Neva Leona Boyd.* Referenced in James, A. "The conceptual development of recreational therapy" In Brasile, F., Skalko, T. K. and burlingame, j. (1998). *Perspectives in recreational therapy: Issues of a dynamic profession.* Ravensdale, WA: Idyll Arbor.

[19] Hospital Service (1919, June 30). *The Red Cross Bulletin*, 3(27), 2–3 Referenced in James, A. "The conceptual development of recreational therapy" In Brasile, F., Skalko, T. K. and burlingame, j. (1998). *Perspectives in recreational therapy: Issues of a dynamic profession.* Ravensdale, WA: Idyll Arbor.

the National Association of Activity Professionals, the National Coalition of Activity Professionals, and the National Association of Social Workers. In order to be well informed and up to date on issues that pertain to your profession, we recommend that you go to the organization's individual websites.

National Association of Activity Professionals (NAAP)

NAAP provides support to activity professionals through education, advocacy, technical assistance, promotion of standards, fostering of research and peer and industry relations.
NAAP, 3604 Wildon St, Eau Claire, WI 54703, 913-748-7288, naappr@gmail.com, www.naap.info

National Coalition of Activity Professionals (NCOAP)

The mission of NCOAP is "To educate and collaborate with health care providers who deliver strong, client-centered services based on dignity and purpose for the empowerment of every generation." NCOAP's vision is to collaborate and align for a stronger future.
NCOAP, 153 Pine Knoll Lane, LaFollette, TN 37766, 423-562-9304, info@NCOAP.org, www.ncoap.org

National Association of Social Workers (NASW)

The National Association of Social Workers (NASW) is the largest membership organization of professional social workers in the world, with 145,000 members. NASW works to enhance the professional growth and development of its members, to create and maintain professional standards, and to advance sound social policies.

NASW, 750 First Street, NE, Suite 800, Washington, DC 20002-4241, 202-408-8600, membership@naswdc.org, www.naswdc.org

American Therapeutic Recreation Association (ATRA)

ATRA represents the interests and needs of recreational therapists. ATRA was incorporated in 1984 as a non-profit, grassroots organization in response to growing concern about the dramatic changes in the health care industry. ATRA has a membership of about 2,000.
ATRA, 11130 Sunrise Valley Drive, Suite 350, Reston, VA 20191, 703-234-4140, national@atra-online.com, www.atra-online.com

Certification and Licensure

There are currently national certification organizations for recreational therapists and activity professionals, along with several state certification, licensure, or registration groups. Social services professionals do not currently need certification. They qualify based on a four-year degree and experience.

For activity professional certification there are two options: the National Association of Activity Professionals Credentialing Center (NAAPCC) and the National Certification Council for Activity Professionals (NCCAP)

NAAPCC, 224 N Millbrook Ct Aurora, CO 80018, 303-317-5682, naapcc.office@gmail.com, www.naapcc.net

NCCAP, 317 Office Square Lane Suite 202A, Virginia Beach, VA 23462, 757-552-0653, info@nccap.org, www.nccap.org.

For recreational therapy certification contact: The National Council for Therapeutic Recreation Certification (NCTRC):
NCTRC, 7 Elmwood Drive, New City, New York 10956, 845-639-1439, nctrc@nctrc.org, www.nctrc.org.

Professionalism

Professionalism is a term that we hear used every day. What does it actually mean to you as an activity professional, social services professional, or recreational therapist? Perhaps the easiest way to define professionalism is to identify individuals whom you regard as professionals. What is it about them that creates that feeling of respect and recognition? Is it something concrete about what they do or just a feeling associated with who they are as a person?

You will most likely answer "something concrete" along with a feeling of confidence that the individual carries with him/her in his/her work. The concrete substance that creates a professional is a combination of purpose, vision, goals, skills, hard work, solid ethics, and constant upgrading of education and skills. Each professional field has its own purpose, vision, goals, ethics, and skills learned through schooling and apprenticeships. While each professional group is unique in many ways, working as a team means that they also need to have much in common.

Professionals share a common goal. That goal is to enhance the quality of life of the people they serve. This creates the vision of how life and programming could be in these settings. It creates a vision of the people we serve coming first and policies being created with considerations of the people we serve coming before concerns about the staff. This sensitivity helps create programs that have a purpose and a goal specific to the quality of life issues we address, regardless of limitations and special needs. We make the positive happen through the use of our skills.

The reality is that this is quite a challenge for the team to meet. Government rules usually mandate that a qualified professional direct these services. This individual needs to be prepared to work hard to educate people about the impact his/her work and programs have and, at the same time, continue to build on his/her own skills and knowledge.

The position of activity director/coordinator is a department head position. This means that not only is this individual responsible for all the duties and services provided by the professionals in his/her department, but s/he is also responsible to every other staff member because of the team emphasis.

Being a professional means taking responsibility. In other words, an area of information forgotten, a resident incompletely assessed, documentation past due, or a lack of appropriate programs reflects on everyone else on the team. If there is a diagnosis that you do not understand or an individual that you don't know how to care for, you must bring this up and work with other disciplines to seek a solution. This obviously goes both ways in that other departments need to work with you in meeting common goals and understanding your goals and priorities.

One sure way of not only being a professional but also feeling that sense of confidence associated with professionalism is to network and be a member of local, state, and national organizations. Not only will you share common issues and concerns, you will also gain important continuing education in the educational meetings, workshops, and conventions as well as a tremendous amount of support. So much of our work is done individually and it is easy to feel "out of the mainstream" as pressures at work mount. Keep yourself balanced by taking care of yourself, your own leisure needs and interests, and professional development. The people you serve will benefit from a well-balanced professional and a happy team.

Activity Professional

There are many types of facilities where activity professionals work. The position description and list of responsibilities in this section shows what an activity professional would be expected to do in a certified long-term care facility. Other facilities, such as assisted living or adult day care, generally have less exacting requirements, but the actual work performed to help the people we serve is quite similar.

The professionals who provide activities for residents in long-term care facilities play many diverse roles within the care facility, but they are all directed at satisfying the goal of creating a homelike environment where the residents have control of their lives. There are administrative responsibilities and resident care duties and plenty of other tasks that keep the work interesting.

The administrative role is as the director of the Department of Activity Services. In that role the activity professional is responsible for creating policies and procedures that lead to programs that meet the needs of the residents and comply with all appropriate government regulations. One of the major areas of responsibility is the development and analysis of quality indicators. Another major area of responsibility is being the supervisor for all of the activity staff and all activity volunteers within the facility.

The resident care role requires the activity professional to act as a member of the interdisciplinary team in assessing residents, writing and carrying out care plans, and updating the plans at appropriate intervals. S/he needs to work with the residents to find out what their capabilities are and to plan activities that maintain and/or enhance those capabilities.

Other tasks like facilitating the Resident Council, publishing a newsletter, coordinating a casino night, helping public relations, conducting community outings, and all the rest are part of the work of providing the best possible environment for the residents of the long-term care facility.

Position Description

Title: Activity Professional

Purpose of the Position

Under the direction of the Administrator, the Activity Professionals, led by the Activity Director, are responsible for the planning, coordination, and implementation of the activity programs. Activities shall be provided on a daily basis and every effort will be made to meet the residents' needs and interests.

Qualifications

A qualified professional who "*Is a qualified therapeutic recreation specialist or an activities professional who is licensed or registered, if applicable, by the State in which practicing; and is eligible for certification as a therapeutic recreation specialist or as an activities professional by a recognized accrediting body on or after October 1, 1990; or has 2 years of experience in a social or recreational program within the last 5 years, 1 of which was full-time in a patient activities program in a health care setting; or is a qualified occupational therapist or occupational therapy assistant; or has completed a training course approved by the State.*"[20]

Duties and Responsibilities

Activity programs are developed within the framework of the facility organizational structure in accordance with federal regulations and the approval of each resident's attending physician. The programs are coordinated in a team effort with related facility services and staff. Programs are to include activities for all residents including residents who are ambulatory, non-ambulatory, and on bed rest. The activities are to be planned for both group and individual participation.

With understanding of the adverse effects of institutionalization, which can promote isolation, sensory deprivation, and dependence, the activity professional shall build into the program a variety of means to counteract these effects. S/he shall:

- Evaluate each resident according to his/her background, interest, leisure, previous lifestyle, physical and cognitive abilities, limitations, and needs. This shall serve as the base from which the individual activity plan shall be developed. After the activity assessment

[20] State Operations Manual, OBRA, Tags F679 and F680 updated November 1, 2017 S&C Memo: Revision to State Operations Manual Appendix PP for Phase 2 (Includes Training Information and Related Issues)

is completed, the activity professional will complete the MDS, Section F.

- Document the individual activity program using the appropriate assessment forms to be placed in the medical record, completing the activity plan within the required time after admission (14 days for federal regulations, 7 days for some states).
- Attend Resident Care Conferences and record in the resident care plan on a quarterly basis (or sooner, as needed).
- Maintain timely progress notes specific to the residents' activity plans, recording at least quarterly in the medical record and more frequently when appropriate.
- Develop appropriate records that indicate resident attendance and participation in the program with reference to residents' response to the program. It is important to note active participation as compared to passive participation. These records also include a bedside log for special programming.
- Develop, implement, lead, and monitor individual and group activities that meet specific needs of the residents.
- Develop activities providing the opportunity for residents to experience sensory input (touch, smell, taste, etc.), group interaction, and personal achievement.
- Include activities that encourage residents to make decisions, participate in planning, and assume a degree of responsibility and independence.
- Develop a method to implement programs within a designated budget allocated by the Facility Administrator. Keep a ledger and inventory of supplies.
- Establish an active volunteer program that includes the screening, orientation, training, supervision, and evaluation of volunteers.
- Develop methods for effective utilization of community resources.
- Serve as a facility liaison to promote positive community support.
- Interpret to residents, other staff members, and the outside community the purpose and achievements of the activity program through at least yearly in-service training and presentations.
- Attend and participate in staff meetings, department head meetings, designated committee meetings, and resident care conferences.
- Develop a method for obtaining current knowledge of federal and state regulations pertaining to activity programs.
- Other responsibilities as defined by the administrator.

The Life of an Activity Professional

A typical day at work may look like this:

9:00–9:30	Check census, resident status, new admissions Change "Today Is" board Change arrow on calendar Check with nursing regarding any changes of condition, discharges, etc.
9:30–10:00	Announce activities Set up room(s) Assist with transporting residents
10:00–12:00	Lead activity groups or supervise other leaders Attend interdisciplinary team (IDT) resident care plan meetings Attend department head meetings Attend MDS meetings Take attendance for groups Attend physical and chemical restraint committee meetings Visit one-on-one
12:00–1:00	Lunch
1:00–1:45	Documentation (new admissions, MDS, care plans, quarterly notes) Interview new residents Coordinate departmental responsibilities Return phone calls Volunteer recruitment, interviewing, and orienting

1:45–2:00	Announce activities Set up for activities Assist with transporting residents
2:00–4:00	Lead activities or supervise leaders Visit one-on-one Take attendance for groups Documentation (assessments, care plans, etc.) Special event coordination Lead a special needs group
4:00–5:00	Organize files and office for next day Write a to-do list for tomorrow Make end of the day farewell visits

OBRA '87 requires that there normally must be some leisure activities in the morning, afternoon, and evening, seven days a week, for all residents. This includes activities for residents who are unable to participate in the group activities. The activity department needs to help facilitate evening and weekend activities whether the activity staff person is there or not.

Some of the specific tasks for activity professionals require them to:

- Assess each resident for individual needs, abilities, and interests.
- Complete an initial activity assessment for each resident.
- Complete the Minimum Data Set (MDS) comprehensive assessment form — Section F (United States). (There may be other areas of the MDS the administrator assigns to the activity professional.)
- Identify a priority care plan need or problem for each resident, if indicated by the assessment, to be included in the individual's care plan.
- Develop a monthly calendar of activities to meet the assessed needs of all residents.
- Plan, organize, and coordinate the activity program.
- Schedule and lead activity groups.
- Supervise adult education instructors while on site.
- Arrange special events and outside entertainers.
- Train staff and volunteers.
- Establish and develop community contacts and resources.
- Manage and supervise the volunteer program.
- Attend the weekly Resident Care Conference meetings.
- Keep a daily record of each resident's involvement in activities.
- Keep a bedside log of date, length of visit, type of visit, and response to visit for all residents in need of one-on-one visits.
- Document the treatment plan in the progress notes at least once a quarter.
- Document and address changes in condition.
- Assure compliance with federal and state regulations and corporate policies and procedures.
- Keep current through national, state, and local professional affiliations to update skills and secure continuing education.
- Edit the monthly newsletter.
- Prepare and keep the budget for the department.
- Evaluate programs to assure appropriateness for the current census of residents.
- Actively engage in evaluating the care given to all of the residents through a quality improvement program.

On a monthly basis the activity professional is responsible for planning and leading activities designed to meet the needs of the residents of the facility. The following pages have samples of activity calendars. The first calendar is for a nursing home, the other for an assisted living facility.

August 2017

Apple Valley Post-Acute Rehab

Sunday	Monday	Tuesday	Wednesday	Thursday	Friday	Saturday
		1 10:00 REHAB FITNESS 11:00 CURRENT EVENTS 2:00 OUTDOORS 3:00 HAVE A LAUGH 3:45 CLASSICAL MUSIC	**2** 10:00 BAG TOSS 11:00 CURRENT EVENTS 11:00 CATHOLIC SERVICE 2:00 REHAB FITNESS 3:00 NAILS 4:00 ARMCHAIR TRAVEL	**3** 10:00 REHAB FITNESS 11:00 OUTDOORS 2:00 J.W. STUDY (E.D.) 2:00 CURRENT EVENTS 3:00 CRAFTS 4:00 LITERATURE GROUP 6:30 SOCIAL HOUR!	**4** 10:00 COFFEE TALK 11:00 UKULELE DEB 2:00 REHAB FITNESS 3:00 BEADING & DOCUMENTARY	**5** 10:00 REHAB FITNESS 11:00 BEADING & DOCUMENTARY 1:45 BINGO! 3:00 MOVIE THEATER
6 10:00 COFFEE SOCIAL 11:00 NAILS 2:00 BINGO! 4:00 CHRISTIAN SERVICE	**7** 10:00 WATERCOLOR & MOVING ART 11:00 CURRENT EVENTS 2:00 REHAB FITNESS 3:00 FREE YOUR VOICE 4:00 AWAKEN YOUR SENSES	**8** 9:00 BOWLING OUTING! 10:00 REHAB FITNESS 11:00 CURRENT EVENTS 2:00 OUTDOORS 3:00 WORD GAME 3:45 CLASSICAL MUSIC	**9** 10:00 NOODLE BALL 11:00 CURRENT EVENTS 11:00 CATHOLIC SERVICE 2:00 REHAB FITNESS 3:00 HARP W/LAURA 4:00 ARMCHAIR TRAVEL	**10** 10:00 REHAB FITNESS 11:00 OUTDOORS 2:00 J.W. STUDY (E.D.) 2:00 CURRENT EVENTS 3:00 CRAFTS 4:00 LITERATURE GROUP 6:30 SOCIAL HOUR!	**11** 10:00 COFFEE TALK 11:00 PICTURE TRIVIA 2:00 REHAB FITNESS 3:00 BEADING & DOCUMENTATRY	**12** 10:00 REHAB FITNESS 11:00 BEADING & DOCUMENTARY 1:45 BINGO! 3:00 MOVIE THEATER
13 10:00 COFFEE SOCIAL 11:00 NAILS 2:00 BINGO! 4:00 CHRISTIAN SERVICE	**14** 10:00 WATERCOLOR & MOVING ART 11:00 CURRENT EVENTS 2:00 REHAB FITNESS 3:00 FREE YOUR VOICE 4:00 AWAKEN YOUR SENSES	**15** 10:00 REHAB FITNESS 11:00 CURRENT EVENTS 2:00 OUTDOORS 3:00 BRAIN GAMES 3:45 UKULELE DEB	**16** 10:00 BAG TOSS 11:00 CURRENT EVENTS 11:00 CATHOLIC SERVICE 2:00 REHAB FITNESS 3:00 CELLO W/DAN 4:00 ARMCHAIR TRAVEL	**17** 10:00 REHAB FITNESS 11:00 OUTDOORS 2:00 J.W. STUDY (E.D.) 2:00 CURRENT EVENTS 3:00 CRAFTS 4:00 LITERATURE GROUP 6:30 SOCIAL HOUR	**18** 10:00 COFFEE TALK 11:00 PIANO W/JOAN 2:00 REHAB FITNESS 3:00 BEADING & DOCUMENTARY	**19** 10:00 REHAB FITNESS 11:00 CHRISTIAN SERVICE 1:45 BINGO! 3:00 MOVIE THEATER
20 10:00 COFFEE SOCIAL 11:00 NAILS 2:00 BINGO! 4:00 CHRISTIAN SERVICE	**21** 10:00 WATERCOLOR & MOVING ART 11:00 CURRENT EVENTS 2:00 REHAB FITNESS 3:00 RESIDENT COUNCIL 4:00 AWAKEN YOUR SENSES	**22** 10:00 REHAB FITNESS 11:00 CURRENT EVENTS 2:00 OUTDOORS 3:00 WORD GAME 3:45 CLASSICAL MUSIC	**23** 10:00 NOODLE BALL 11:00 CURRENT EVENTS 11:00 CATHOLIC SERVICE 2:00 REHAB FITNESS 3:00 NAILS 4:00 ARMCHAIR TRAVEL	**24** 10:00 REHAB FITNESS 11:00 OUTDOORS 2:00 J.W. STUDY (E.D.) 2:00 CURRENT EVENTS 3:00 CRAFTS 4:00 LITERATURE GROUP 6:30 SOCIAL HOUR!	**25** 10:00 COFFEE TALK 11:00 FOOD COMMITTEE 2:00 REHAB FITNESS 3:00 BEADING & DOCUMENTARY	**26** 10:00 REHAB FITNESS 11:00 BEADING & DOCUMENTARY 1:45 BINGO! 3:00 MOVIE THEATER
27 10:00 COFFEE SOCIAL 11:00 NAILS 2:00 BINGO! 4:00 CHRISTIAN SERVICE	**28** 10:00 WATERCOLOR & MOVING ART 11:00 CURRENT EVENTS 2:00 REHAB FITNESS 3:00 FREE YOUR VOICE 4:00 AWAKEN YOUR SENSES	**29** 10:00 REHAB FITNESS 11:00 CURRENT EVENTS 2:00 OUTDOORS 3:00 WORD GAME 3:45 UKULELE DEB	**30** 10:00 BALLOON TOSS 11:00 CURRENT EVENTS 11:00 CATHOLIC SERVICES 2:00 REHAB FITNESS 3:00 HARP W/LAURA 4:00 ARMCHAIR TRAVEL	**31** 10:00 REHAB FITNESS 11:00 OUTDOORS 2:00 J.W. STUDY (E.D.) 2:00 CURRENT EVENTS 3:00 CRAFTS 4:00 LITERATURE GROUP 6:30 SOCIAL HOUR!		

Religious: Chaplain by request, Beauty Shop on Friday, Pet visits, and more...1035 Gravenstein Hwy S, Sebastopol, CA 95472 (707) 823-7675 Activities Subject To Change.

AgeSong University
From Assisted to Community Living

June 2017

LR AU Living Room
SR AU Sun Room
Ch AU Chapel
G AU Garden
DR AU Dining Room

Sunday	Monday	Tuesday	Wednesday	Thursday	Friday	Saturday
				1 9:30 Ch AgeStrong Exercise **10:30 SR Rhythms (GERO)** 11:00 G Morning Stroll! 1:00 LR Piano & Prayer 1:00 LR Crossword 6:00 SR Evening News/Movies!	2 9:30 Ch Pilates/Yoga Fusion! **11:00 Ch Drama Therapy! (GERO)** **1:00 Ch Express Emotions** 2:00 LR Happy Hour/Live Music 3:30 SR Afternoon Stroll 6:00 SR Evening News/Movies! 6:30 Ch Family Council	3 9:30 Ch AgeStrong Exercise 2:00 SR Crossword! **3:00 G Social Hr/Board Games** 3:30 G Afternoon Stroll 6:00 SR Evening News/Movies!
4 **9:00 LR Eldership Course** **9:30 Ch Exist Movies (GERO)** **11:00 LR Live News** **1:30 SR Infinity Gospel Church** 2:30 SR Sports 6:00 SR Evening News/Movies!	5 **9:30 Ch Mindful Movement (GERO)** 10:00 LR News & Politics **11:00 SR Harp Lessons w/Greg** **1:00 G Garden Club (GERO)** **3:00 LR Resident Council** **4:00 LR Eldership Course** **6:00 SR Therapeutic Yoga (GERO)** 6:00 SR Evening News/Movies!	6 9:30 Ch AgeStrong Exercise 11:00 LR Tasty & Nutritious **1:00 SR Art W/ Elders** 1:00 LR Crossword **2:00 Ch Therapeutic Touch! (GERO)** **3:00 Ch St. Elizabeth** 6:00 SR Evening News/Movies!	7 9:30 Ch AgeStrong Exercise 10:00 SR Holy Communion **11:00 SR Harp Lessons w/Greg** **11:00 SR Tech Mobile** 1:00 LR Crossword! 6:00 SR Evening News/Movies!	8 9:30 Ch AgeStrong Exercise **10:30 SR Rhythms (GERO)** 11:00 G Morning Stroll! 1:00 LR Crossword 2:00 LR Music through the Decades 6:00 SR Evening News/Movies!	9 9:30 Ch Pilates/Yoga Fusion! **11:00 Ch Drama Therapy! (GERO)** **1:00 Ch Express Emotions** 2:00 LR Happy Hour/Live Music 3:30 SR Afternoon Stroll 6:00 SR Evening News/Movies!	10 **8:00 DR Omelet Bar W/ Steve!** 9:30 Ch AgeStrong Exercise **10:00 SR Mindfulness (GERO)** 2:00 SR Crossword! **3:00 G Social Hr/Board Games** 3:30 G Afternoon Stroll 6:00 SR Evening News/Movies!
11 **9:30 Ch Exist Movies (GERO)** 10:30 G Garden Stroll **11:00 LR Live News** **1:30 SR Infinity Gospel Church** 2:30 SR Sports 6:00 SR Evening News/Movies!	12 **9:30 Ch Mindful Movement (GERO)** 10:00 LR News & Politics **11:00 SR Harp Lessons w/Greg** **1:00 G Garden Club (GERO)** **1:00 LR Crossword!** **3:00 G Evening Stroll!** **4:00 LR Elders Academy** 6:00 SR Evening News/Movies! **6:00 SR Therapeutic Yoga (GERO)**	13 9:30 Ch AgeStrong Exercise 11:00 LR Tasty & Nutritious 1:00 LR Crossword **1:00 SR Art W/ Elders** **2:00 Ch Therapeutic Touch! (GERO)** 6:00 SR Evening News/Movies!	14 9:30 Ch AgeStrong Exercise 10:00 SR Holy Communion **11:00 SR Harp Lessons w/Greg** 1:00 LR Crossword! 1:00 LR Bookmobile 6:00 SR Evening News/Movies!	15 9:30 Ch AgeStrong Exercise **10:30 SR Rhythms (GERO)** 11:00 G Morning Stroll! 1:00 LR Crossword 2:00 LR Music through the Decades 2:00 LR AU Elders "Got Talent"! 6:00 SR Evening News/Movies!	16 9:30 Ch Pilates/Yoga Fusion! **11:00 Ch Drama Therapy! (GERO)** **1:00 Ch Express Emotions** 2:00 LR Happy Hour/Live Music 3:30 SR Afternoon Stroll 6:00 SR Evening News/Movies!	17 9:30 Ch AgeStrong Exercise 2:00 SR Crossword! **3:00 Ch Summer Salute with Music/Dance/Poetry** 4:00 G Afternoon Stroll 6:00 SR Evening News/Movies!
FATHER'S DAY 18 **9:30 Ch Exist Movies (GERO)** 10:30 G Garden Stroll **11:00 LR Live News** **1:30 SR Infinity Gospel Church** 2:30 SR Sports **3:30 Ch Grace United Church!** 6:00 SR Evening News/Movies!	19 **9:30 Ch Mindful Movement (GERO)** 10:00 LR News & Politics **11:00 SR Harp Lessons w/Greg** **1:00 G Garden Club (GERO)** **1:00 LR Crossword!** **3:00 G Evening Stroll!** **4:00 LR Elders Academy** **6:00 SR Therapeutic Yoga (GERO)** 6:00 SR Evening News/Movies!	20 9:30 Ch AgeStrong Exercise 11:00 LR Tasty & Nutritious 1:00 LR Crossword **1:00 SR Art W/ Elders** **2:00 Ch Therapeutic Touch! (GERO)** 6:00 SR Evening News/Movies!	**SUMMER SOLSTICE** 21 9:30 Ch AgeStrong Exercise 10:00 SR Holy Communion **11:00 SR Harp Lessons w/Greg** **11:00 LR Tech Mobile** 1:00 LR Crossword! 6:00 SR Evening News/Movies!	22 9:30 Ch AgeStrong Exercise **10:30 SR Rhythms (GERO)** 11:00 G Morning Stroll! 1:00 LR Crossword 2:00 LR Music through the Decades 6:00 SR Evening News/Movies!	23 9:30 Ch Pilates/Yoga Fusion! **11:00 Ch Drama Therapy! (GERO)** **1:00 Ch Express Emotions** 2:00 LR Happy Hour/Live Music 3:30 SR Afternoon Stroll 6:00 SR Evening News/Movies!	24 **8:00 DR Omelet Bar W/Steve** 9:30 Ch AgeStrong Exercise 10:00 SR Mindfulness (GERO) **2:00 Ch St. Boniface** 2:00 SR Crossword! **3:00 G Social Hr/Board Games** 3:30 G Afternoon Stroll 6:00 SR Evening News/Movies!
25 **9:30 Ch Exist Movies (GERO)** 10:30 G Garden Stroll **11:00 LR Live News** **1:30 SR Infinity Gospel Church** **2:00 LR Piano & Cello** 2:30 SR Sports 6:00 SR Evening News/Movies!	26 **9:30 Ch Mindful Movement (GERO)** 10:00 LR News & Politics **11:00 SR Harp Lessons w/Greg** **1:00 LR Crossword!** **1:00 G Garden Club (GERO)** **3:00 G Evening Stroll!** **4:00 LR Elders Academy** **6:00 SR Therapeutic Yoga (GERO)** 6:00 SR Evening News/Movies!	27 9:30 Ch AgeStrong Exercise 11:00 LR Tasty & Nutritious 1:00 LR Crossword **1:00 SR Art W/ Elders** **2:00 Ch Therapeutic Touch! (GERO)** **2:30 G Afternoon Stroll** 6:00 SR Evening News/Movies!	28 9:30 Ch AgeStrong Exercise 10:00 SR Holy Communion **11:00 SR Harp Lessons w/Greg** 1:00 LR Crossword! **2:00 SR Monthly Birthdays** **2:30 SR Memorial (GERO)** 6:00 SR Evening News/Movies!	29 9:30 Ch AgeStrong Exercise **10:30 SR Rhythms (GERO)** 11:00 G Morning Stroll! 1:00 LR Crossword 1:00 LR Piano & Prayer 2:00 LR Music through the Decades 6:00 SR Evening News/Movies!	30 9:30 Ch Pilates/Yoga Fusion! **11:00 Ch Drama Therapy! (GERO)** **1:00 Ch Express Emotions** 2:00 LR Happy Hour/Live Music 3:30 SR Afternoon Stroll 6:00 SR Evening News/Movies!	**All events are subject to change at any time.**

Calendar of Events

Activity Consultation

Each state has different state laws that regulate the skilled nursing setting. These are adhered to along with the OBRA '87 Tags F679 and F680 interpretive guidelines. Some state laws address the need to have an activity consultant under contract to assure that the department and staff is in compliance with state and federal guidelines. In addition, many companies have their own corporate consultants that work with the activity professional. A consultant is an individual who specializes in an area of expertise, has years of experience in the field, and keeps up with ever-changing regulations and trends in the field.

Be sure that you are working with a consultant who not only has the professional qualifications, but also has a strong communication style and works with you as an advocate and trainer. The consultant's goal should be to teach the activity professional as much as s/he can so that the activity professional grows in the position and continues to create new and vital programs.

If you are working with a consultant on a regular basis, be sure that you feel that your needs, interests, and concerns are listened to and acted on. Keep a list of things that you want to learn during these visits. Ask about new ideas and resources so that you are getting the most out of your time.

A consultant completes a report regarding the areas reviewed. This is given to the administrator and activity professional. Keep these on file as they document your work together. They also are good references to areas previously reviewed. The administrator, consultant, and staff member meet at the end of the visit for an exit review. This is the time to discuss issues and areas covered. Remember that this consultant is now a member of your team. You should feel refreshed, educated, and energized after meeting with your consultant. If you feel as though your time has been wasted, something is missing.

The new interpretive guidelines require more and more from the activity professional. A qualified activity consultant can help you grow and succeed. This success is translated into better programs and services for your residents.

Social Services Professional

This section describes the work of a social services professional in a long-term care facility. Similar job descriptions would apply to other places where social services professionals work.

While most of the professionals on the health care team draw their information about a resident from concrete information (such as a health history), social services is a bit different. We deal with communication and emotion, helping the residents and guardians to express their feelings about what is happening and what is being planned. It makes our perspective different from the others. Social services is a soft science, therefore a bit unpredictable, as is human behavior.

The social services professional's main responsibilities as part of the resident care team can be summarized as follows:

- Assess resident needs
- Update resident status etc.
- Develop a discharge plan
- Interpret observed behaviors
- Counsel residents and families
- Field grievances from residents and families
- Ensure resolution of grievances
- In-service other staff and members of the community
- Role-model professional attributes

Assess Resident Needs

Any resident assessment must be preceded by a complete reading of the history and physical and, if available, the discharge summary from the acute hospital. The social services professional must know, before meeting the resident, why s/he was hospitalized and what made it necessary for him/her to come to this facility. The history and physical may also give you clues as to lifestyle issues which influenced the initial hospitalization.

Take special note of any diagnosis of mood or behavior or any diagnosis which might impact mood or behavior, such as depression, dementia, schizophrenia, a new amputation, a new terminal diagnosis. Also, look for medications that address mood and behavior diagnoses. You must be aware of diagnosis and medications as you will be responsible for bringing them into the assessment interview. If the resident is unable to participate fully in the assessment process, involve the family/responsible party as much as possible.

Some of the talents that are useful in this aspect of a social services professional's work are natural curiosity, genuine interest, consistent tact, and the ability to be persuasive. During the initial assessment, the resident moves from the one-dimensional person written about in the chart to the three-dimensional person with a past, present, and future. Background information such as birthplace, siblings, education, marriage, children, occupation, lifestyle, religion, retirement, and hobbies emerge to paint a picture of a person in society — his/her past. Next, we find what the circumstances were which brought him/her to need to use the facility — what series of illnesses, failures in the living situation, or changes in health status necessitated placement — his/her present.

By combining past and present, the social services professional should be able to develop an idea of how the resident may react to illness: how s/he will live with it, be controlled by it, or develop and use a sick role.

According to the latest survey guidelines, the initial assessment must include the following questions about psychological issues:

- Do you use psychiatric medications such as Paxil, Celexa, or Zyprexa?
- How long have you been taking the medications?
- Why are you taking the medications? (This may take some probing with questions such as: Why do you think your doctor prescribed this medication? Were you depressed? What did you do when you were depressed?)
- Have you ever had special care or treatment for a mental health condition, such as a hospitalization or psychiatric treatment?
- Have you ever tried to commit suicide? Have you ever thought of harming yourself?
- Do you have a history of substance abuse or are you currently taking alcohol, smoking, or using any other controlled substance? The history and physical might provide some of this information but it is not always accurate.

These questions might be difficult to ask at first but as you become more skilled as an interviewer, you will find your own way of asking without feeling that you are imposing on the resident. The people we serve are being asked these questions in order to establish a baseline for care and to determine if special measures must be initiated to assure that the person is safe and not a threat to himself/herself.

Other goals of the assessment include evaluating orientation. Is the resident alert and aware of time, place, and events (also referred to as oriented x3, but it is better to state the specific orientations for clarity) or only alert and able to answer simple questions that do not test the memory? Do sensory impairments (especially deafness) impact orientation? Who visits? Who tends to concrete needs? Is the relationship loving or dutiful? What are the resident's special identifying traits? Does the resident always wear hats? Like to wear certain colors? Grab at all passersby?

There are several factors that work in your favor as you approach an assessment interview:

- Most people like to talk about themselves.
- Families of residents also enjoy reminiscing about the past and equate your gentle inquiries with caring about the well-being of the resident and their family.
- This is an opportunity to acknowledge the pain of separation (family from resident

and/or resident from what had been his/her world) and to divide the facts of the past from the reality of the now and the uncertainty of the future.

A positive experience at this point can disarm the resident's anger as well as decrease the family's sadness and confusion that had arisen from the unnecessary guilt of placing someone in a long-term care facility. The assessment can set the tone for all future interactions.

Why should assessment — developing the case history — be so important? Do the "who, what, where, when, and why" of a person's past make a difference?

Assessment is important because unless we develop an image of the resident as a complete person, we will always be taking care of faceless sick folks. We will never learn to take care of people. The sadness for social services professionals is that we will never know the residents in the context of their previous lifestyle. We will never see them become well. We can, however, glimpse a person's totality if we ask questions appropriately and use that information to help plan the resident's future.

Once the initial assessment interview has been completed with the help of the resident, family, and medical database, it is necessary to complete the Minimum Data Set (MDS) if the resident is in a nursing home. Combing through the information you have gathered should provide the information for the MDS. Essentially the MDS distills what you have learned. But, because it is only a summary of all the facts you have at your fingertips, it would be wise to record the salient data that has not been used for the MDS on another assessment form or as a narrative statement so that nuances of the resident's personality and behavior do not become lost to you.

Depending on the information recorded on the MDS and aided by your fact gathering, you will make an entry on the resident care plan. We have sometimes gone into an interview thinking that we know what a person's care entry will be and have been very wrong. One must never assume.

Generally, just rewriting what you have learned will crystallize the problem, need, and concern without any need for preconceptions. At the end of this assessment/MDS process, the social services professional will know what follow-up each person requires. For example, is discharge back home or to a lesser level of care of primary concern? Is the resident in the long-term care facility for terminal care (i.e., related to illness) as opposed to custodial care? Is the resident having problems adjusting to the change from home to a long-term care environment? Or is the resident unable to give you any clues (because of inclination or disease state) and will the social services professional have to use his/her skills to repeatedly assess needs? In any case, there is a job to do.

Develop a Discharge Plan

The community of residents in most facilities has changed to reflect the communities from which they have come — and to which they might return. Our society and its problems mean that we no longer see the same type of residents that we saw 20–30 years ago when we really were the "old folks home." Now we see younger people with complicated, often chronic, health care issues that require a lot of community support in order for them to be safe in their chosen environment.

In many cases, we cannot plan discharges without family input. The questions for both resident, if able, and the family, remain the same:

- Where were you living?
- How much help did you need for your ADLs?
- Did you use any equipment: walker, wheelchair, etc?
- Did you have any support at home, such as preparing meals, bathing, dressing, laundry, shopping, transportation, or cleaning help? Who provided the help?

- What is your functional goal for discharge? What must you be able to do for yourself?
- What is the family's functional goal for discharging the resident?
- Where is the planned discharge location?
- What additional supports might be required after this discharge, such as equipment, home care, Meals on Wheels, transportation?

The complications in discharge planning include:

- Safe placement (sometimes this is not back to the home).
- The financial resources of the resident to afford additional care at home or in an assisted living situation.
- Capability to make independent health care decisions.

Update Resident Status

Things change! A resident might suffer a health crisis that impairs orientation. A husband or a child might die. Teeth might get lost. Financial circumstances might be altered. The resident might return to the previous higher level of functioning.

A change in condition or social status must be noted so that this information is available to all members of the care team. Never forget that people who are ill in a long-term care facility live in a well-controlled balance. Many outside influences have been removed from their lives or have been altered or diminished. As a result, changes that are more easily absorbed by a well person can greatly influence the physical and emotional status of a resident. Obviously, illness will make a difference, but even something as subtle as a change in the visiting pattern of a family member, an argument, or the switch from private payment to Medicaid can result in behavior change. Whatever it is, a social services note is important. This will lead to a more accurate interpretation about the resident, as described below.

Interpret Observed Behaviors

We help interpret the psychosocial needs of the resident for other members of the care team. These needs are based on a resident's personality, his/her reaction to illness, and his/her reaction to outside influences. Anger, aggression, passivity, and anxiety: these are responses. As a social services professional, you have the information to assist the resident care team with interpretation: determining the most likely reason why the resident is giving this response to his/her environment. The key to the puzzle is why this response is being used, not the response itself. Use every opportunity (resident care conferences, rehab meetings) to share what you know, especially if it will have a positive effect on resident care.

Counsel Residents and Families

We are in the facility, first and foremost, to assist the resident. However, most residents come to us with a family, and the family often also needs our care. The social services professional forms a bridge between community and facility. S/he provides important resource information but, even more importantly, emotional information. If we are successful at interpreting behavior, facility policies, and bureaucratic requirements, the resident and the family will find it easier to accept the placement. If their concerns are not dealt with, they will resist and may never deal with feelings of abandonment, guilt, loss, and defeat. This is true for both the resident and the family. Every facility has rules and regulations. We think it is best to give this information to the resident (if well enough) or to the responsible party at the time of admission.

The problem is that so much emotional baggage is being brought into the facility during admission that most of the information cannot be comprehended, no matter how clearly conveyed or sincerely received. Therefore, advise the resident and family members that they are not expected to know and understand everything. Advise them to observe, make lists, and ask questions. There is usually a very good explanation for everything, but one must be in a receptive state of mind to understand it. The initial intake discussion is an excellent opportunity for the resident, family/responsible person, and social services professional to become connected. From then on, you will often be sought out because you are a constant in an ever-changing environment.

Follow up on all reasonable requests. One premise of OBRA '87 is that the residents and families have the right to make reasonable requests for change and the facility has the responsibility to act on the request in a reasonable manner. Find good answers for things you don't know. Always be willing to listen to a frustration or a sorrow. You will find that your interest in and information about current concerns will ease worried minds — and help establish good communication with the resident and the family/responsible person.

Field Grievances from Residents and Families

Never forget that the long-term care facility is a new bureaucracy to most people. It is an emotional experience that may create barriers to understanding as well as feelings of impotence. The social services professional has a major role in interpretation: complaints and grievances are often not what they seem to be. Frequently they are a form of communication, a way of entering into conversation and eliciting assistance in a foreign and not always welcoming milieu.

Listen with compassion, not judgment. Seek to sort out the real complaint and refer it to the appropriate department unless you are able to deal with it yourself. Listen; write down key words, dates, and times; make a list of concerns; and tackle them one at a time. Then, return with your follow-up information.

You should expect to hear more complaints at the beginning of a placement. This has a great deal to do with resident's and family's personal pain and with misunderstandings or miscommunications. Are clothes being lost in the laundry? Has the family been informed about the facility policy for marking them?

Never assume that someone is simply a chronic complainer. Listen, try not to be defensive, and remember that any attempt at a solution goes a long way toward establishing good relationships.

Sometimes, in order to diffuse a volatile situation, we will listen, try to relate to all concerns, and ask, near the end of the interview, if the family feels the resident is cared for, liked, and responded to. We feel that putting things at this very basic level will sometimes produce a more satisfying outcome — especially if the response is yes. We don't forget about the lost slippers, but their importance takes its appropriate place in the list of "what comes first."

Occasionally when we ask a resident if all is going well, s/he won't want to say that it is not for fear of getting someone in trouble. The same is true of families. Both resident and family may feel very vulnerable in these instances and are afraid of reprisal: physical or emotional abuse heaped onto the resident by a vengeful employee. It is important to describe the grievance procedure early in the new resident/family relationship and to impress upon them the importance of the correct process.

To summarize the grievance procedure:

1. Establish this avenue of communication with residents and families early in the relationship.
2. Reassure the timid that you will take action and there will be no reprisal.
3. Follow up on all concerns.
4. Report back to the individual who initiated the grievance.

Ensure Resolution of Grievances

Facilities must post the grievance procedure. In cases when the consumer is not satisfied with your response, s/he should be instructed and encouraged to see your administrator. If this is still not satisfactory, the state ombudsman should become involved. An ombudsman is a representative of a government (usually state) program who is appointed to receive and investigate complaints of abuse made by individuals in licensed and certified facilities.

The ombudsman program was mandated and funded by the Older Americans Act amendments of 1975. Acting as an advocate for the patient, the ombudsman assesses and verifies each complaint and then seeks a way to resolve it. An ombudsman must report findings to the appropriate agencies, including law enforcement and Department of Health Services, and help to achieve equitable settlements of issues.

The concept of ombudsman programs originated in Scandinavia in the 1800s. The ombudsman is often looked on as an enforcer but, actually, they are meant to be neutral and available to assist both residents and families and the facilities. Because of their increasing involvement in the survey process, it behooves us to educate ourselves about who they are and what they can do to help us.

If you have not already established a relationship with your area's or state's ombudsman office and your facility ombudsman, do it now. You will find that familiarity will break down barriers of mistrust and fear of the ombudsman.

In-service Other Staff and Members of the Community

Although there is no actual mandate which says what or how many in-services social services professionals are responsible for, it makes sense that we focus on those topics that we know best. The reason that social services professionals are reluctant to give in-services is that often we don't have confidence in what we know. Yet, our perspective is unique in the facility and we have a special feeling about residents and their feelings.

An in-service about your role in the facility is a good start! Or, there may be a particular topic you have learned a great deal about and feel comfortable sharing. (Alzheimer's disease and its impact on resident and family interest us a great deal.) Talk about resident rights and our responsibilities toward meeting them. Discuss the psychosocial needs of the elderly. Demystify the needs of the dying resident. Speak of resident dignity and privacy and the right of confidentiality. If you still feel stumped for a topic, examine the elements of communication and what a difference it can make to communicate efficiently.

Prepare three to four topics for discussion so that when you are asked to present, you will be ready and confident. It will be invigorating to share your knowledge and elicit responses from the group, especially if you are speaking about something with which you are very comfortable.

Role-Model Professional Attributes

This is the social services professional's most subtle activity in the facility. If you are doing it well, some things you normally do will get done even when you are not there.

Nothing that a social services professional does is either secret or magic — it only seems that way. By being open and friendly with other staff members at all levels (from the administrator to the certified nursing assistants to the housekeeping staff) you are modeling, teaching, and being an example of how to do your work so that your absence does not create a void — as it shouldn't.

Always answer questions honestly; discuss such things as how to talk with residents who are dying or how to respond to bereaved family members. Your example may give courage to others to offer solace and support.

Be proud of your professional approach to your work and you will be role modeling and influencing behavior. And even though you will not always be in the facility, your social services skills, your being-there-for-people skills should pervade the entire facility and create a positive atmosphere.

You will know you have succeeded when a staff member comes up to you and says, "When you weren't here the other day, I remembered that you always take Lucy to a quiet spot and speak calmly to her when she is upset. I tried it and it worked for me, too."

Position Description

Title: Social Services Professional

Purpose of the Position

Under the direction of the Administrator, the social services professionals, led by the Social Services Director, are responsible for assuring that high-quality social services are provided to residents and their families, assisting them with the social and emotional aspects of illness and disability. The professional also promotes a therapeutic community including residents, families, and the entire staff so that supportive relationships will be developed, thus enhancing the care given.

Qualifications

In the new guidelines, 483.40 Behavioral health encompasses a resident's whole emotional and mental well-being. This includes, but is not limited to, the prevention and treatment of mental and substance use disorders and the use of non-pharmacological interventions. Staff must have appropriate competencies and skills.

A qualified social service professional may come from many backgrounds and educational degrees. As this job increases with expectations, this staff member needs strong skills and a qualified social work consultant as a guide.

A qualified Social Worker (Tag F850) (required by OBRA '87 law in a facility with more than 120 beds) is an individual with "*a bachelor's degree in social work or a bachelor's degree in a human service field including but not limited to sociology, special education, rehabilitation counseling and psychology; and one year of supervised social work experience in a health care setting working directly with individuals.*"[21]

[21] OBRA Tag F850.

Duties and Responsibilities

Provide social services to attain or maintain the highest practicable physical, mental, and psychosocial well-being of the resident as discussed below:

- Complete a psychosocial assessment, a social history, and a discharge planning assessment within the required time after admission. A Medicare assessment must be completed by day 5; others by day 7. You then have up to 14 days to complete the MDS and the care plan. It is advised that you write a discharge care plan along with the initial assessments.
- Process all social services paperwork required by managed care systems in a timely manner.
- Make an entry in the resident care plan if there is an identified social services problem.
- Always chart when a social services intervention is indicated.
- Complete a quarterly social services progress note.
- Update the discharge plan annually for long-term care residents and at least quarterly for residents who display a potential for discharge to a lesser level of care.
- Reassess the social services entry on the resident care plan at least quarterly, updating problems, goals, and approaches as appropriate.
- Interpret psychosocial needs, strengths, goals, and plans to appropriate staff.
- Counsel residents and families during orientation and adjustment to the facility and during other times of crisis or trauma.
- Participate as part of the interdisciplinary team in resident care conferences, presenting the psychosocial components of the resident's needs, and formulating a coordinated plan.
- Identify changes in responses, behavior, or personality, such as depression, anxiety, withdrawal, or aggressiveness and discuss

this with the interdisciplinary team. Document this in the chart.

- Maintain a file of community resources, including community social and mental health agencies. Appropriate referrals are made when necessary.
- Maintain knowledge of current facility, state, and federal regulations, policies, and procedures as they apply to social services.
- Facilitate and convene a Family Council as indicated by facility need.
- Attend and participate in staff meetings, department head meetings, designated committee meetings, and resident care conferences.
- Participate in the facility in-service education program, especially as it applies to the psychosocial needs of the resident; this is coordinated with the Staff Development Director.
- Other responsibilities as defined by the administrator.

The Life of a Social Services Professional

We'd like to think when we go to work in the morning that our day will end up the way we had imagined it would. This almost never happens. Chores we had expected to tackle first may remain undone, sometimes until tomorrow or the next day. People we needed to phone may have been unavailable, so our task is incomplete. Paperwork finished — well, that rarely happens.

By its very nature, the work of a social services professional is full of distractions and unanticipated emergencies. It is rare to go from Resident A to Resident B in a straight line! Some days it will feel that your feet don't even touch the floor and that nothing has really been accomplished. This actually means that you abandoned your game plan sometime in the first hour of the day and never returned to it. Remember, though, that unanticipated work is still work!

It is best to begin with a plan of action. This can actually be broken down into segments. Having the full picture, specifying a month's worth of responsibilities, will bring focus to each day.

Daily

Upon arrival in the morning, check in with the Director of Nursing or the Nursing Supervisor. Ask about:

- Anticipated admissions
- Anticipated discharges
- Emergency discharges
- MDS schedule for the day, including CAAs and care plan updates
- Room changes
- Deaths

Check with the staff nurses and aides about:

- Behavior changes
- Change of condition
- Resident needs
- Lost dentures or glasses

Make a list and decide how you will follow up.

Weekly

- Do new resident assessments
- Write quarterly and annual updates for the week
- Chart on new residents, checking for adjustment or progress toward discharge
- Attend resident care plan meetings
- Attend rehabilitation meetings
- Attend behavior management and chemical restraint review committee meetings
- Attend physical restraint review committee meetings
- Attend weight management committee meetings
- Attend falls prevention committee meetings

Monthly (if applicable)

Send out notices for next month's resident care conferences to family members, guardians, and other appropriate individuals.

Ongoing

Resident and family contact — the real reason we go to work every day.

Every day is a new day. Remain hopeful that you will "finish," but accept the challenge of a changing environment, while trying not to become too frustrated.

Recreational Therapist

All nursing homes in the United States are required to have an activity director to provide activities for residents. Being credentialed as a recreational therapist (CTRS) is one of the five educational backgrounds approved for the position of activity professional. The recreational therapist who is certified through the National Council for Therapeutic Recreation Certification is able to fill one additional position that is different from that of the activity professional. The recreational therapist may also fill a position as one of the therapists on the rehabilitation treatment team. Unlike the position of activity professional, nursing homes are not required to have a recreational therapy position.

This section contains a sample job description for a recreational therapist who is working as a member of the rehabilitation team. The types of services provided by the recreational therapist, separate from the activity professional position, are limited and covered under only one section on the multi-disciplinary MDS (Section O). Following the sample job description is an article on the types of services that a recreational therapist might provide in a nursing home setting.

Position Description

Title: Recreational Therapist

Purpose of the Position

Under the direction of the Director of Rehabilitation Services, or the administrator, the recreational therapist is responsible for implementing recreational therapy interventions as part of the treatment team. This therapist may also be responsible for supervising the activity staff and overseeing the general recreation program.

Qualifications

Credentialed as a Certified Therapeutic Recreation Specialist (CTRS) through the National Council for Therapeutic Recreation Certification (or equivalent state licensure); has experience working as a member of a rehabilitation treatment team; and has an understanding of the needs of geriatric populations.

Duties and Responsibilities

The recreational therapist is responsible for providing the necessary rehabilitation treatment interventions required by residents and within the therapist's training and credential. Treatment will be provided in both groups and one-on-one sessions. Regular and ongoing communication with the rest of the treatment team and adherence to all local, state, and federal laws and standards of practice is expected.

- Provide diagnostic and resident management services in the following areas: community integration, Advanced Activities of Daily Living (AADL), aquatic therapy, adaptive equipment, and cognitive rehabilitation.
- Participate in the multidisciplinary team in the development, implementation, and evaluation of the care plan.
- Monitor resident response to treatment. Modify care plan or approach to treatment as indicated by resident needs.
- Demonstrate good communication skills in documentation in the medical chart, in working with the other team members and family members, and in other required areas of communication.
- Maintain regular, ongoing, and timely records of contacts with residents; documentation is expected to be per occurrence.
- Other responsibilities as defined by the administrator.

Recreational Therapy Services Separate from the Activity Director Position

A Certified Therapeutic Recreation Specialist (CTRS) is sometimes hired as a member of the rehabilitation treatment team (along with the physical therapist, occupational therapist, and speech pathologist) and is not hired to be the activity professional. In this case the recreational therapist's (CTRS's) job description would be different than if s/he were working in the position of activity professional.

The professional service model of recreational therapy includes three components of service: **Recreation** (which in long-term care settings is the activity program, MDS 3.0, Section F), **Leisure Education, and Physician Ordered Recreational Therapy** (which in long-term care settings is MDS 3.0, Section O, Part F). The recreational therapist may oversee all aspects of this model in skilled nursing as department head. Or, the therapist may be working as an adjunct therapist on the team.

In either scenario, the recreational therapist needs to determine candidacy for therapy vs. general recreation needs. The diagram on the next page shows the six-step process that the therapist goes through to determine who will be receiving recreational therapy with physician orders. When providing physician-ordered therapy, MDS 3.0, Section O, Part F is completed by a recreational therapist who is CTRS certified.

Recreational therapy treatments are more than activities, as can be seen in the following examples.

Aquatic therapy is more than just exercising or playing in the water (although these activities are very beneficial in and of themselves). For recreational therapists who have specialized training in aquatic therapy, using techniques such as Bad Ragaz in pools with the appropriate water temperature for the resident's diagnosis should clearly be seen as specialized treatment and procedures.

Adaptive computer equipment (assistive technology) may only be a specialized treatment and procedure if the recreational therapist is evaluating the resident for specialized devices that will be used exclusively by that resident to improve function. The following are considered conventional equipment and are not likely to be considered specialized devices: cell phones, cable, CD drives, computer CPUs, disk drives, disk operating or system software, keyboards, microphones, modems, scanners, monitors, mice, printers, software programs (or application programs), and trackballs. Assistive technology usually includes the following equipment: abbreviation expansion and macro programs, access utilities, arm and wrist supports, Braille embossers, electronic pointing devices, interface devices, joysticks, keyboard additions, menu management programs, monitor additions, optical character recognition and scanners, pointing and typing aids, reading comprehension programs, refreshable Braille displays, screen enlargement programs, screen readers, speech synthesizers, switches and switch software, talking and large-print word processors, touch screens, voice recognition, and writing composition programs. Once the equipment is available, the recreational therapist would provide treatment sessions to help the resident learn how to use the equipment.

Community integration is more than taking a resident out into the community to enjoy community resources, even if this involves teaching the resident some new skills in the process. Moving back into the community, even if it is just for a few hours instead of permanently, requires many complex skills. Often, after acquiring a new disability, an individual will need training in the use of adapted techniques and equipment to successfully make the transition. The recreational therapist works on advanced activities of daily living to help the individual return to a less restrictive environment.

Cognitive therapy is the therapist's use of words to teach and counsel the resident to bring about the desired change. Of all four types of specialized treatment and procedures, this may be the most difficult to truly separate out from required and expected activities. The primary difference here is the scope (usually more limited in nature than reality orientation) and intensity (greater intensity). For example, interventions related to increasing executive functions (initiation, self-monitoring and awareness, planning and organization, problem solving, mental flexibility and abstraction, and generalization and transfer) using the assessment process and intervention strategies as presented in *Vision, Perception, and Cognition, Fourth Edition* (Zoltan, 2007) may well qualify as specialized treatment and procedures because of their scope and intensity.

The Six-step Process to Determine Candidacy for Recreational Therapy in LTC

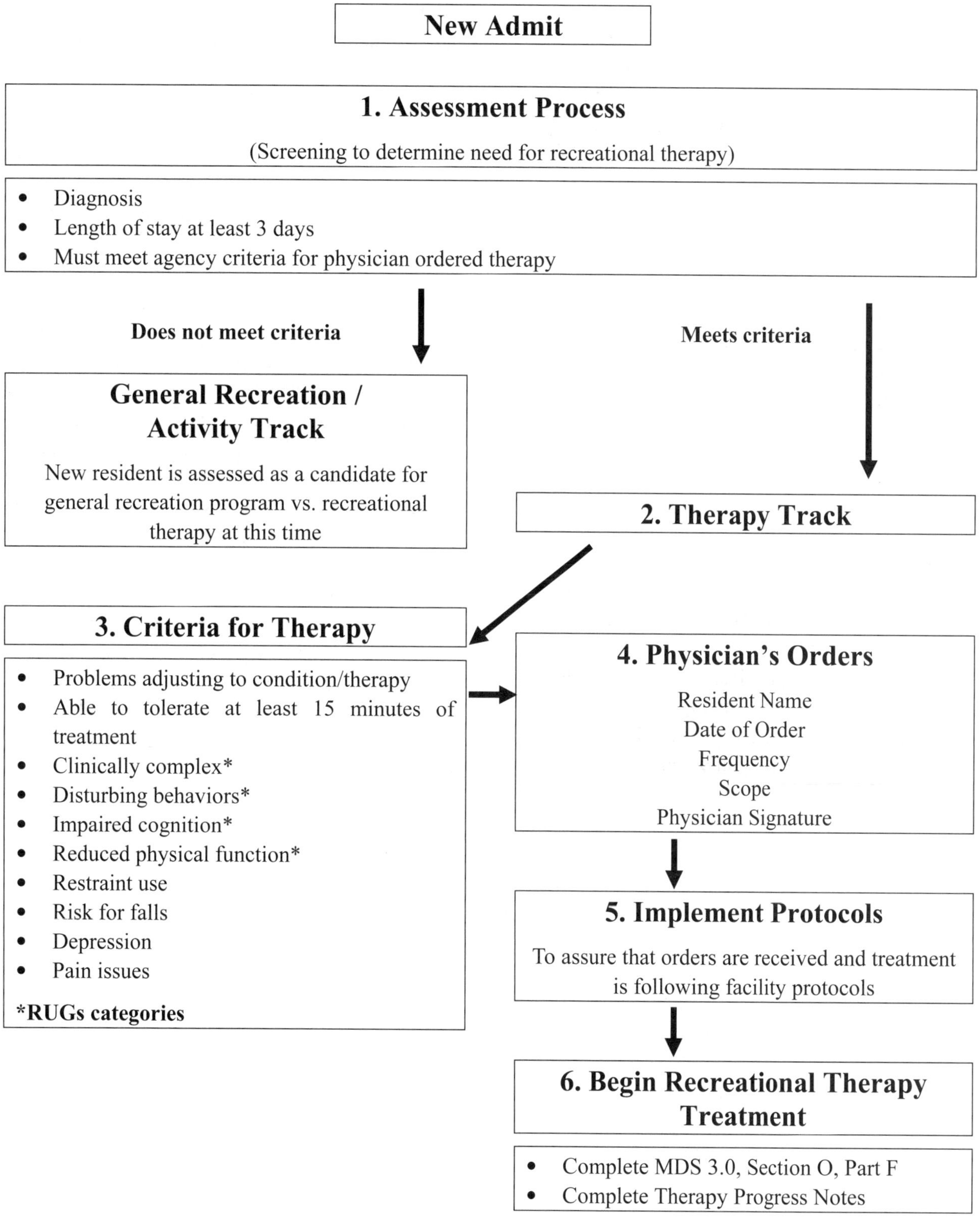

New Admit

1. Assessment Process

(Screening to determine need for recreational therapy)

- Diagnosis
- Length of stay at least 3 days
- Must meet agency criteria for physician ordered therapy

Does not meet criteria →

General Recreation / Activity Track

New resident is assessed as a candidate for general recreation program vs. recreational therapy at this time

Meets criteria →

2. Therapy Track

3. Criteria for Therapy

- Problems adjusting to condition/therapy
- Able to tolerate at least 15 minutes of treatment
- Clinically complex*
- Disturbing behaviors*
- Impaired cognition*
- Reduced physical function*
- Restraint use
- Risk for falls
- Depression
- Pain issues

***RUGs categories**

4. Physician's Orders

Resident Name
Date of Order
Frequency
Scope
Physician Signature

5. Implement Protocols

To assure that orders are received and treatment is following facility protocols

6. Begin Recreational Therapy Treatment

- Complete MDS 3.0, Section O, Part F
- Complete Therapy Progress Notes

Teamwork

The moment you walk into a facility, you have joined a team. It is not just you, the residents, and the families. The team also includes all of the other workers in your facility:

- Nursing (including aides)
- Activity staff
- Social services staff
- Therapists
- Dietary workers
- Administration
- Business office staff
- Physicians
- Housekeeping staff

Using the data presented to the health care team by each member of the team and input from the resident and his/her family, we develop a resident profile. We are working together to figure out what is best for the resident. Mutual goal setting is a powerful tool for finding the best care plan. It involves give and take of ideas and is stimulating for everyone. With the resident's good in mind and with the resident and/or responsible party being involved to the maximum extent possible, we find that the plans we make usually work well when we implement them.

All members of the team have a valuable voice in creating the culture of the health care setting. Certified nursing assistants (CNAs) are an invaluable source of information. They are with the residents in a much more intimate way than we are and are sometimes in a far better position to recognize and describe mood changes. CNAs see a lot of visitors, view interactions, share confidences. They know when a resident needs new clothing, is upset by a roommate, or just doesn't seem the same. All disciplines can profit from information the CNAs have. Make sure you solicit information, pay attention, and then follow up. Make the CNAs your allies. Respect and respond to their inquiries and their requests.

With the new emphasis on the Tag F680 OBRA '87 interpretive guidelines, it is more important than ever that we use all available sources to assess the residents' needs. It is essential that we either know or can anticipate what a resident is capable of and of his/her frailties and needs. Using this information, we must have a plan that everyone knows and, to an extent, in which they all participate. These guidelines clearly state that all staff members are accountable and responsible for following through with the wishes and interests of each resident.

4. Resident and Facility Environment

This chapter will look at the environment, as it is perceived by the people we serve, and the environment in which you will be working. If a professional is not aware of the profound importance and significance of a person's personal environment, s/he needs only look around his/her own home or room. Objects and mementos that could be easily overlooked by the rest of the world have special meaning. They give comfort and joy. They help create a place where a person enjoys spending time.

Friendships and feeling like part of the community are important aspects of our lives. Our friends and our culture help us know who we are. Our ability to express our spiritual feelings is vital for understanding the purpose of our lives. The physical layout should assist all the people in the environment in accomplishing their goals. The working environment should lead to the best care for the people we serve.

This chapter talks about all these aspects of designing an environment so that each of the people we serve will have the best opportunity for a high quality of life. At the end of the chapter you will find a set of forms you can use to evaluate the environment of your facility.

Cultural Competency[22]

Our health care populations are becoming increasingly diverse. It is important that all health care professionals, including activity professionals, social services professionals, and recreational therapists learn the skills required to provide culturally competent care. This section will look at what is required.

In long-term care settings, it is the role of activity professionals to provide an ongoing schedule of group and individual activities that reflects the cultures, needs, interests, and preferences of the people they serve. Accomplishing this goal can be a challenge for activity professionals because residents are from increasingly varied ethnicities and many different cultures. To provide appropriate resident-centered care, activity professionals must develop a clear understanding of cultural competency, cultural humility, and its implications for designing, developing and providing culturally accessible activities.

Social services professionals play an important role in understanding the cultures of people in their settings. They are often in the best position to learn about problems that cultural differences cause. Often they can act as outside advisors for residents, families, and staff to explain and smooth over differences of understanding about the health care system. In the best case, they can increase the positive connections between caregivers and the people we serve.

Recreational therapists, in their rehabilitation role, need to be aware of how culture affects their treatment modalities and goals. Treatment is not the same for all people. Culture plays a role in the types of therapy that are appropriate for a particular resident.

Cultural competency, defined as a set of behaviors, attitudes, or practices that allow individuals to work effectively across cultures, is a necessary part of all health care professionals' continuing education and practice. It is extremely important for all activity professionals to have a clear understanding of cultural competency, cultural humility, and its implications for designing, presenting and conducting culturally

[22] Information on Cultural Competency was written by Tameka Battle

accessible activities. Culturally accessible activities are specific activities that are familiar and acceptable to residents from a particular culture.

All members of the health care team, including activity professionals, should be aware of their own culture and how it interacts with the cultures of the people we serve. Knowledge gained through the resident assessment process lets us develop culturally accessible activities. Awareness of our culture with respect to the diverse needs and interests of the cultures of the people we serve is required for effective delivery of services.

Cultural competency viewed from the perspective of the health care professional is delivering care that is non-threatening, genuine, and meets the cultural and linguistic needs of each of the people we serve. Cultural competency is concerned with what we learn from other individuals in addition to learning more about ourselves and our beliefs. The basic goal is that resident-centered care should be unbiased and free from stereotypes and misconceptions. For the activity professional the goal is to provide meaningful activities that reinforce the dignity and humanity of each person and support their growth and healing by engaging them emotionally and intellectually.

In this section, we will discuss cultural competency, the six stages of cultural competency, and steps we can follow to achieve personal cultural competency.

A Diverse Nation

The United States will become more racially and ethnically diverse in the coming years. According to US Census Bureau data from 2015, by the year 2030 one in five Americans is projected to be 65 and over. By 2044, more than half of all Americans are projected to belong to a group that is not non-Hispanic White. By 2060, nearly one in five of the nation's total population is projected to be foreign-born.

As of July 1, 2015, in the US there were 55 million Hispanic people from Spanish-speaking cultures, representing 17.6% of the nation's total population. The Hispanics were once the nation's fastest growing population, but they are now behind the Asian population (Colby & Ortman, 2014). In 2015, Americans from Asian backgrounds constituted 20.3 million of the nation's population and are predicted to become a larger percentage in future years. Americans from African nations have shown remarkable growth in the United States during the last 40 years, doubling each decade from about 80,000 in 1970 to about 1.6 million in the period from 2008 to 2012, according to the US Census Bureau. Along with increasing racial and ethnic diversity in our nation, there is also a growing multiracial population (Jones & Bullock, 2012).

Long-term care populations reflect the increased diversity of American life. Although, people may come from cultures with a tradition of caring for the frail elderly and the family member with complex medical needs at home, there are fewer available family members to provide this care on a long-term basis. Unless current health care trends change, the low reimbursement for home care services and the lack of availability of home care assistance in some communities means that the cultural diversity of the long-term care population will continue to rise. Now more than ever, it is important that we develop an awareness of cultural competency and its impact on the delivery of activities, therapy, and social services in the long-term care setting.

Professional Organizations' Statements on Diversity

Studies show that there is a need for all health care professionals — physicians, social services professionals, occupational therapists, nurses, CNAs, activity professionals, recreational therapists, dietary staff, and everyone else — to understand culturally competent care. Culture and health will have an impact on how health care services are delivered. Cultural competency needs to be an ongoing part of continuing education and practice. National organizations that represent the professionals discussed in this book have all made statements related to cultural competency.

The Centers for Medicare and Medicaid Services (CMS), the federal agency that administers the nation's health care programs, has designed a case study curriculum for health care providers on cultural and linguistic competencies for minority and diverse communities.

The National Association of Activity Professionals (NAAP) has clearly outlined in its mission, values, and vision that "the strength of NAAP lies in the diversity of its members. NAAP recognizes the rich cultural and educational backgrounds of its members and values the variety of resources represented."

The National Association of Activity Professionals Credential Center (NAAPCC) follows the standards and requirements established by the National Commission for Certifying Agencies (NCCA). NAAPCC accepts any continuing education workshop or session on cultural competency and/or diversity. As an organization, NAAPCC understands the importance of activity professionals working with diverse populations and its code of ethics states: "the NAAPCC certified professional shall strive for professional competence, maintain and advance their knowledge of the field of activities, respect the body of activity accomplishment, and contribute to its growth."

The National Certification Council for Activity Professionals (NCCAP) includes two content areas in their body of knowledge that relate to cultural competency. They are "Cultural Attitudes and Culture Change in the Continuum of Care" and "Effective Cross Culture Communication." Both are part of the Modular Education Program for Activity Professionals (MEPAP, 2nd Edition).

The National Association of Social Workers (NASW) has two standards related to cultural competency. In Standards and Implications for Cultural Competence in Social Work Practice, Standard #1 (Ethics and Values) says, "social workers shall function in accordance with the values, ethics, and standards of the NASW (2008) Code of Ethics. Cultural competency requires self-awareness, cultural humility, and the commitment to understanding and embracing culture as central to effective practice." Standard #2 (Self-Awareness) says, "Social workers shall demonstrate an appreciation of their own cultural identities and those of others. Social workers must also be aware of their own privilege and power and must acknowledge the impact of this privilege and power in their work with and on behalf of clients. Social workers will also demonstrate cultural humility and sensitivity to the dynamics of power and privilege in all areas of social work" (NASW 2015).

To highlight the importance of cultural competency and clinical practice in the field of recreational therapy, the American Therapeutic Recreation Association (ATRA) has an ongoing commitment to advancing diversity in recreation therapy. In 2011, the ATRA Board revised their Statement on Diversity to include "The Association values the role that diversity plays in every aspect of service delivery, recognizing that diversity is vital to all elements of recreational therapy practices and education" (ATRA, 2011). In addition, ATRA, through its Code of Ethics and Standards of Practice, promotes "diverse and inclusive participation by its leaders, members, and affiliates" (ATRA Code of Ethics, 2009).

The National Council of Therapeutic Recreation Certification (NCTRC) addresses cultural competency as a skill set that should be self-evident in all certified therapeutic recreation specialists. The NCTRC Certification Standards in the 2014 NCTRC National Job Analysis states, "cultural competency (e.g. social, cultural, educational, language, spiritual, socioeconomic, age, and environment) is required for competent practice by the therapeutic recreation professional" (NCTRC, 2016).

These professional organizations highlight the importance of cultural competency for activity professionals, social services professionals, and recreational therapists. It is important for all of us to develop a level of cultural competency in order to provide culturally accessible activities based on the cultures of the resident population in long-term care settings.

The Concept of Culture

Before developing cultural competency, we must have an understanding of what culture means. "Cultural competency begins with having knowledge of different cultures or aspects of social diversity" (Hohman, 2013). According to the US Department of Health and Human Services Office of Minority Health, culture is defined as "integrated patterns of human behavior that include the language, thoughts, communications, actions, customs, beliefs, values, and institutions of racial, ethnic, religious, or social groups" (Egede, 2006). When taking an introspective view on how one views culture, culture includes the language one speaks or expresses, the thoughts one may incorporate in their daily lives, actions; the things one does and the reason behind the motives of one's actions, customs, beliefs, values, communication, and places or institutions that embrace or develop one's culture. The iceberg analogy of culture, developed by Dr. Gary Weaver, (American University's Executive Director of the Intercultural Management Institute), looks at culture as a submerged iceberg in deep waters. At the bottom of the iceberg are the invisible aspects of culture. Still below the surface are beliefs and values, styles of verbal and nonverbal communication, how one handles emotions, ethics, notions of modesty and time, and feelings about physical space. These concepts are the things that are not readily observed by people. These deep and unrevealed characteristics are personal and guarded by individuals.

On the other hand, there are visible aspects of culture, the tip of the iceberg that can be seen. These include how one dresses, foods, language, music, games and rituals, and engagement and interaction in festival and visual arts. These outward expressions of culture are the proud representation of who people are and how they are regarded within their culture. As the health care professional acquires a definition of cultural and its implications on the delivery of health services, they develop a strong foundation for cultural competency.

Six Stages of Cultural Competency

According to the National Center for Cultural Competence, "Cultural competence is a set of values, behaviors, attitudes, and practices within a system, organization, program, or among individuals that enables them to work effectively across cultures" (Cross 1989, Isaacs & Benjamin 1991).

The most significant work on cultural competency comes from *Toward a Culturally Competent System of Care,* Volume I, by Cross, Bazron, Dennis, and Isaacs (1989) and Volume II by Isaacs and Benjamin (1991). The original monograph looks at the provision of services provided to children of color who are severely emotionally disturbed. In that volume, cultural competency is developed into a framework that serves as a foundation for examining how care-providing organizations can effectively deal with cultural differences related to patient care and treatment issues. Terry L. Cross, a licensed clinical social worker and his colleagues, Barbara J. Bazron, Karl W. Dennis, and Mareasa R. Isaacs first looked at cultural competency in 1988 as members of the Child and Adolescent Service System Program (CASSP) Minority Initiative Resource Committee, a project funded by the National Institute of Mental Health in conjunction with the Georgetown University Child Development Center in Washington, DC.

Cross and his team felt that the cultural strengths of the four target groups — African Americans, Asian Americans, Hispanic Americans, and Native Americans — provided a platform for learning how to deal with differences. The rich diversity found among the cultures was important in developing the framework that provided insight into the roles culture plays in the lives of individuals. It showed the role of culture in the way people think, behave, and make choices. While being aware of the dangers of stereotyping, Cross et al. viewed cultural competency as a developmental process with six stages of responses to cultural differences. The six stages form a continuum from cultural destructiveness to cultural proficiency. We'll look at each stage with examples that show how the activity professional can display this type of competency in a long-term care facility.

Cultural Destructiveness. Someone in the first stage, cultural destructiveness, displays deliberate and intentional denying, rejecting, or ostracizing of another person's culture. An activity professional who is at this level of cultural competency provides activities based on the dominant culture in an attempt to impose its values and traditions on other cultures.

Cultural Incapacity. Someone in the second stage, cultural incapacity, is aware of other cultures and displays the ability to accept different cultures. However, the person is unable to effectively provide activities within those cultures.

Cultural Blindness. Someone in the third stage, cultural blindness, assumes that the diverse cultures of their clients are all the same and may ignore the strengths and weakness of the cultural differences. Activities are based on a universal approach.

Cultural Sensitivity. Someone who has reached the fourth stage, cultural sensitivity, begins to be aware of the cultural values of their clients along with their own cultural values. That person displays a willingness to learn about and understand thc values of all cultures. This is the beginning of cultural humility, which we will look at later in this section.

Cultural Competency. Someone in the fifth stage, cultural competency, has the ability to work effectively across cultures. By researching and understanding different cultures of the people we serve, the activity professional provides culturally accessible activities that reflect the cultures of the diverse resident population and needs of the residents.

Cultural Proficiency. Someone in the sixth stage, cultural proficiency, takes a proactive approach to providing culturally accessible activities by collaboratively working with clients, families, and staff to promote cultural diversity. When activity professionals understand the importance of diversity, they continuously look for ways to increase their knowledge of culturally competent practice.

Reaching Cultural Proficiency

Cross's model describes practitioners in a different setting, but it seems to apply well to activity programs. In the field of long-term care it is important that activity professionals determine the stage of cultural competency for their current practice. Then they need to develop a level of cultural competency and cultural humility that enables them to provide culturally appropriate, resident-centered activity programs.

This conceptual model has been used in various settings to assist new and seasoned health care professionals develop personal cultural competency and deliver culturally competent patient care. There are several steps to achieving personal cultural competency.

Recognition. Recognize your personal cultural biases and preconceived ideas that you have regarding individuals.

Desire. Find reasons to learn about other cultures and to become involved with them.

Seeking. When you recognize and develop a desire to learn more about other cultures, be proactive in increasing your knowledge of other cultures.

Developing. Culturally competent communication and interpersonal skills are developed over time. Developing personal cultural competency is ongoing and always evolving.

Cultural Humility

The concept of cultural humility was first introduced as training for physicians. Over the years, training has expanded to other allied health professions, such as nursing, occupational therapy, recreational therapy, social work, and activities. Personal biases and stereotypes often affect a person's conception of another's culture, which leads to cultural chauvinism — a person's own culture is valued over other cultures.

Cultural humility is a term that acknowledges our knowledge of another person's culture is limited. As activity professionals, it is impossible to know everything about another's culture just as it is impossible to fully understand another race, gender, sexual orientation, age, class, status, or disability. When practicing cultural humility, we accept our limitations and actively engage in self-evaluation and self-reflection.

As activity professionals think about designing quality inclusive activities, they should learn about the cultures of residents newly admitted into the facility. The readily available information on the web makes this an easy task. The more difficult challenge is to understand what kinds of information we need to appropriately provide culturally accessible activities.

Cultural competency can be viewed as the knowledge the activities staff needs in order to provide culturally accessible activities. Cultural humility goes beyond that to understand that we need to put the knowledge into practice. It involves looking deep within yourself to acknowledge that we all hold inherent biases and stereotypes based on our own life experiences. Cultural humility helps us master cultural competency with knowledge of diverse cultures and provide services that enhance the resident's quality of life. There are three basic steps to achieve cultural humility.

The first step is to acknowledge that developing cultural humility is a lifelong process that requires an open and honest evaluation of yourself. You will see that we all have biases and stereotypes that can hinder growth towards cultural competency.

Step two involves looking for places in the facility where there could be more cultural sensitivity and competency. In long-term care activities this might involve celebrating cultural holidays. Pictures used in activities should be familiar to each ethnic group. The health care requirement to use the resident's language should be extended to activities as much as possible.

The third step is to work on developing partnerships with different disciplines and team members who are advocates for the needs and concerns of residents. In long-term care it would be ideal to involve every interdisciplinary team member as an advocate. The team could share ideas, knowledge, and ways to improve cultural competency.

Chapter 6 contains more information about culturally accessible activities, including an activity for exploring cultural differences.

Cultural Environment

To develop the skills of cultural competency, we need to put what we have learned into practice. Developing an awareness of the unique needs, beliefs, and practices of individuals from a different culture is an ongoing process. Culture refers to a sense of belonging to a group or community that holds significance and value for its members. In order to provide a sense of belonging and meaningful life, it is imperative to create and enhance a sense of culture. Culture, in this context, can go a long ways toward giving purpose to the people we serve, employees, and volunteers in a specific setting. The feeling of being part of a larger whole can be empowering, particularly for individuals who may feel wrenched from familiar settings, values, or capabilities.

Culture contributes to the sensation of life in the environment. It can create:

- A sense of belonging
- A feeling of security and safety
- An affirmation of individuality, autonomy, and personal accomplishments
- Respect for diversity
- A sense of purpose and involvement

- Enhanced independence as opposed to learned helplessness
- Opportunities for new and pleasantly surprising experiences
- Growth
- Enjoyment
- A nurturing community

The professional can nurture the creation of a setting that celebrates the cultures of the people we serve by:

- Encouraging all of the people we serve, employees (professional, non-professional, and volunteers) to think about and evaluate ideas about lifestyle, leisure, and potential
- Encouraging innovation
- Adding the element of appropriate risk-taking for both staff and the people we serve
- Looking for the uniqueness of each person and promoting that quality
- Encouraging leadership
- Becoming a facilitator in as many situations as possible
- Finding the child within ourselves and recognizing that playfulness is a necessary component of growth
- Listening well and communicating clearly
- Lending support in as many ways as possible
- Sharing the control
- Giving everyone responsibility for a positive environment

Working on all of these aspects of culture improves the lives of our residents and demonstrates our commitment to cultural competency.

Personal Environment

One of the most important elements of our personal environment is the space around us. The facilities we work in do not have much space, usually providing less personal space than the people we work with had in their own homes. The lack of space makes personal space all the more important. This space is one's territory. The amount of territory a person believes to be his/her own is defined by him/her alone. We need to respect the individual's concerns about that space, his/her territory, and guard it as s/he does. It may be one of the few things left in the world that remains personal. This space is territory and must be respected with vigor to give dignity to each individual.

For example, you are sitting and talking to one of the participants in your adult day care program and suddenly you hear someone yelling out, terrified. You look up and see nothing unusual. The individual who is yelling remains in her wheelchair, holding her book. She is surrounded by others in their wheelchairs and all of them seem to be oblivious to her. However, if you know her well, you have learned to identify, through ongoing interactions with her, what triggers her yelling. In this case, someone in one of those wheelchairs is just a little too close to her!

How will you know that this is true? By asking her and using her verbal and nonverbal messages to verify what she is telling you. You have already heard her verbal message and the panic in her expression confirms it. She needs more personal space. It is your responsibility to see that she gets it.

All people establish their own definition of personal space. The more disabled they are, the more vulnerable they may feel and the wider the personal space they are likely to need. The people we serve have little enough left that is personal; losses abound. But our person, our body, always belongs to us despite the physical and emotional insults it has incurred. We always need to control our physical space.

Culturally, we define this space, these invisible boundary lines. Intrusion into them is a violation of us personally. In the United States, we serve people from many different cultures. Some desire a personal space that does not allow touching or hugging. Others may be uncomfortable if we stand too far away. Finding the right personal space is another aspect of cultural sensitivity.

Personal space must be respected wherever it exists. Meeting the personal space needs of each individual is a requirement for a good personal environment.

The personal environment also includes the things we put in the space around us and in our rooms. The interpretive guidelines for environment in long-term care settings check for Individuality and Autonomy (OBRA '87 Tags F550 to F586 covering a variety of resident rights). We can improve a resident's personal environment by seeking out ways to celebrate the resident, his/her life, family accomplishments, and interests. Any touch from home that adds a personal touch to the environment is important. Self-expression enhances quality of life. This expression can change a residence from an institutional setting to a warm environment.

Being surrounded by familiar possessions serves another function — the stirring of memories. For those who have very limited access to the physical environment, memories provide a safe and comfortable dwelling place. Even a resident with dementia may be refreshed and reminded of family and events if given photos or memorabilia that provide entrance into a long-ago past.

Spiritual Environment

The spiritual aspects of the environment involve the questions of purpose and meaning of life. This involves personal values and belief systems. For many, it also involves special routines and religious social contacts. For some residents the day of worship was different from the other six days of the week. The pace was different and frequently offered extra time for family and friends.

Another aspect of spiritual environment has to do with a feeling of reverence toward God or other deities. Staff or other residents who make fun of another person's beliefs or who use swear words decrease the quality of a resident's spiritual environment. Empowerment of, and respect for, the resident increases it. Making a better spiritual environment for each resident is one of your responsibilities.

Physical Environment

How the environment should be designed depends somewhat on the type of facility in which you work. Long-term care facilities need to take great care to make sure that the residents' rooms are personalized. Assisted living facilities can rely more on the people living there to bring in personal items. Day care facilities are, of course, not concerned with living space, but other ideas about the physical environment discussed in this section still apply. Most of the rest of the ideas about making the people we serve comfortable and developing a supportive working environment apply to all types of programs and facilities.

The physical plants of most long-term care facilities were originally designed in the early 1960s when the philosophy for long-term care facilities was focused on the bedroom and not the living space or environment. It was believed that most long-term care residents would be spending most of the day in bed in frail health and eventually die, and thus they did not need a living space or larger environment. This was a damaging myth. Unfortunately for those resilient individuals who helped prove this myth false, there were no areas designated for resident activities. The places in which residents did congregate had to be shared with at least two other services in the long-term care facility.

With many adaptations and remodeling over the years, the industry has tried to work within the original structure of the long-term care facility while being sensitive to personal needs for space. The goal is not to remodel the long-term care facility, but rather to affect change within the existing structure.

Luckily, most other facilities have been designed with more appropriate concern for the people we serve. However, it is still important to ask the question: How do we create an environment around the people we serve to stimulate them? Here are some answers.

Begin with all of the orientation tools available. Ideally each room should have a clock, a calendar, and large-print room numbers. The room itself should have aesthetically pleasing pictures or mobiles. For an individual who enjoys pets, provide animal visits, or, at least, opportunities to read or look at books and posters about animals.

For someone who is restricted to bed, place the bulletin board within visual range. If they can only focus up towards the ceiling, place an easy-to-see poster on the ceiling. Mobiles are also effective for residents who are restricted to bed. (Before placing any object on the ceiling, be sure that it is allowed by local fire codes.)

When there is a special event occurring in the facility, bring theme props to the room so that everyone has the opportunity to feel a part of the community.

Remember that, as people age, they require more light to see clearly. Be sure that there is enough light for the resident to see all of the things in his/her room.

Give the residents the opportunity to request and be involved in changes that will enhance further independence and involvement (bookshelves for reading, opening doors or windows, reading lights, calendars, and clocks) in accordance with OBRA '87 or other appropriate standards. (OBRA '87 Tag F558, Accommodation of Needs: "*A resident has the right to reside and receive services in the facility with reasonable accommodations of individual needs and preferences, except when the health or safety of the individual or other residents would be endangered...*")

In the United States there are laws that outline minimum measurements for objects and structures in the resident's environment — the Americans with Disabilities Act (ADA). The next four pages provide you with a sample of the requirements. The first two pages are a checklist for permanent signage — those signs that would stay up year after year. The sign for the activity room, residents' lounge, and potentially the sign for the bulletin board used for the monthly calendar would all fall into this category.

The other two pages show diagrams for minimum clearance for rooms and hallways. Remember, any object placed in the hallway reduces the space available. Minimum clearances do not mean from wall to wall but the actual space available. Fish tanks and wheelchairs "parked" along the wall make it harder for residents to get around. Chairs and couches, while homelike, may place the facility in violation of the ADA.

Remember that the ADA is a civil rights law. Any violation of this law is a violation of someone's civil rights and civil rights laws are considered more important and more significant than Medicare or Medicaid laws.

Survey Form 19: Signage

Facility Name: ______________________ **Facility Location:** ____________________

From: ________________ **To:** _______________

Section	Item	Technical Requirements	Comments	Yes	No
4.1.2(7) 4.1.3(16) 4.30.1	**Directional and Information Signs**	Do signs that provide direction to or information about functional spaces of the building comply with 4.30.2, 4.30.3, and 4.30.5 (See below)? **EXCEPTION: Building directories, menus, and all other signs that are temporary are not required to comply.**			
4.30.2	Character Proportion	Do the letters and numbers on such signs have a width-to-height ratio between 3:5 and 1:1; and a stroke width-to-height ratio between 1:5 and 1:10?			
4.30.3	Character Size	Are the characters on such signs sized according to viewing distance with characters on overhead signs at least 3 inches high?			
4.30.5	Finish	Do the characters and backgrounds on such signs have a non-glare finish?			
	Contrast	Do the characters contrast with their background (light-on-dark or dark-on-light)?			
4.1.2(7) 4.1.3(16) 4.30.1	**Room and Space Identification Signs**	Do signs, which designate permanent rooms and spaces comply with 4.30.4, 4.30.5, and 4.30.6 (See below)?			
4.30.4	Raised and Braille Characters	Are the characters on such signs raised and accompanied by Grade II Braille?			

Section	Item	Technical Requirements	Comments	Yes	No
	Pictograms	If a pictorial symbol (pictogram) is used to designate permanent rooms and spaces, is the pictogram accompanied by the equivalent verbal description placed directly below the pictogram? (The verbal description must be in raised letters and accompanied by Grade II Braille.) (If the International Symbol of Accessibility or other information in addition to room and space designation is included on the sign, it does not have to be raised and accompanied by Grade II Braille.)			
		Is the border dimension of the pictogram at least 6 inches high?			
	Character Size	Are the raised characters on such signs between 5/8 inch and 2 inches high and raised at least 1/32 inch?			
	Upper Case	Are the raised characters on such signs upper case and sans serif or simple serif?			
4.30.5	Finish	Do the characters and background on such signs have a non-glare finish?			
	Contrast	Do the characters on such signs contrast with their background (light-on-dark or dark-on-light)?			
4.30.6	Mounting Location	Are such signs mounted on the wall adjacent to the latch side of the door? (At double-leaf doors, are the signs placed on the nearest adjacent wall?)			
	Mounting Height	Are such signs mounted with their centerline 60 inches above the ground surface?			
	Approach	Can a person approach to within 3 inches of such signs without encountering protruding objects or standing within the swing of the door?			

Survey Form **19–2**

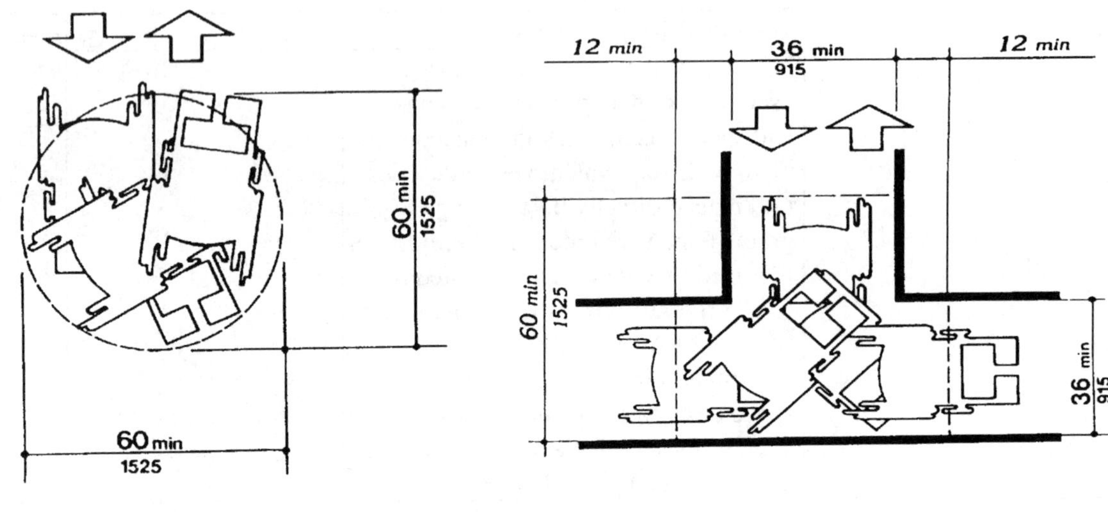

(a) 60-in (1525 mm) Diameter Space

(b) T-Shaped Space for 180° turns

Figure 3: Wheelchair Turning Space

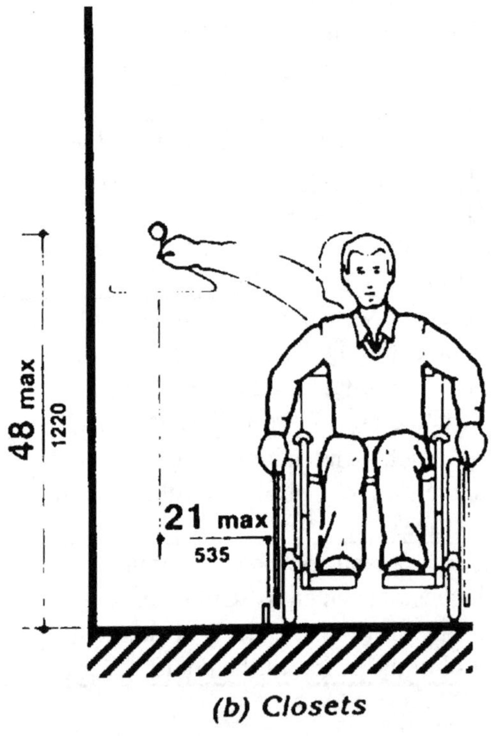

(b) Closets

Figure 38: Storage Shelves and Closets

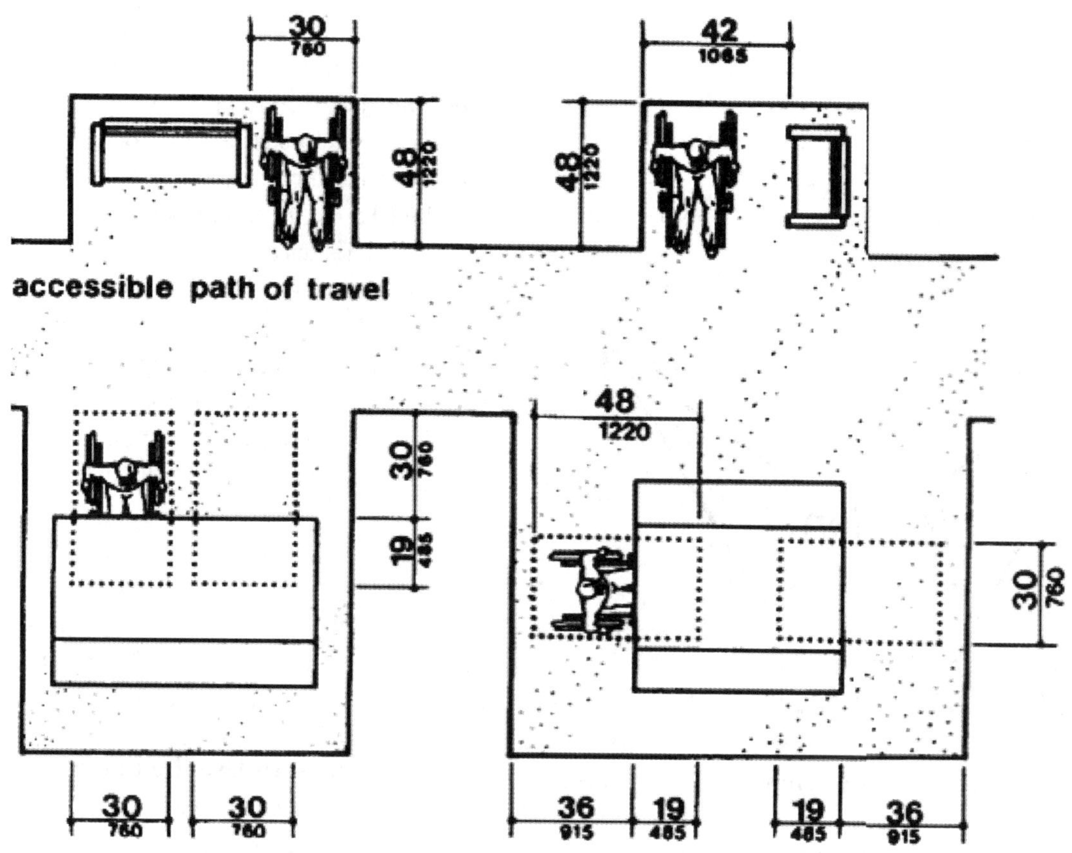

Fig. 45
Minimum Clearances for Seating and Tables

Working Environment

The working environment involves at least four different groups of people who are concerned about a resident's health and well-being. If we could view these interactions from above, this is what we might see:

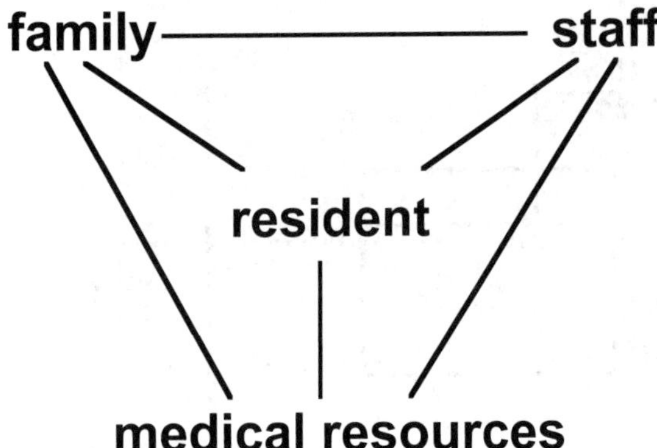

These interactions are complicated and complex and if all parties involved are not scrupulously careful, they will shortly resemble a game of gossip, with a "he said/she said" mode of communication, which may lead to misinterpretations of facts and volatile situations. No one wants to lose control and no one — from the people we serve to family to medical staff — wants to be the last to know! We cannot state clearly enough that communication between all of the interested parties is one of the most important components in quality care.

Environmental Assessment Form

The **Environmental Assessment Form** is designed to encourage us to not only assess the environment of our facility, but to then act to remedy situations that need improvement.

Part I — Psychosocial/Supportive presents specific beneficial characteristics of a positive environment. Commonly found obstacles are included to help sharpen the focus on problems and point to interventions.

Part II — Physical Factors presents physical characteristics of the facility and obstacles in the same format as Part I.

Part III — Department Environment looks at some of the requirements of the work environment for professionals.

This form represents a generic version of an instrument that, hopefully, will become individualized and specific to the setting in which it is used. Use of this form on a regular basis can serve as an ongoing progress report on the environmental state of the facility and the level of cooperation among staff members and residents for the benefit of all.

How to Use the Form

Step One: Read the characteristic in column one.

Step Two: Read the obstacles in the middle column. Do these obstacles exist? Are there others?

Step Three: Use this blank column to identify solutions that work for both the people we serve and staff. Think about human and physical resources needed. Think about what is on hand and how it can be used. Be creative.

Step Four: Repeat steps one through three until all items have been covered.

Step Five: Add concerns not noted on the form and continue the process until all items have been addressed.

Environmental Assessment Form

Psychosocial/Supportive

Stimulating Environment	Obstacles	Interventions
Reality Awareness Objects	No clocks. No calendars.	
Sense of Surprise/Newness	No change in schedule or activities offered — every day is the same.	
Variety/Diversity	Lacking programs that meet individual needs.	
Promotes Independence	No opportunity to engage in individual leisure interests. No opportunity for decision-making.	
Curiosity	No build-up to an event. No one seems to care.	
Communication	No feeling of inclusion. Confusion about changes without being informed first.	
Meaningfulness	Feeling of being disenfranchised. No individualization. No feeling of being needed or of a sense of purpose.	
Normal Schedule	Schedule changes with little notice. Canceled activities.	
Motivation	No desire to try something new. Lack of stimulating curiosity. Preferred activities not offered.	
Education	Too advanced/intimidating. Too simple.	
Welcoming	Lack of social interaction between staff and the people we serve or between the people we serve.	
Attitudes	Staff failure to see the individual and his/her potential. Unrealistic expectations.	
Community	Sense of isolation.	
Involvement	Lack of intergenerational programs. Lack of opportunities to help.	
Normal Life Setting	Lack of plants/animals. Lack of normal structure of the daily routine.	
Cohort Factors	No provision of design appropriate to the familiar themes of past lives.	
Multi-Cultural	No diversity in cultural beliefs, customs, and environment.	

Environmental Assessment Form

Physical Factors

Factors	Obstacles	Intervention
Light	Privacy curtains pulled near window — no light. Dining room too bright. Bedroom too dark — want to read at night. Amount of light in hallway significantly different than light in rooms.	
Sound	Roommate's TV too loud. Radio on all day — wrong station.	
Available Space	Can't maneuver with chair in room. Too much furniture in living room or dining room.	
Accessibility	Controls out of reach. Bulletin boards behind bed. Can't get to clothes in cupboard.	
Decor	Beautifully decorated, BUT not functional for daily use. Lack of contrast in colors and design. No personal belongings in the room.	
Quiet Spaces	No place to go for privacy.	
Orientation Objects	Disorientation due to lack of clocks and calendars for individual use. Poor signage — not appropriate size or placement. Facility name not available.	
Color	Light shades of color hard to discern if visually impaired. Too bright — hard to relax.	
Visibility	Calendar too small. Room numbers unavailable.	
Adaptability	Need board lower on wall. Light above bed hard to reach. Light switch too small.	
Odors	Persistent strong smells. Soiled linen containers.	
Activity Space	Lack of small areas for individuals to sit and watch activities with opportunity for physical distancing from others to avoid over-stimulation.	
Technology	Inappropriate level of technology. Too high-tech or too antiquated for age group of resident.	

Environmental Assessment Form

Department Environment

Factors	Obstacles	Intervention
Supply Space	No space for supplies and materials needed to run programs.	
Meeting Space	Inadequate private space to meet with the people we serve for assessments and/or discussions.	
Meeting Space	Inadequate space for meetings with volunteers. Lack of space for other community integration activities.	
Meeting Space	Inadequate space or privacy for meetings with families.	
Work Areas	No private areas for each staff member to keep his/her work materials.	
Work Areas	No quiet areas for making phone calls, doing planning, and conducting interviews.	
Quality of Life Services	Department doesn't reflect the facility philosophy for quality of life.	

Plan of action to improve environment:

5. Meaningful Person-Centered Activity Programs

This chapter looks at the specifics of matching the assessed needs of the people we serve with activities and other care program ideas. It is referred to as Person-Centered or Person-Appropriate Programming according to the new OBRA '87 Tag F679 interpretive guidelines. In this model, you provide the most appropriate care to each individual person.

Assessment is the process of discovering who the person is and what their physical and psychosocial needs are for optimum care and functional status. After the assessment, a care plan is created for each person that outlines the path the staff will take to meet the person's needs. Every goal listed on the care plan should be linked to a need identified on the person's assessments.

After assessing individual needs, you take a more global view of the population of the people you serve as a whole. This is done by summarizing the individual programming needs of each person and finding individual and group activities that help meet all the needs. While doing this, you can evaluate your current program offerings and make changes to meet the needs of your current population.

Some of the basic ideas that you will want to keep in mind as you assess and design your activity program include:

- Look at the entire population and its diversity. This is the framework of your program.
- Be sensitive to the needs of all the cultures you are programming for.
- Have a philosophy written for your department and program.
- Form a committee of the people being served to give input into the program. This is their program and should be designed around their interests — not just your own.
- Identify the talents and leaders in your community and draw them out.
- Wellness, prevention, and creativity should be reflected in all activities.
- Find opportunities to give to the community outside of your own setting,
- Provide social opportunities that include and invite everyone.
- Offer specialized groups that do not include everyone so that there is a balance.
- Create an environment of respect, dignity, and accessibility.
- Consider what you would want if you lived in this community.
- Identify percentage of population with varying levels of dementias. Add memory enhancement programs and memory aids to your cognitive programs. These should be included in the program rather than additional services.
- Each resident's life is a story to be told and celebrated.

The Wellness Tree of Life

The Wellness Tree of Life is a wellness model developed to show how people can live better lives. Some individuals living in assisted or skilled nursing will recover and improve from their diagnosis — such as a fractured hip or pneumonia. Many others will live their lives with one or more chronic disorders. Quality of life for many really means how well they can live and continue their lives regardless of their disability or limitation. Because of this reality, our programs need to be created from a wellness model. This will help the activity professional better provide for a diverse population. It will help the residents or clients by teaching them and assisting them to focus on the abilities and joys that they still have. This creates resiliency and enhances quality of life, along with bringing more meaning to life. Wellness is a state of mind and a lifestyle. Wellness does not mean the absence of disease or illness.

> People say that what we're all seeking is a meaning to life. I don't think that's what we're really seeking. I think that what we're seeking is an experience of being alive, so that our life experiences on the purely physical plane will have resonances within our own innermost being and reality, so that we actually feel the rapture of being alive.
>
> *Joseph Campbell, The Power of Myth*[23]

> Wellness is a life-growth process that embodies the philosophy of holistic health. It is the integration of mind, body, and spirit throughout life's journey. Simply stated, what you do, think, feel, and believe has an impact on your health and well-being…The desire for optimal health as we age — to be functionally able for as long as possible — has people embracing the concepts of wellness as a leading model of health management. The wellness model promotes self-responsibility for health and well-being within all areas of a person's life. This model incorporates a holistic perspective: The whole is greater than the sum of the parts. It integrates, balances, and blends the six dimensions of wellness (emotional, social, intellectual, physical, spiritual, and vocational) into individualized programming. Research shows that for many aging individuals, participation in whole-person health programs slows the aging process and promotes independence.
>
> *Jan Montague, MGS*

When wellness is the philosophy of an activities department, all of the programs should reflect this concept. Consider this as the tree's root system. Preventing loss (or further loss) of independence and function is incorporated and supported through education and in the everyday lifestyle of the community. The community culture includes diversity, respect, dignity, and attention to the uniqueness of each individual and his or her life. The combined lives of everyone are the community's story. The recreation program helps to interpret these stories through the activities provided and created by all who live and work there.

As of January 2010, The International Council of Active Aging (ICAA) has added another dimension of wellness, environmental wellness. "Why? Because research shows that the environment in which we live, work or play, has a significant impact on our health and well-being. The environment influences the way we exercise, engage our minds and spirits, and socialize; it can also affect participation levels. It is crucial, however, to look at environmental wellness as not just about the outdoors, but also about the environment that we create for wellness, both indoors and out."[24]

---

[23] Campbell, J. 1988. *The power of myth.* Doubleday. p. 3.

[24] Colin Milner, CEO, ICAA. 2010. *The Journal on Active Aging,* 9(1), 8. www.icaa.cc

The Wellness Tree
Dimensions of Wellness

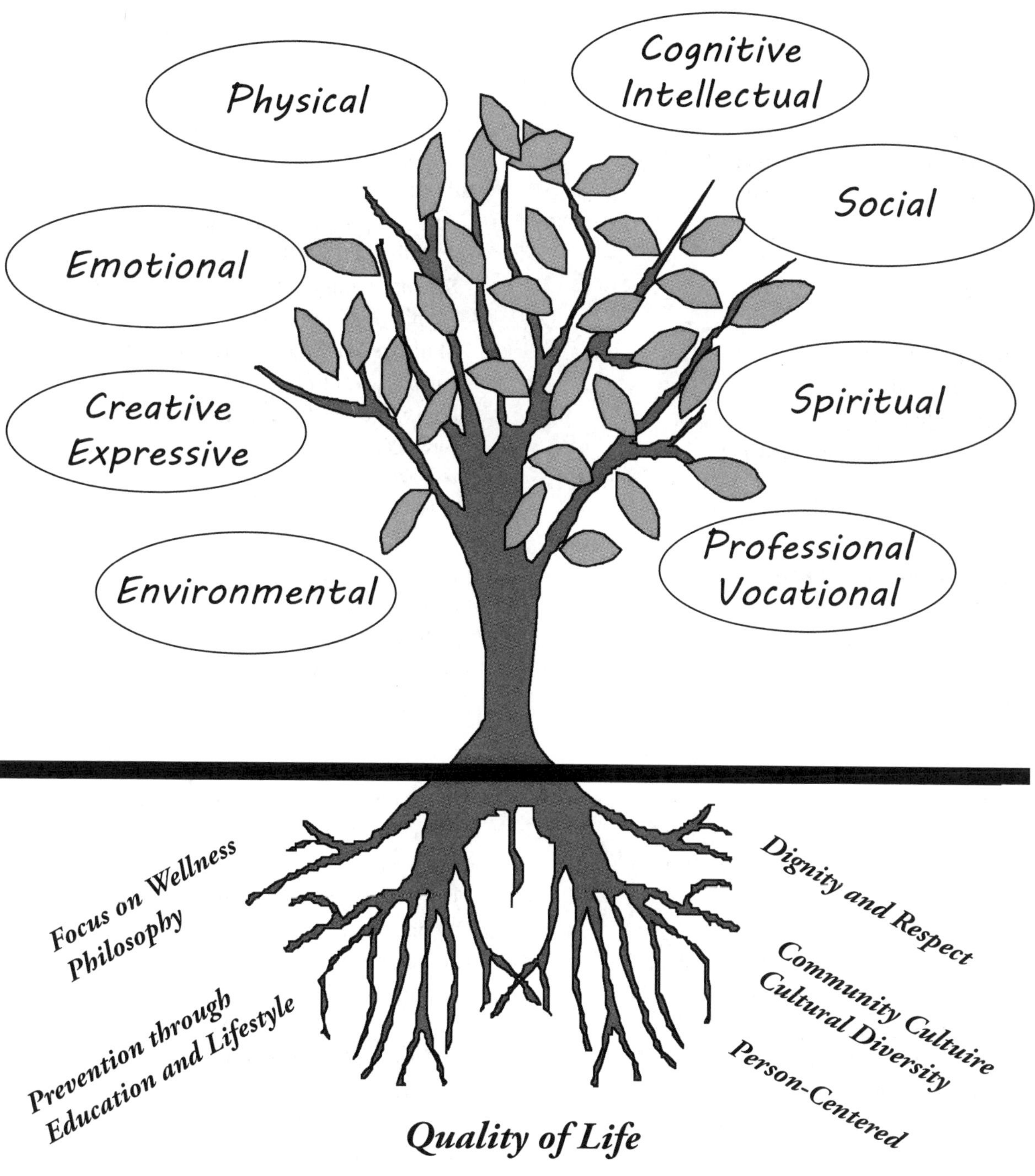

Categories from The International Council of Active Aging. Illustration © Betsy Best-Martini 2018.

Wellness Elements that Translate into Program Ideas

Physical
Exercise
Education
Strength training
Movement and music
Yoga
Tai chi
Relaxation
Stress reduction
Adaptations for special needs and limitations
Prevention and focus on wellness
Wii

Emotional
Social support
Sense of community
Ability to help others
Ability to teach others
Share experiences and expertise
Having a voice in decision making (Resident Council)
Work-related experiences
A sense of humor and fun

Creative Expressive
Creative expressive opportunities
Self-expression of thoughts
Life-long learning
Life review
Gardening
Pets
Creative writing

Environmental
Awareness of resources in environment
Encouraging green processes
Nature and light in the physical setting
Places for people to gather together outdoors
Walking paths
Gardens, labyrinths, bird feeders, wind chimes

Cognitive/Intellectual
Intellectual stimulation
Community involvement
Current events groups
Political involvement
Available newspapers, magazines, and journals
Community speakers' bureau
Disease-prevention lectures
Memory-enhancement programs
Volunteer opportunities
Leadership opportunities
Mentoring opportunities
Life-long learning
Library outreach
Computer programs and training
For individuals with dementias:
- Sensory stimulation and reality awareness for cognitive stimulation
- Skill-based activities and life skills to maintain current level of function

Cognitive brain fitness programs such as Dakim (www.dakim.com)

Social
Interaction with peers
Community involvement
Interaction with people of all ages
Adult education classes
Family involvement
Service clubs

Spiritual
Philosophical reviews and readings
Opportunity and accessibility to practice religious beliefs
Inspirational readings and discussions
Opportunities to help those less fortunate
Life review
Support for grief and loss issues

Professional/Vocational
Work-related activities
Focus on skills and talents
Helping others
Sharing expertise
Speaker series
Volunteer opportunities

Person-Centered Activity Programming

If the programs are to truly meet the diversity of needs of the current population, professionals must design and provide programs that meet all levels of functional and cognitive needs. Activity programs need to be designed to encourage and enhance success and positive leisure experiences regardless of level. This might occur individually, in a small special needs setting, or in a large group setting, depending on the treatment goal and resident's personal needs.

Person-Centered Program Levels

Person-Centered Activity Programming

Each level will have varying types of groups and goals. An individual may move from one level to another on an upward or downward path and consequently require different and specialized person-centered programs to meet his/her current needs, as shown in the diagram below.

This chapter provides you with a general overview of levels of programming. After we discuss other important aspects of running programs we will return again to these levels of service.

Chapter 7 will review ideas on how to work with individuals with significant impairments. Because these residents tend to be challenging to work with, we will also provide you with many activity ideas.

Chapter 8 will talk about working with individuals with moderate to mild impairments. Again, you will be given many activity ideas to use with this group. That chapter has a special section on working with men and also an extensive section on cognitive stimulation. The majority of individuals you will work with will fall into this level of impairment.

There are many levels of programming depending on the cognitive and functional ability level of the individual along with his/her interests and preferences. You need to assess individual needs, what level of program or intervention each needs, and then what type of setting is best: one-to-one, small group, or large group. It all depends on the goals created from the assessment process.

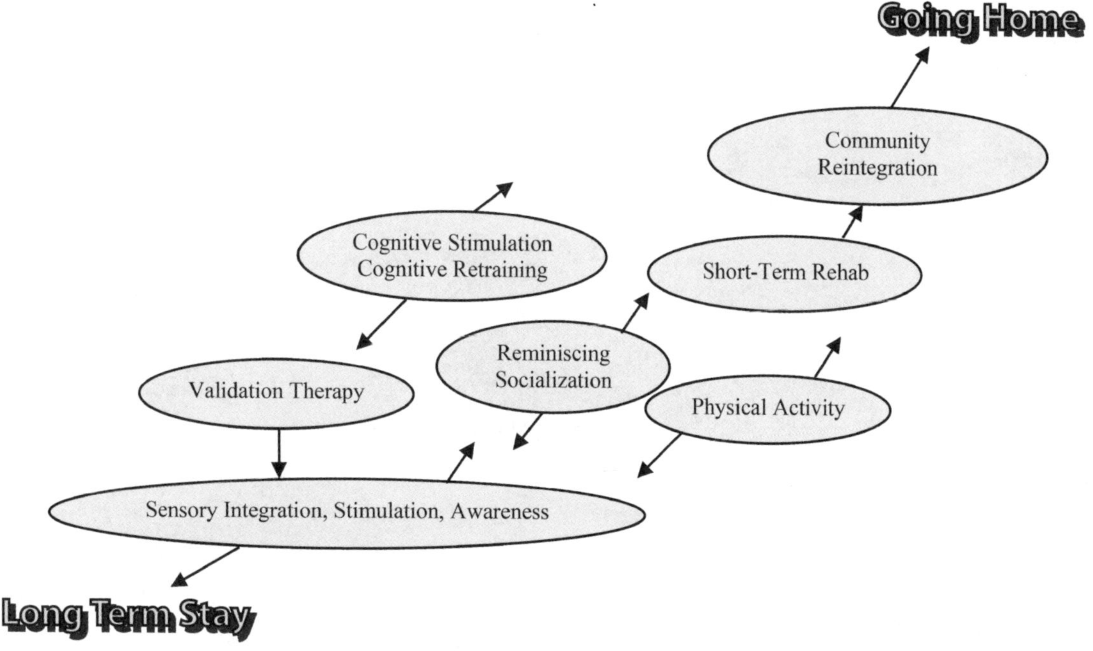

Some of these activities will be designed for all residents and others created for those with specific needs depending on long-term stay or short-term stay.

Chapter 9 discusses working with and providing activities for individuals who may have the potential to regain function and move to a less restrictive environment.

Some individuals will move from level to level. Use this with the Activity Needs Assessment (described later in this chapter) to be sure that you have programming which is appropriate for all of the people you serve.

Discovering the Person

The first step in creating person-centered programs is to discover the person. The following two forms will help you understand more about the person you are working with.

The first form will help you discover who the person is, what they respond to best, and what brings meaning and quality to their day-to-day life. I like to refer to this as "finding the key" to this person. The key is the discovery process. The sociogram will help you in this discovery process. It is also a good way to train all staff in individual, person-centered programming. You start with identifying the individual and adding in as much information as you all know as a team. As you continue adding to the information, appropriate interventions will become very clear.

The second form will help you create a profile for each resident. You can make this available for all staff so they can become better acquainted with each resident's treatment plan. A sample of how to fill out the form follows the blank form. This profile form can be reduced to fit on one side of a 4" x 6" card. The resident picture can then be placed on the opposite side. The profile form is for staff use only.

Person-Centered Sociogram

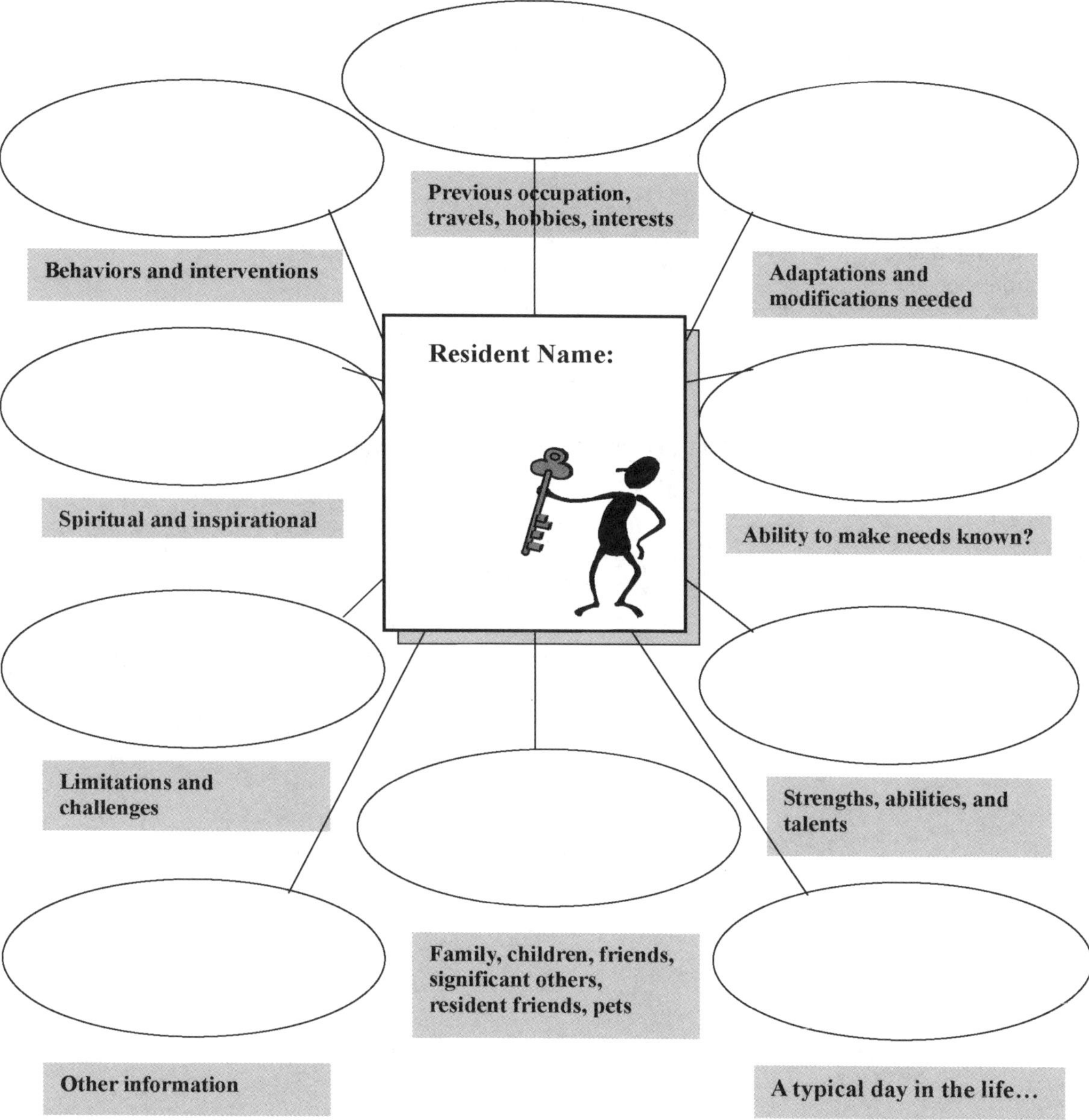

What do we know about this person? Add all the information you know. Then add information from other colleagues and family members. You will be amazed how much you know about each individual. Emotional, Social, Intellectual, Physical, Spiritual, Goals, Hopes, Successes, time they like to get up, favorite foods, roles that increase self-esteem. What do they respond best to? **Find the key.**

Person-Centered Programming

Resident Name: ______________________________ **Date:** ______________________

List at least ***two*** abilities and ***two*** limitations to be aware of:

Abilities and Strengths	
Limitations and any adaptations needed	

Activity Interventions: (activities identified as interests and interventions on the care plan)

1.
2.
3.
4.

Comments:

Person-Centered Programming (SAMPLE)

Resident Name: Barbara Best **Date:** 3/24/18

List at least *two* abilities and *two* limitations to be aware of:

Abilities and Strengths	1. Makes good eye contact when aroused 2. Responds to conversation, familiar music, and hand holding
Limitations and any adaptations needed	1. Unable to communicate needs 2. Repetitive verbalizations 3. Needs a calming environment with limited sensory, social stimulation

Activity Interventions: (activities identified as interests and interventions on the care plan)

1. Music on CD player in room: classical, show tunes, relaxation
2. Sensory Group 3x weekly, bring to small dining room at 10 AM — M W F
3. 1 to 1 visits 3x weekly — S T Th for pet visits, hand massages, memory book

Comments: Keep environment calming and quiet so that she can respond to stimuli at highest level possible within her ability.

Cognitive Activity Levels

One of our greatest problems is finding appropriate cognitive challenges for each of the people we serve. Here are some ideas to help you find appropriate challenges for different levels of ability.

Cognition is the brain's ability to process information. Remember that:

- You need to use it or you lose it. Keep the brain active in its many and marvelous mysteries and highways.
- Cognitive deficits such as memory loss are not a part of normal aging.
- An individual should never be termed low-functioning or high-functioning. S/he may be exhibiting signs and symptoms of decline in intellectual or cognitive functioning. The decline is not the whole person —it's just one area of weakness. There are always areas of strength present that need to be discovered through comprehensive assessments. The person is not the deficit.

Components of Cognition

Cognition is made up of:

- Attention
- Concentration
- Planning
- Sequencing
- Initiation
- Problem solving
- Reasoning
- Memory
- Orientation
- Communication
- Awareness and ability to interpret one's environment and world

Cognitive Loss

According to the RAI manual (MDS 3.0), a cognitive loss or dementia problem is suggested if one or more of the following are present:

- Short-term memory loss
- Long-term memory loss
- Impaired decision making
- Problems understanding others

The Cognitive Loss guidelines look at cognitive losses that are reversible (10% of skilled nursing residents) along with interventions. The guidelines also look at chronic cognitive losses and how we can provide the best quality of life for these residents through environment, activities, and sustaining current functional capacities and strengths. These three areas should be goals for the programs that we provide.

Some contributing factors to cognitive losses could be

- Depression
- Lack of motivation
- Medications
- Diet
- Sensory impairments
- Malnutrition
- High fever
- Fluid imbalance
- Meningitis
- Anemia
- Hyperthyroidism
- Anxiety
- Traumatic brain injury
- Stroke
- Substance abuse
- Dementia due to HIV
- Neurological disorders
- Pain
- Need for task segmentation
- Communication disorders
- Lack of involvement in surroundings and ability to make decisions
- Low self-esteem and lack of self-confidence
- Excess disability (decline related to environmental stimuli that exacerbate any current deficits)

Cognitive Strengths

Older adults have particular skills in the areas of Crystallized Intelligence (the accumulated life skills such as vocabulary or social and conversational skills). All of these crystallized areas can be utilized as compensatory skills. This is a strength to work with. Sensory memory is the first and most captured memory for all of us. Because of this, sensory stimulation programs enhance cognitive functioning at the most basic and profound level.

> The sensation of smell is 'wired' to the reticular activating system of the brain, the system responsible for general arousal and alertness. It is the first sense to develop in infants and occupies a larger area of the brain than any other sensory system.
>
> *Rosenbloom & Morgan, 1986*

Intelligence and Perceived Intelligence Equals Independence

Creating Cognitive Challenges at All Levels

Finding the best set of activities for different levels of cognitive abilities can be a challenge for you. Here are some thoughts to help with your person-centered programming.

III. Maintaining and Sustaining Cognitive and Functional Ability Level

In considering this goal, one must take into account the progression of diagnosed disorders. These residents have little or no potential for reality orientation and score moderately to severely impaired on cognitive skills for daily decision-making (MDS 3.0 Section C1000 = 2 or 3). Appropriate activities include:

- Sensory stimulation
- Aroma therapy
- Pet therapy
- Sensorimotor activities
- Physical movement and games
- Body awareness
- Name identification
- Object identification
- Sorting games, matching skills
- Focus on long-term memory skills (trivia, reminiscing, multi-sensory)
- Looking at and/or reading the daily paper or magazines
- Creative writing, group poems
- Singing and music making
- Range of motion
- Cooking skills, life skills, basic money management, shopping skills, motor skills
- Task segmented activities for all of the above
- Sensory boxes
- Photo albums and picture albums of familiar objects and things
- Completion of familiar sayings such as "Too many cooks spoil the _________."
- Humor and laughter. People remember better and respond at their potential when they feel safe and are smiling and feeling good about themselves (self-fulfilling prophecy).
- Validation therapy
- Reading out loud or being read to

II. Restoration of Cognitive and Functional Ability Level

These residents have potential for reality orientation and score modified independence to moderately impaired on cognitive skills for daily decision-making (MDS 3.0 Section C1000 = 1 or 2). Ideas for these residents include:

- Daily reality orientation including date, weather, location, and daily events
- Memory aids. Use visual aids to reinforce information.
- Repetition is very important. Allow more time for responses and for individuals to be as independent as possible.
- Memory book
- Games that promote attention and expression
- Reading out loud, word games, simple crossword puzzles, Scrabble
- Creative writing beginning with writing the date and individual's name

- Activities that enhance and reinforce social skills. From re-orientation, the leader works on re-motivation and re-socialization skills.
- Activities that require a certain level of active participation in speaking and answering questions
- Problem solving games. This could be as simple as starting by reading the advice columnist in your paper or on line and asking how each individual would resolve the problem and then moving on to more advanced questions and games. This creates a cluster of skills and allows the leader to build on more advanced cognitive skills of understanding, abstract thought, and communication.
- Life skills such as grooming issues, money management, social skills, cooking, writing lists, sequencing events
- Reminiscing groups
- Geography classes, including completing a USA map puzzle for visual and tactile reinforcement
- Physical movement and exercise activities
- Musical activities that demand a greater level of active participation or assisting other residents in need
- Activities that require a higher level of social interaction and perhaps require teamwork and cooperation
- Resident Council
- Card games and board games
- Current events, cultural activities, newspapers, magazine review

I. Improvement or Retraining of Cognitive and Functional Ability Level

These residents have potential for orientation and score independent to modified independence on cognitive skills for daily decision-making (MDS 3.0 Section C1000 = 0 or 1).

Remember that according to the diagnosis and contributing factors, individuals may fluctuate from level to level and documentation must reflect these changes. An example would be working with an individual who is recovering from a CVA or a recent head injury.

In addition, many of these individuals will not want to participate in the general activity program as they may wish to be seen as a short-term-stay patient rather than as a resident. Having them in small groups with other individuals at this level will prove more successful. The activity professional must work very closely with the therapy staff in addressing therapy goals specific to the treatment plan.

With the new Electronic Data Submission (EDS) and the Prospective Payment System (PPS) being implemented as the final final rule of OBRA '87, the interdisciplinary team will want to assess and capture a resident on Medicare Part A at the lowest level of function, mood, and behavior in order to fully assure coverage for the services needed towards rehabilitation goals.

Some thoughts on creating activities for these people include:

- Activities designed by the therapist and supported by the activities department
- Physical and movement activities
- Creative writing
- Crossword puzzles or word and board games specific to cognitive functions
- Memory aids to enhance individual strengths
- Adaptations to prepare for independent living and a lesser level of care
- Community reintegration skills. Learning the skills and resources needed to be reintroduced to living outside of the facility
- Memory book
- Pursuing independent leisure interests (reading, painting, crafts, letter writing, movie watching)
- Communication enhancing activities

Designing Physical Activity Programs[25]

Physical activity and exercise programs are provided to all residents regardless of functional levels. We need to adapt the physical activity to the present ability level of the individual so that it is a success-oriented experience. Functional fitness helps maintain individuals at their present level of function as long as possible. It is also a great indicator as to how independent s/he may be. As physical function declines, all other aspects of one's quality of life are altered — sometimes forever.

Exercise programs can be tailored to special needs, or you may teach a general warm-up program. Sometimes teaching a small, specialized exercise group adapted to residents, such as those with arthritis, is easier because all of your safety precautions will be similar. In each class, however, residents will have a variety of functional levels along with special needs. Here are some general safety precautions for exercise:[26]

- Be sure to have physician orders for exercise. These may also include physical therapy recommendations and restrictions.
- Remind participants to always follow the physician's and therapist's recommendations to stay within their safe and pain-free range of motion.
- Never skip a warm-up period. If a participant is late for class, s/he is at higher risk for injury. Warm ups increase the core body temperature and help lubricate the joints to prepare for movement. See the box to the right for a warm-up routine you can use.
- Warm ups should last at least ten minutes. You may extend this time when the entire exercise class is warm-up exercises.

[25] Used with permission, Adapted from B. Best-Martini, 2006. "Let's get moving." *Creative Forecasting*, October, 2006.

[26] Best-Martini, E. & Botenhagen, K. 2003 *Exercise for frail elders.* Human Kinetics. Champaign: Ill. Pages 61–62

A Safe and Effective Warm-Up Routine[27]

Seated Lower-Body Range of Motion

Hips

- Seated up-and-down leg march
- Seated out-and-in leg march
- Seated hip rotation

Knees

- Seated best foot forward and backward

Ankles

- Seated toe point and flex
- Seated ankle rotations

Seated Upper-Body Range of Motion

Spine

- Seated side reach
- Seated torso rotation
- Seated twists

Cervical Spine (neck)

- Seated chin-to-chest ("Yes") movement
- Seated chin to shoulder

Shoulders

- Seated arm swing
- Seated butterfly wings
- Seated shoulder rotation
- Seated stir-the-soup
- Seated shoulder shrugs

Shoulders and elbows

- Seated rowing
- Seated close-the-window

Wrists

- Seated wrist flexion and extension
- Seated wrist rotations

Fingers

- Seated hands open and closed
- Seated sun rays
- Seated piano playing

[27] Best-Martini, E. & Botenhagen, K. 2003 *Exercise for frail elders.* Human Kinetics. Champaign: Ill. Pages 65–82.

- The back should be warmed up in a vertical position before twisting or bending the trunk sideways.
- During upper- and lower-body range-of-motion (ROM) exercises, participants should lift arms and legs only as high as comfortable while maintaining an erect posture.
- Participants should avoid hyperextending (locking or extending a limb or part beyond the normal joint ROM). When standing, they should avoid locking the knee of the supporting leg and keep the knee soft, not bent.
- Always encourage good posture and breathing throughout the exercise. Holding your breath while exercising increases blood pressure.

Identifying person-centered physical activity needs

The following are the steps you need to take to identify person-centered physical activity needs described in OBRA '87 Tag F679 interpretive guidelines.[28]

Assessing Individual Needs. Everything starts with a comprehensive assessment process. Be sure that your activity assessment includes specific information regarding previous lifestyle and customary routine, especially as they relate to physical activity. What types of physical activity did this individual enjoy: dancing, gardening, walking, going to the gym, swimming, golfing…?

MDS 3.0 Section F. Interview the resident and ask, "While you are in this facility, how important is it to you to have books, newspapers, magazines, music, pets, news, group activities, outdoor opportunities, participate in religious activities, etc."

MDS 3.0 Section G. Review MDS Section G. Physical Functioning and Structural Problems to better understand an individual's functional limitations and abilities for ADLs and balance/range of motion issues.

MDS 3.0 Section O, Part F. For recreational therapists providing physician-ordered therapy, you may be focusing your treatment on mobility issues, gross motor function, balance skills, community reintegration skills, and/or co-treatment groups with PT or OT.

Care Planning. Activities should be linked to an MDS-generated care plan under the approach column. You do not need a separate activity care plan unless you set off a trigger on Section F or you have identified an activity need not addressed by the MDS, such as sensory stimulation. Of great importance is how specifically you write your approaches. The approaches need to be very specific: mention who is providing the service, how often the service is provided, and exactly what the intervention is. By doing so, you can better document follow-through with the care plan approaches.

Examples: 1. AC will walk with Res. to exercise class 2x weekly to increase endurance. 2. Res. will follow through with two flexibility movements to music 2x weekly as seen by moving scarf with both hands from side to side. 3. Res. will breathe in and blow on a pinwheel to improve breathing techniques and stay focused on leader.

Adaptations

Adaptations are as individualized as the residents you work with. Table 1 highlights all of the identified special-need categories listed in the interpretive guidelines along with recommended adaptations.

[28] Used with permission, Adapted from B. Best-Martini, "Let's get moving." *Creative Forecasting*, October, 2006. revised 8/22/2010

Table 1: Adaptations for Exercise Activities

Special Need	Adaptation
Visual Impairment	Be especially aware of the room set-up, placement of supplies for exercise, and lighting. This resident may achieve better success in physical activity being seated next to the leader. You may also want to have large visual cue cards or pictures for him/her to see.
Hearing Impairment	Seat resident near or next to the leader. Be demonstrative in your visual cues on exercising and give positive feedback to encourage self-esteem and sense of belonging.
Language Barrier	Have cards made that are bilingual, including pictures of the exercises or body parts being exercised. Teach other participants some words in this resident's language. Exercise can be taught by watching and following vs. giving verbal cues to this individual. Ask family or staff members to help translate as needed.
Use of one hand	Encourage resident to move the affected arm or leg with the help of their other hand. Add body awareness activities to place a greater focus on the affected side. Use Velcro hand mitt and ball to include resident in physical games. Also use handballs to manipulate and work both hands for muscle strengthening and motor skills.
Terminally Ill	Relaxation CDs and music along with breathing exercises to reduce pain and tension, as requested.
Pain Issues	Always check to see how an individual is feeling before starting exercise of any kind. Work with nursing to determine if anti-inflammatory or other types of medication can be given a short time before the individual begins to exercise. This resident is a good candidate for a short and slow-moving range-of-motion warm-up routine.
Short-term Stay	Review the therapy goals established by the PT, OT, RT, or ST and create an intervention that enhances the same goals. The resident may prefer a relaxation CD or slow-moving CD such as seated tai chi for individual use in his/her room.
Younger Residents	Check for preferences in music and current exercise interests. They may want to attend a college exercise class or community event.
Cognitive Impairments	Break down movements into simple steps. Use lots of repetition and praise. Add colorful props for motivation and sensory stimulation and integration.
Behaviors Related to Dementias	Remember that physical ability and strength are the talents that someone dealing with dementia still has available to them. Highlight this and give lots of positive feedback. The guidelines include many recommendations such as dancing, physically resistive activities (punching balls, kneading clay, hammering, and tapping), being outdoors, walking, gardening, rocking chairs, and drumming. Be creative and know your resident's needs and abilities.

Physical Function and Common Medical Disorders[29]

The table above looks at adaptations based on physical or mental conditions. Sometimes it is useful to consider the diagnosis of the people we serve to provide better person-centered exercise programs. In this section we present a list of the more common conditions encountered, with brief descriptions and suggestions about the best way to personalize exercise. Although every disorder has a basic description, remember that every person you see will present himself or herself in a unique manner.

Preventing loss of function and mobility is a primary goal of physical therapy and is greatly enhanced by exercises in a group setting or one-on-one basis provided by other members of the health care team. With the increasing constraints of insurance companies, many individuals are no longer able to receive the extended therapy they need. This is resulting in greater numbers of people who depend on the activity professional and other staff to continue the focus on therapy goals. You need to have not only a basic knowledge of diagnoses but also the ability to blend this understanding with movements and exercises to help maintain and enhance functional skills.

Heart and Circulation

Individuals with cardiac disorders may have sustained a myocardial infarction or have undergone open-heart surgery for valve replacement, coronary artery bypass, or even a heart transplant. Clinically, they may present varied appearances, from no outward signs to shortness of breath with minimal activity.

Have the individual monitor his/her pulse before, during, and after the sessions with caution not to exceed 20–30 beats above his/her resting heart rate. Some medications modify the individual's responsive heart rate so that this target heart rate will not be appropriate. If in doubt, ask the individual's physician or the nursing staff for assistance. Many areas also have a local cardiac rehab group, which can provide the facility's staff with additional good information.

Suggestions for exercise:

- Limit upper extremity activity, thus reducing stress on the heart. Do not use arm weights.
- Encourage activities that involve walking.
- Encourage stationary bicycles.
- Encourage dance activities.

Musculoskeletal

Many individuals with total hip replacement (THR) or total knee replacement (TKR) come for short-term rehab and may not be interested in participating in social activities. But many residents also have to undergo procedures and are quite willing to participate in activities.

Total Hip Replacement

If your person is between one and eight weeks following a total hip replacement, s/he must follow some very important precautions.

- S/he cannot bend at the hip greater than 90 degrees. Therefore, s/he must be in a semi-reclining position with a firm seat. (No low-seated chairs.)
- The knees need to be up in a V-position, with pillows below both knees.
- The foot on the operated leg may not turn inward.
- S/he will ambulate with either crutches or a walker. No canes at this point. S/he may not be able to bear full weight on the affected leg, so no standing exercises or leaning forward.

Note: After his/her hip has healed (six to eight weeks post-op), s/he may return to full weight bearing ambulation with no bending restrictions.

Total Knee Replacement

An individual with a total knee replacement may have restrictions as to his/her weight

[29] This section on was written by Mary Kathleen Lockett, RPT.

bearing ability, but many are full weight bearing. S/he will use either a walker or crutches and, depending on his/her physician's request, may or may not be wearing a leg brace. Compared to an individual with a total hip replacement, there are fewer restrictions but s/he may have a bit more pain.

Suggestions for exercise:

- Encourage sitting exercises with the brace removed.
- There is no limit to upper extremity exercises.

Weight Bearing Status

The following abbreviations are frequently used:

FWB Full Weight Bearing

NWB Non-Weight Bearing

PWB Partial Weight Bearing (refers to bearing 25% to 75% of weight on leg)

TTWB Toe Touch Weight Bearing (allows individual to rest leg on floor, but no weight may be put on it)

Neurological Groups

Cerebral Vascular Accident — CVA

A CVA is a neurological disorder also known as a stroke. Whether an individual has sustained a right CVA with resulting left-sided weakness or a left CVA with right-sided weakness will determine the cognitive and physical deficits present. It is important to remember that individuals can be affected very minimally with excellent recovery or have extensive damage with poor recovery.

Left Hemiplegia (Right CVA). While language is mostly intact, beware of impulsive behavior and neglect of the left side. Encourage the person to keep his/her head centered in midline. Encourage left-sided activities and movements. Be aware that reasoning with an individual with left hemiplegia is often difficult.

Right Hemiplegia (Left CVA). Language is often affected resulting in aphasia, which may be receptive, expressive, or global. Establish a communication task and expect the individual with a right hemiplegia to have fair reasoning skills.

Suggestions for exercise:

- The muscle tone in the individual's extremities may vary from flaccid to spastic.
- Be alert for painful shoulder syndromes seen with either type of tone.
- If the individual is in a wheelchair, make sure that his/her upper body is supported in the midline.
- Be sure the affected arm is supported and have the individual use the non-affected leg to propel the chair.
- Lapboards are strongly encouraged by therapists. Because they are considered to be a kind of physical restraint, interdisciplinary team approval is required in a long-term care setting.
- If the individual is ambulatory, balance may still be affected, so encourage sitting exercises. If standing, have the individual hold on to a secure surface.
- Expect frustration and occasional inappropriate behavior, especially with an individual who is aphasic. Ask his/her therapist for suggestions if you are having difficulty with a particular individual.

Multiple Sclerosis — MS

MS is a neurological disorder affecting more women than men. It can be very mild or very severe. There can be remissions for years or no remissions. It can allow a person to remain ambulatory or cause them to need a wheelchair for mobility. Common clinical presentations are tremors and sensory losses in the extremities, visual disturbances, unsteady gait, and occasional personality disorders.

Suggestions for exercise:

- It is important for these individuals to exercise with the goal of increasing strength and range of motion.
- Of equal importance is the need to avoid getting overly fatigued.

- Allow frequent rest periods.
- Encourage sitting exercises if balance is affected. Otherwise, allow standing exercises with support.

Parkinson's Disease

This chronic neurological disorder can present a range from mild rigidity with no cognitive deficits to severe rigidity with cognitive deficits.

Suggestions for exercise:

- Start the exercise session with head rotations to the right and left.
- Follow with reciprocal arm exercises and trunk rotation to the right and the left.
- Marching in place is an excellent activity, either standing or sitting.
- Have the individual keep time to a metronome.
- Reciprocal and rotational activities are felt to help to decrease rigidity.

Note: Be very alert to the possibility that these individuals will lean or fall backwards and have trouble initiating movements.

Head Injury

Many individuals who are in their teens, twenties, and beyond are being admitted to long-term care facilities with head injuries. It is highly recommended that these individuals be screened for appropriateness by their therapist prior to entering your activities. This is due to their variable cognitive status and a decreased ability to tolerate certain levels of stimulation.

Suggestions for exercise:

- Limit auditory and visual stimulation to reduce the possibility of over-stimulation.
- Try to work on a one-on-one basis and gradually incorporate individuals into a group setting, small group first.
- A calm and firm voice works best. Avoid yelling or speaking too loudly.
- Be patient but do not tolerate any aggressive behavior.
- Ask the therapist for appropriate interventions.

Pulmonary

Chronic Obstructive Pulmonary Disease (COPD) results in the individual's decreased ability to breathe normally. Many of the people with this condition need low-flow portable oxygen.

Suggestions for exercise:

- Sitting exercises
- Decrease the number of upper extremity/arm exercises.
- Stop all exercises if the individual becomes winded.
- Pacing all activities is the key to functional independence for the individual with COPD.

Note: The individual will be most comfortable with the head and shoulders forward. Continue to encourage activities to lengthen the trunk such as one-armed overhead stretches.

Activity Needs Assessment

After you have assessed each of the people you serve to find out what needs each one has, you must design a program for your facility that meets the needs of all of them. To do that you need to know the current needs, interests, cognitive abilities, and functional levels of the individuals who are present today. Perhaps the activity program was designed for last year's needs and many of those people are no longer here. Federal law mandates that activity programs in long-term care facilities must *"provide, based on the comprehensive assessment and care plan and the preferences of each resident, an ongoing program to support residents in their choice of activities, both facility-sponsored group and individual activities and independent activities, designed to meet the interests of and support the physical, mental, and psychosocial well-being of each resident, encouraging both independence and interaction in the community."*[30] Even without

[30] *State Operations Manual*, OBRA Tag F679

the mandate of the federal law, it still makes sense to be sure your program meets the needs of the people you serve.

Ask yourself how many of the people benefit from the activity program. Does the program seem to cater to those able to attend large groups and classes? Are many of the people you serve uninterested in attending? Are many residents in need of supportive activities (special-needs and one-on-one programming)? Why do the alert, short-term rehab residents refuse to go to group activities? What do we offer to them as alternatives? Review the guidelines for the *Activity Needs Assessment Form*, take a current census sheet, and complete this form.

In F-Tag 838, the facility is responsible for completing a facility assessment form. Information from the activity-needs assessment will help provide information for the facility assessment.

Guidelines for Completing the Needs Assessment Form, Step 1

Each of the people we serve needs to be listed in a single category. The group selected represents the level where the individual functions *most* of the time. For example, if an individual is *mostly* active but occasionally passively involved, s/he goes under "actively involved." Place an asterisk (*) next to each name, as they also need to be assessed for specialized programs. Add the cognitive level after the name so you can be sure your mix of activities matches the cognitive functioning level of the people you serve.

This assessment form needs to be updated with names of newly admitted individuals so every individual is reflected on the assessment. The form itself should be updated as often as the admission and discharge schedule changes the census—as often as once a day Keeping this form on your department's computer will help to make updates easier.

- Individuals in Actively Involved are actively participating in group activities.
- Individuals in Passively Involved are present at group activities but are passive observers — "fringe participants." Determine if they are passive by nature, or under- or over-stimulated in a group setting.
- Individuals in Mild to Moderate have mild to moderate cognitive impairments.
- Individuals in Advanced Stages have dementias that have progressed to the point of possible disturbing behaviors.
- Individuals in Alert and Independent include residents who are both in individual and group leisure pursuits. They attend activities at least two to four times a week but not on a regular basis. They keep involved in individual leisure interests, occasionally attend events or special presentations, and receive visits from families and friends. They may be in short-term rehab. If so, these individuals are receiving therapy with the intent of being discharged as soon as possible. For the most part, they do not wish to enter the residents' world and thus tend to avoid social settings and contact with most of the residents who will be staying in your program indefinitely. Their needs and goals are very different from those of an individual in long-term care. Many of these individuals are being served through Medicare or an HMO for whom the PPS system of reimbursement applies.
- Individuals in Refuse decline all activities. These individuals are alert but do not involve themselves in any individual or group leisure interests. They spend their days in their rooms or in the hall. They do not seek out companionship or activities.
- Individuals in Profound Multiple and Singular Sensory Losses include a large percentage of the population. They fit into this category because this is the most pronounced need addressed at this time. Be specific as to type and severity of individual sensory losses.
- Individuals in Critically Ill may be in hospice, on dialysis, dependent on ventilators; have naso-gastric (NG) or other enteral feeding tubes, and/or have a critical illness. Each facility varies greatly, so use this column as needed to keep track of individuals who require mostly one-on-one activities.
- Individuals in Traumatic Head Injuries or Comatose. These two categories have separate needs but are grouped together in this form.
- Individuals in Other include other identifiable subgroups that have special needs including smokers, younger participants, and residents with developmental disabilities. They generally have a low attendance at group activities. These groups are under the same column but obviously have nothing in common in terms of disabilities and program needs.

Activity Needs Assessment Form

Activity Professional ______________________ **Date** __________

Take a current census list and add the name of each individual in one column only.

Individuals actively involved in group activities and individual leisure interests	Individuals passively involved in groups with limited individual leisure interests	Mild to moderate cognitive impairments and mild dementias	Advanced stages of dementia with some disturbing behaviors (including apathy)	Alert and independent in both individual and group leisure interests Could be short-term stay	Refuse all activities and not involved in independent leisure interests	Profound multiple and singular sensory losses Be specific with type and severity of sensory loss	Critically ill, comfort care, hospice, pain issues, IV, NG, wound care, dialysis, ventilator dependent	Traumatic head injury Comatose	Younger residents Develop-mentally disabled Other:

Guidelines for Completing the Needs Assessment Form, Step 2

After the activity professional completes the needs assessment form, s/he must now take a closer look at each category to further assess the population's programming needs.

Actively Involved

Individuals in this group attend and participate in leisure activities. Do they need to be better connected to functions outside the facility? Are they physically overexerting themselves by this high level of participation?

Passively Involved

Individuals in this group choose not to initiate interactions and/or engage in leisure activities that require more skills or energy than they may possess. Determine why these individuals are passively involved. Is it due to sensory losses or because they cannot tolerate a large group setting because they shut down due to sensory overload? Is this passivity a long-standing personality trait, which would not be expected to change?

If these or other reasons make them poor candidates for group activities, their needs may be better met in another group. If they can be more actively involved, the ideal is to find ways to make that possible and therefore include them in more social activities. Individuals experiencing cognitive losses may be disoriented, but respond successfully to reality awareness and remotivation groups. Help facilitate their involvement to the maximum level of their functional ability.

Mild to Moderate Cognitive Impairments and Mild Dementias

Individuals in this group have moderate to severe inability to make decisions and make themselves understood. (Review MDS, Section C C1000) The types of programs appropriate to this level are listed under cognitive challenges on page 103.

Advanced Dementias with Some Disturbing Behaviors (Including Apathy)

Individuals in this group have severe inability to make decisions and make themselves be understood. They are in more advanced stages of dementias and are dependent on others for all ADLs. Apathy is included as a disturbing behavior, as some individuals at this level need frequent arousal and stimulation to decrease the level of apathy.

Alert and Independent in Leisure Interests

Individuals in this group are able to participate in their own leisure activities, and do so most of the time. If there is an activity of interest to them, they will usually join in. These individuals make choices about their leisure time. Be sure to clearly document their involvement in the activities that are not listed on the standard activity list so you can show that their leisure needs are being met. These individuals may be in the facility for short-term rehab. The professional's role with these individuals is often that of a resource person or an adjunct therapist to enhance the rehab goals. Separate groups of activities designed for rehab residents may be very appropriate.

Refuse All Activities

Individuals in this group consistently refuse to engage in any leisure activity, either facility-sponsored or of their own choosing. This may reflect the lifestyle they were accustomed to before admission. If so, be sure to document this and define how you came to this determination. Other causes for refusal could be depression, fear of groups, distrust, lack of culturally appropriate activities, or lack of motivation. Obviously these people need assessment to determine why they are making the choices that they are making. They may eventually become more involved after they develop a trusting relationship. They may be in need of specialized one-on-one programs. Or they may simply be making a personal choice not to be involved — which is their right. Be sure that programs are available for them and document that they were informed about those programs, and chose not to attend,

Profound Multiple and Singular Sensory Losses

Individuals in this group have individual needs based on the level and severity of their sensory loss. Many of the individuals in other categories are also dealing with these types of losses, so be sure that individuals listed here are those with a profound sensory loss.

Critically Ill, Comfort Care, Hospice, Ventilator Dependent, Dialysis, Pain Management

Individuals in this group have a very high level of acuity. Many are unable to leave their rooms and/or to become engaged in activity groups. These individuals' needs are very diverse and personalized. Many or most will be provided with services on a one-on-one basis. For professionals working in units in an acute care hospital, this is the major resident profile. The challenge is in creating a theme-oriented and individualized program that can be offered on a one-to-one or small group basis if there are a few individuals present in the day room.

Traumatic Brain Injury, Comatose

Individuals in this group may eventually progress to leisure groups, but they primarily need specialized one-on-one experiences. The individuals with head injury and in a semi- to full-comatose state are quite a challenge and demand a special understanding of what they can and cannot tolerate in terms of activity programming. Remember that these two groups have extremely different needs in programming. As with all individuals, be familiar with and use the interdisciplinary approach and always feel comfortable asking questions of other team members to increase your understanding of the person and her/his diagnosis.

Your interactions with the individual in a comatose state will vary according to his/her level of consciousness. Individuals with head injuries will usually be much younger people. Depending on the length of time since the injury and the physical healing of the injured area, this individual will need different types of programming interventions. Be sure to read the therapy notes and talk to the physical, recreational, occupational, and speech therapists. They will be happy to help you use your time with the individuals to meet specific therapy goals.

Cognitive retraining and cognitive stimulation are appropriate during progressive therapy and, again, require a team approach to identify what is needed. In terms of group activities, be cautious with these individuals. A group may be over-stimulating for them — may cause agitation and combativeness or even seizure activity. It is normal for individuals with head injuries to have fluctuations in their tolerance level. Observe them closely and be aware of their reactions to and tolerance of stimulation. Keep them at a safe distance from commotion and other residents until they have been fully assessed and evaluated for this level of involvement.

Others

Individuals in this group choose not to attend most or any of the groups but do spend most of their leisure time in a social network with others they feel comfortable with. (This may be especially true of smokers.) Their attendance does not reflect specifics about them. Be sure to document their social skills as demonstrated within the group as well as other information regarding interests, strengths, and lifestyle.

Person-Centered Quality Assurance Review

F-Tag Guidelines — Adaptations	Interventions listed in guidelines	Met Y/N	Comments
Adaptations for visual impairments	Increased lighting, magnifying glasses, light-filtering lenses, large print.		
Adaptations for hearing impairment	Speakers, amplifiers, headphones, less background noise, written instructions, gestures, adapted TV.		
Adaptations for physical limitations	Placement of supplies to enhance visual interaction, upper extremity function, range of motion, hand dexterity (large handles, large needles), ability to manipulate items based on weight, use of one hand, (provide holders, clamps, vise, etc.)		
Cognitive limitations	Task segmentation, programs encouraging long-term memory, length of activity appropriate to needs.		
One-to-one programming	Sensory stimulation, cognitive therapy, validation therapy, aromatherapy, social engagement, walks, spirituality, creativity, task-oriented and self-directed activities, pet therapy, letter writing, puzzles.		
Language barrier	Translation tools, translators, publications, audio/video materials in resident's primary language.		
Terminally ill, hospice	Life review, quality time with family, spiritual support, music, relaxation CDs, reading.		
Pain	Spiritual support, relaxation groups, music, massage, aromatherapy, pet therapy, touch, breathing.		
Prefers room or unable to leave room	In-room visits, touch and sensory activities, access to art materials, access to technology of interest (computer/electronic media, DVD, video games, radio and TV programs, audio books).		
Short-stay residents	Offer choice of activities: books, cards, movies, hand-held games, computers, CDs.		

F-Tag Guidelines, Problem Behaviors	Interventions listed in guidelines	Met Y/N	Comments
Walking difficulties Walking without purpose	Provide objects that can be manipulated, aromatherapy, validation therapy, reality awareness, and space and environmental cues that encourage physical exercise and reduce extraneous stimulation.		
Name calling, hitting, kicking, biting, sexual behavior, compulsive behavior	Structured activities, exercise, movement, exchanging self-stimulatory activity for more socially appropriate behaviors in public places.		
Disruptive social behavior	Offer activities that resident can succeed at, small groups or one-to-one, familiar occupation/life skills activities, physical activity, slow exercises.		
Rummaging	Life skill/normalizing activities such as folding laundry, sorting socks, stacking cans.		
Withdrawn or isolated (apathy)	Activities before and after meals, tasks that need to be completed out of room, activities that feel useful and purposeful, outdoors, gross motor exercise to improve mood.		
Attention seeking	Leadership jobs and roles, small groups, social activities, and service projects.		
Lacks awareness of personal safety or is self-destructive	Observe closely in groups and avoid use of potentially dangerous objects. Use emotionally soothing activities, physical activities, small group or one-to-one activities.		
Delusions or hallucinations	Decrease stress and increase awareness of actual surroundings, offer verbal reassurance.		

Facility Standards

Facility Standards	Met Y/N	Comments
Activity assessment addresses interests and needed adaptations.		
Care planning needs are based on measurable objectives with desired outcomes, not just attending activities.		
Care plan identifies the disciplines responsible for carrying out transportation and needed assistance to successfully participate.		
All staff members provide functional assistance, adaptive equipment to accommodate leisure requests.		
Schedules for therapy and treatment are arranged to meet individual activity preferences.		

Planning Activities

After you have identified the needs of the people you serve from the list above, plan a set of activities that meets the needs of all of the individuals. Some ideas for activities are included in the chapters that follow. If you work in a nursing home, it is a good idea to check the activity plan against the Person-Centered Quality Assurance Review forms on the following pages to see if it meets the OBRA '87 requirements for activities. Mark yes or no to indicate whether each item is addressed and add comments about the items that need to be improved.

Activity Review Forms

The purpose of these forms is to assure program compliance with the interpretations and terminology of the OBRA '87 regulations. In addition, they will assist you in designing person-centered programming. All of the following areas are within the regulations and should be a part of your activity program. While this form was developed for use in long-term care settings, it is appropriate for assisted living and other types of settings.

After reviewing how to use the form for your department, take your monthly calendar and write down each activity in the first column. In the second column use the list below to describe which part(s) of the OBRA '87 requirements are covered by the activity. For example, a fishing trip might cover outdoor, male-oriented, and an activity for all ages. In the third column write the component of wellness covered (physical, cognitive, spiritual, etc.). The fourth column says whether the activity is basically active (e.g., dancing) or passive (e.g., listening to music).

This is a quality review exercise to evaluate the programs you currently offer. (If you want to practice this evaluation on someone else's schedule, you can use the schedules in the section on *The Life of an Activity Professional* in Chapter 3.)

After the form is filled out, analyze each of the columns to make sure you offer activities that cover each of the OBRA '87 areas, all aspects of the wellness model, and provide a balance of active and passive activities as appropriate for the current list of people you are serving. Part two of the form allows you to make notes on what you discover and considers other aspects of your activity program.

OBRA '87 Activity Types

The following types of activities are required by the OBRA '87 Interpretive Guidelines.

Stimulation Activities. Activities designed with the goal of offering input and stimulation to one or more of the senses. Examples: music, tactile activities such as pet visits, and multi-sensory experiences such as themes that incorporate touching, tasting, smelling, seeing, and hearing within the activity.

Solace Activities. Activities that by their nature provide solace. These are offered to residents who are critically ill, dealing with pain, have limited endurance, and are spending most of the time in bed or in their room. Examples: relaxation CDs, pain management CDs, slides and videos, being read to, pet visits, memory book writing, creative and expressive opportunities.

Physical Health. Activities that promote physical well-being. These should be offered to every resident. Examples: exercise class, movement to music, reinforcement of therapy goals, obstacle courses, wheelchair management, breathing exercises, walking, and relaxation exercises.

Cognitive Health. Activities that provide intellectual stimulation to maintain and enhance awareness and cognition. Cognitive activities should be provided for all levels of ability. Examples: current events, discussion groups, values clarification discussions, problem-solving scenarios, life management skills, trivia, reminiscing, reality awareness, stress management techniques, and orientation.

Emotional Health. Activities that promote a sense of self, life review, and empowerment. Examples: all activities that bring out the individual either in a group or one-on-one situation, reminiscing, "this is your life" games, opportunities to discuss emotional concerns and needs in a supportive environment, socialization activities which assist in helping individual residents feel a part of a community or group.

Self-Respect. Activities that support individual views and beliefs. Activities that promote respect in content and participation and at all levels of needs and abilities. Examples: cultural activities that introduce different customs and beliefs, all activities that focus on the individual and previous lifestyle and accomplishments, Resident Council.

Male-Oriented Activities. Activities that are designed to meet the special interests and needs of the men at your facility. These groups and activities are offered according to the percentage of men in the facility. Examples: see the Resocialization section of Chapter 8 for program ideas.

Task-Segmentation. Activities that take into account a resident's need to have the task broken down into subtasks in order to successfully engage in and complete the activity. Task segmentation is addressed on the MDS form and should be reviewed by everyone who supervises activities. Examples: art projects, breaking the tasks down step by step: pick up the brush, dip brush into the paint, place brush onto the paper that is taped to the table, etc.

Seasonal/Special Events. In order to enhance quality of life, staff need to be very aware of the normalization concept. Because many individuals cannot easily continue their previous lifestyle and routines after being admitted to your setting, it is the responsibility of all staff members to assist in keeping life as normal as possible. Seasonal celebrations and acknowledgments of special events must be offered and reinforced in activities. Examples: birthdays, holidays, religious occasions, voting issues and elections, national, state, community, and facility events.

Indoor/Outdoor. Activities that are offered outdoors, weather permitting, or indoors in different locations for variety. Examples: picnics and barbecues, outdoor walks, outings, opportunities for individuals to be outdoors in a safe and secure area.

Community Based. Activities that help connect the resident with the surrounding community so they still feel a part of their community. Examples: outings into the community to the library, lectures, restaurants, fairs, stores. It is also important to provide the reverse so that community members, organizations, and groups come into the facility to visit the residents.

Cultural. Activities that identify and honor all cultures. These include activities that bring culture to the resident. Examples: museum docent visits, slide shows of famous painters and artists, painters coming into the facility to paint while residents watch or to lead an art class for residents, special activities that honor other cultures and traditions.

Religious. There should be a special group or presentation for all identified religious beliefs. These can be services, presentations, individualized room decorations that are theme specific, family involvement in sharing the event and beliefs.

Adaptations/Special Needs. Activities that are adapted as required so that all residents can participate according to their individual needs and abilities. This could be an adaptive device, special seating arrangement, visual cues, an interpreter, etc.

Activities for All Ages. Assurance that all age groups identified in the population have meaningful and age-appropriate activities available to them. Examples: special outings for young residents to concerts, restaurants, and parks; intergenerational programs; staff involvement with activities so that there are people of all ages involved. This also refers to activities that are familiar to an individual according to his/her age, not the age of the staff designing the program. Involve the residents in identifying what would be appropriate.

In-Room Activities. Activities that are brought to the individual if they are not able to or interested in joining a group. Examples: bringing a seasonal theme to the room along with decorations; providing specialized sensory programs to those in a semi-comatose state; including residents who remain in their rooms on the Resident Council by discussing topics individually in the individual's room after the meeting.

Activity Program Review Form

Facility ______________________________ **Date** ____________

Write down each activity listed in the current calendar. Write what area of OBRA '87 regulations it meets, what component of wellness, whether it is an active or passive activity (always keep a balance), and any comments

Tag F679 — Activities (OBRA '87 Nursing Home Regulations)

"...An ongoing program to support residents in their choice of activities, both facility-sponsored group and individual activities and independent activities, designed to meet the interests of and support the physical, mental, and psychosocial well-being of each resident, encouraging both independence and interaction in the community"

Activity	OBRA '87 Tag F679	Wellness Model	Active Passive	Comments

Activity Program Review Form — Part 2

Questions to ask in reviewing the program (List examples for the "yes" answers and ideas for the "no" answers):

Yes/No

Do you cover each of the OBRA '87 activity areas?... _____
Notes:

Do you provide activities for all parts of the wellness model? .... _____
Notes:

Are active and passive activities balanced? .... _____
Notes

For individuals who do not attend group activities, do you provide individual projects? .... _____
Notes:

Do individuals give input about the design of the program? .... _____
Notes:

Is transportation assistance by nursing staff allowing all interested individuals to attend?..... _____
Notes:

Are individuals informed of opportunities? .... _____
Notes:

Is the schedule of activities acceptable to the schedule of individual needs?............................ _____
Notes:

Do individuals have a choice in regards to activities? .... _____
Notes:

Do you provide varied programming to meet the diversity of individual needs and abilities? _____
Notes:

Social Services Review Form

OBRA '87 regulations require a set of actions related to social services for the people we serve. The Social Services Review Form summarizes the requirements and provides a checklist to review the quality of social services provided to the people we serve. Even if there is no official social services professional, the tasks listed in this form must be provided be someone at the facility.

In Part 1 of the form, mark whether the required service is provided to every person in the facility. Note cases where the requirement is not met in the first question in Part 2. The rest of Part 2 looks at other aspects of the social services professional's job and provides space to note where improvement is required.

Social Services Review Form

Facility ______________________________ **Date** ______________

Tag F745 Social Services (OBRA '87 Nursing Home Regulation)
483.40(d) "The facility must provide medically-related social services to attain or maintain the highest practicable physical, mental, and psychosocial well-being of each resident."

Requirements	**Interpretation**	**+ = Met - = Not Met**
Identify the need for medically-related social services and provide these services	Maintaining or improving ability to personally manage everyday physical, mental, and psychosocial needs.	
Adaptive equipment	Assuring provision of special devices and equipment to enhance functional and emotional independence.	
Restraint reduction	Providing alternatives to drug therapy or restraints by understanding and communicating to staff why individuals act as they do, what they are attempting to communicate, and what needs the staff must meet.	
Clothing and personal needs	Assisting with identifying and purchasing needed supplies and items.	
Maintaining contact with the family about changes	Informing family about changes that occur in current goals and discharge plans. Attending care plan meetings.	
Referrals and outside services	Assisting with accessible transportation, talking books, and absentee ballot forms.	
Financial and legal matters	Providing assistance with requests for attorney, pension information and updates, funeral arrangements.	
Health care decisions	Assisting individuals with information about current health status and decisions pertaining to treatment. Requesting others to be a part of this decision-making process.	
Discharge planning	Assisting with living situations, home health services, transfer agreements with other facilities.	
Counseling services	Providing opportunity for individuals to discuss concerns or assisting with obtaining outside counsel.	
Grief counseling	Meeting the needs of individuals who are grieving.	
Support individual needs and interests	Keeping staff informed of individual interests and preferences to enhance a sense of self and self-esteem.	
Building staff and resident relationships	In-service training to continually assist understanding and support of individual needs.	
Self-determination and choices	Empowering the individual to make his/her own choices about lifestyle in the long-term care facility.	
Promoting staff awareness of dignity and individuality	Role modeling, in-service training, family council, resident council.	

Social Services Program Review — Part 2

Questions to ask when reviewing the program (List examples for the "yes" answers and ideas for the "no" answers):

Yes/No

Are all the requirements in Part 1 of this form met? .... _____
Notes:

Do facility staff implement social services interventions to assist the individual in meeting treatment goals? .... _____
Notes:

Do staff responsible for social work monitor the individual's progress in improving physical, mental, and psychosocial function? .... _____
Notes:

Has goal attainment been evaluated and the care plan changed accordingly? .... _____
Notes:

Does the care plan link goals to psychosocial functioning and well-being? .... _____
Notes:

Have the staff responsible for social work established and maintained relationships with the individual's family or legal representative? .... _____
Notes:

OBRA '87 Interpretive Guidelines Tips

The overall OBRA '87 federal interpretive guidelines were revised in September 2010 and further revised and enhanced in 2017. Some of the federal laws and regulations changed along with the interpretive guidelines to assist surveyors in determining compliance with the law. Review and become very familiar with these guidelines if you are working in skilled nursing. These interpretive guidelines are created for surveyors to follow during their survey process. The guidelines are also helpful for activity professionals working in other settings, as they establish high standards for the profession. The following information provides tips for administrators and activity coordinators to help them understand the interpretive guidelines.

The form on the next page helps you follow the interpretive guidelines.

Administrator Tips

Non-traditional settings and programs such as the Eden project may appear different and this is taken into account and encouraged.

Activities can occur at any time and do not need to be offered only by activity staff.

If there is a conflict in scheduling services when a resident wishes to attend an activity, the team needs to alter therapy or bath schedule, modify meal schedule, assist in dressing, toileting, and transporting.

Focus less on large groups and more on reality orientation; the focus needs to be on each resident's history, preferences, strengths, and needs.

All staff must provide visual, hearing, physical, and cognitive adaptations as needed to enhance the individual's success.

All staff need to be trained in how to identify behavioral patterns and then intervene before the behavior occurs or intervene when symptoms present themselves.

All staff need to assure that residents are provided timely transportation. Transportation is a facility program, not just the activity department's program.

Surveyors will interview residents, CNAs, nurses, activity staff, and families to hear their opinions about the activities offered.

Care planning needs to be fully individualized and measurable, with well-written and specific interventions.

Quality Assessment and Assurance need to be ongoing and well documented.

Activity Coordinator Tips

Be creative in designing types and times of groups, services, and environments.

Look at trends in population and needs and offer opportunities according to the individuals currently residing in the facility.

Listen to what the resident requests and bring resident's needs and requests to the whole team. Everyone is accountable to assure accommodation of needs.

Work with adult education teachers to assure attendance while meeting requirements.

Be aware of eyeglasses, hearing aids, and seating arrangements. Use visual aids, and microphones and other auditory aids. Break tasks into segments.

Train all staff to identify and chart times and reasons for behaviors. Individualize interventions.

Encourage physical activity, organizational tasks, and social opportunities.

Identify needs and interests, and help assure that staff schedule resident involvement in areas of interest and abilities. In-service staff that this is a facility-wide program.

Activities staff will not be the only ones interviewed by surveyors about the activity program and services.

Be aware of each care plan. Assure follow-through on and documentation of each intervention.

Quality Assessment and Assurance is your best way to evaluate how well your department is doing.

QA Form for Interpretive Guidelines

Interpretive Guideline	Current Opportunities Offered	Met
Person-centered, person-appropriate		
Useful and purposeful activities		
Pursuits that increase self-esteem		
Pursuits that bring pleasure and comfort		
Pursuits that provide for individual talents and creative expression		
Pursuits that promote success		
Pursuits that promote independence and functioning at the highest level possible		
Active vs. passive opportunities		
Physical activity		
Community outings		
Weekend programs		
Behavioral symptoms and interventions		
One-to-one interventions		
Teaching new skills		
Spirituality		
Adaptations for special needs		
Quality assessment and assurance		
Facility accommodates schedules and provides supplies to meet resident interests		
Create a sense of belonging		
Resident assistance and transport from all staff to and from programs		

For each resident, we provide:

Individualized activity assessment including history, preferences, strengths and needs, choices, patterns	
Goals that are specific and measurable as well as individualized	

Surveyors will review care plan and then observe selected residents to determine if the interventions are occurring.

Surveyors will interview residents, activity staff, CNAs, social services, and nursing staff.

6. Meaningful Person-Centered Activities

This chapter looks at several aspects of providing meaningful person-centered activities. Included are suggestions for providing a good overall environment, working with a group, and developing a special place for leisure. We will also look at how to analyze the aspects of each activity and provide a set of basic activity ideas to use as the core of your program.

According to both federal and state regulations, and to meet the needs of the people we serve, each setting is required to provide a meaningful and purposeful program of activities. This program should serve each and every individual regardless of ability or limitation. The intent is to assure that leisure and recreation needs are being met for people who no longer live at home or who have lost the ability to move about in the community. Therapeutic activities within a clinical setting are provided in order to meet specialized and individualized needs. The activity program and services need to be person-centered.

Activity Suggestions

This section discusses the overall requirements for activities. If an activity program is going to be successful, it must provide all of these elements at the level appropriate for each individual:

- Orientation and direction
- Reassurance
- Physical contact
- Consistent routine
- Choices that can be understood
- Appropriate levels of stress
- Verbal cues
- Movement
- Past identity
- Socialization
- Reminiscence

How do we accomplish this? Perhaps the best place to start is by modifying the environment. Decreased functioning can lead to situations in which the individual feels trapped in an environment that poses an apparently unsolvable problem and the person is unable to change or influence the situation.

- Reduce noise and visual distractions
    - Limit group size
    - Limit number of people giving instructions
    - Decrease background noises (TV, intercom, etc.)
    - Show resident sound sources
- Increase environmental cues
    - Use color (or shapes, animals, flowers, food, etc.) for identification
    - Reduce glare (carpet floors, move light sources, seat residents with their back to light source)
    - Eliminate prints and patterns on floors, walls, and furniture
    - Choose strong, contrasting colors for backgrounds
    - Allow time to adjust from outdoor to indoor lighting
- Redirect wandering behaviors
    - Camouflage doors with barriers or room dividers
    - Increase staff awareness of the impact of their own entering and exiting
    - Try to schedule activities to use shift change as distraction
    - Place two doorknobs on each door leading from the unit. Individuals with moderate to severe dementias usually

cannot figure out how to open a door if they need to turn two doorknobs.

- Maintain each person's normal schedule as much as possible (this helps the person feel in control)
  - Clothing/dressing
  - Bathing/showering time
  - Reading/buying newspaper
  - Church services

Participant, Activity, and Leader

The Participant. Know the individuals before programming for a group. Focus on individual needs, interests, and abilities. How do you mix levels of ability and functioning in a group? How do you help each person be at the top of his/her game?

The Activity. Is the activity appropriate for the audience? What are your goals (seasonal, theme-based, normalizing, interesting, challenging, fun) for this activity? Do you have a back-up idea if this activity does not work as planned?

The Leader. Are you changing leadership styles to meet the needs of the audience and activity? Do you know how to deal with behavioral and personality challenges? Are you a good role model and teacher? How are your communication skills and techniques?

Culturally Accessible Activities

Activity professionals have an obligation to provide activities that reflect the cultures, needs, interests, and preferences of the people we serve. This requires cultural competency, as described in Chapter 4. Activities must reflect the cultural needs of a diverse resident population.

The activity professional must know the cultures of the residents to provide culturally accessible activities. The activity professional should consider the following:

- Which cultures are represented in the activities?
- What cultural motivations affect each resident?
- Which types of activities, experiences, and attitudes reflect the different cultures of your resident population?

The activity professional should consider all of the culture variables that have an effect on activities, such as ethnicity, race, language or preferred dialect, spirituality or religion, and holiday rituals and traditions. Other, implicit cultural variables that can have an effect on activities include gender orientation, political viewpoints, experiences with oppression or discrimination, family roles and structure, and socioeconomic factors.

When developing an activity program, the activity professional must provide activities for residents who do not want to participate in the majority culture. The requirement for person-centered activities includes providing alternative activities based on cultural differences.

As the activity professional develops a level of cultural competency regarding a diverse resident population, it will become easier to provide appropriate activities. There are three areas of culture that are especially important to consider when providing culturally accessible activities.

Cultural linguistic differences. The staff should consider the use of idioms, when "yes" may mean "no," when the same language may be used with a different meaning, or even when the same word is used with a different language. Appropriate touching, gestures, eye contact, and the use of interpreters for different languages should be considered for the activities provided. Remember that people who are deaf or hard of hearing often consider themselves to be part of a different culture with a different language.

Religious differences. Cultural competency requires understanding the resident's religious practices. You should be aware if sexual segregation is required by a resident's culture. This practice may be a religious requirement. In some cultures, there is a strong belief that illness is a direct result of some supernatural force beyond the person's control. Other cultures believe it is a divine punishment. Prayer, as an inward ritual to express gratitude to the divine, is often an important part of recovery from illness. It may be difficult for the medical staff to totally accommodate religious beliefs about illness, but activity professionals can design activities that will feel comfortable for all of the people we serve. A resident should be supported in celebrating holy days, with appropriate rituals, sacred symbols, and garments as part of culturally accessible activities.

Dietary practices. When activity professionals provide culturally accessible activities, they should be aware of the dietary practices of their residents. Different cultures have different food preferences and restrictions. The activity professional should consider whether there are any traditional foods that could be harmful to a resident's health based on their current medical condition. Even more important is understanding that residents are often misdiagnosed as non-compliant because they refuse to eat the food offered. Often the residents are not refusing all food. Because they come from a different culture, they may not like the taste of food that is new to them. Even more important is recognizing that food may be forbidden due to cultural or religious holidays or observances.

The following activity is one way to continue developing your cultural competency. It will also help your residents understand the cultures of other residents in your facility.

Exploring Cultural Differences

This activity explores the basic concepts of cultural diversity and how to embrace the commonalities found in different cultures. This activity can be adapted to the degree of function, such as cognition and physical limitations.

The goal of the activity is to find the commonalities between cultures. It shows that culture has influenced our identity no matter what our differences are. This culturally accessible activity provides residents with a deeper understanding of the cultures in the group. And it can be very useful when the activity professional is designing future activities based on the residents' cultures, needs, interests, and preferences.

At the beginning of the activity, the residents are informed of the purpose of the activity and are provided with an index card and a large-print list of personal descriptors. The list of personal descriptors includes characteristics that describe the residents' personality or are influenced by their culture. A list of descriptors is shown on the following pages.

The residents are then asked to choose three personal descriptors.

In groups of four they share these descriptors and explain how their culture influenced these aspects of their identity.

After sharing, each of the small groups can report to the larger group about different cultural influences that led to the same characteristics.

Personal Descriptors

Able
Achiever
Active
Adaptable
Aggressive
Alert
Aloof
Ambitious
Analytical
Animated
Articulate
Attractive
Beautiful
Bold
Bright
Calm
Carefree
Caring
Certain
Challenger
Cheerful
Clever
Cocky
Competent
Competitive
Confident
Conforming
Conscientious
Controlled
Challenging
Cooperative
Courteous
Creative
Decisive
Dependable
Determined
Dignified
Disciplined
Direct
Diplomatic
Discreet
Do-gooder
Doer
Domineering
Driver
Effervescent
Efficient
Emotional
Energetic
Enterprising
Enthusiastic
Expressive
Extrovert
Fair
Flexible
Follows through
Follower
Forceful
Free
Friendly
Gentle
Giving
Glib
Gregarious
Hard worker
Honest
Honorable
Humorous
Imaginative
Independent
Ingenious
Innovative
Inspiring
Intellectual
Intuitive
Introvert
Judgmental
Kind

Knowledgeable
Leader
Lively
Logical
Loyal
Mature
Methodical
Meticulous
Noncommittal
Observant
Optimist
Organized
Organizer
Original
Overweight
Patient
Perceptive
Perfectionist
Personable
Persuasive
Pessimist
Pleasant
Practical
Pragmatic
Precise
Progressive
Punctual
Questioning
Quiet
Rambler
Rational
Realistic
Reasonable
Relaxed
Reliable
Respectful
Responsible
Secure
Selfish
Self-confident
Self-reliant
Self-starter
Sensitive
Serious
Sharp dresser
Shy
Sincere
Skillful
Speaker
Social
Soft-spoken
Sophisticated
Stable
Striver
Superficial
Supervisor
Supportive
Systematic
Tactful
Tenacious
Tolerant
Traveler
Trustful
Trusting
Tough
Wise
Workaholic
Writer
Youthful
Zestful

Challenges and Techniques of Group Work

One of the most challenging and ever-changing roles that the professional plays is that of group leader. Many factors come into play in determining the overall composition and capacities of the group and, therefore, appropriate activities for that group. For example:

- When the majority of participants are frail and dealing with sensory and cognitive losses, the professional must radiate confidence and fine-tune activities to the capabilities of the group.
- When there is a high level of confusion or disorientation among group members, the leader will need to provide a high degree of structure and direction for the group.
- When the majority of the participants are cognitively aware and otherwise capable, the leader will need to be able to step back and allow the residents to assume natural leadership roles.

The following list presents some issues and needs that the professional should consider when leading a group. Each requires a constructive and compassionate response from the leader whether through action or attitude.

- Passivity
- Lack of purpose
- Behavioral issues
- Anxiety
- Apathy
- Communication disorders
- Confusion
- Dependency
- Depression
- Anger
- Loneliness
- Wandering
- Lack of response
- Short attention span
- Hyperactivity
- Feelings of uselessness
- Sensory losses
- Low self-esteem
- Cognitive losses
- Embarrassment regarding condition

Here are some tools and techniques that have proven helpful in working with groups:

- When setting expectations and goals for the group, be sure to be realistic about what this group of individuals can successfully achieve.
- Structure each member's environment within the group to enhance his/her abilities and thereby increase involvement in socialization, improve attention span, and provide a positive and successful experience.
- Always focus on the group member *today* and the abilities that s/he has *today.*
- Acknowledge the efforts and accomplishments of each group member individually.
- Offer time within each session for individuals to share past memories and experiences.
- Verbally acknowledge any information acquired through conversation regarding past occupations, accomplishments, and interests of group members.
- Introduce the familiar themes of family, pets, foods, holidays, and nature regardless of group members' cognitive levels.
- Remind the group of pleasurable experiences that are familiar to everyone.
- Allow opportunities to demonstrate what has been learned. Repetition and visual cues enhance learning.
- Remember that we all need to be needed. This can be a goal for a group — to be of help to others. Projects and gifts can be made for staff, visitors, entertainers, and each other.
- Adults like to know that they are held accountable for their role in the group. Feedback from the leader is very important.
- Use touch to motivate and to help refocus attention in the group. For individuals who do not have family visiting regularly, their

only touch may be during therapy or activities. Never forget how strongly one is affected and nurtured by holding hands, hugging, or just touching another in a loving and appropriate way.

Groups are important socially and are clinically used as a means of assessing one's social functioning. Social functioning tells us a great deal, as it is always impacted by physical and mental changes. We can begin to see changes in how an individual responds to others. Some of these changes will be directly correlated to depression, change in medical condition, cognitive changes, and/or sensory changes.

Because being with others enhances our ability to cope with changes in our lives, we are always in the business of encouraging an individual to spend time with others. The phrase "friends can be good medicine" has been clinically researched — friends do profoundly impact one's sense of well-being and the ability to cope and build resiliency.

Leisure, Leisure, Leisure

For most individuals the concept of leisure brings to mind *time* that is available to pursue hobbies and interests. The experience may be for relaxation or rejuvenation. It may be therapeutic or just recreational. Some individuals view leisure as a *state of mind*, having little to do with blocks of time. For these individuals almost any activity, including work, can be viewed as a positive leisure experience. The way leisure is perceived is an important part of each person's personality.

The amount of free time available to individuals who are institutionalized is much greater than at any other time in their adult lives. In order to understand individuals, we need to understand their era and values. This is known as the "cohort factor." A cohort is a group of people who share a common characteristic, life event, or interest. Men who grew up in the United States during the Depression, who fought together in World War II, then engaged in similar activities after the war (e.g., fraternal organizations) is a cohort. Many people, particularly those growing up in the early 1900s, give very little importance to this thing called leisure. Their work ethic usually made them value their work over the rest of their activities. The Baby Boomer generation generally regards leisure as being very important.

Often people view leisure as free time away from occupation or survival, but it can be so much more than that. Leisure is as much a state of mind as it is the availability of time. The people we serve tend to have a great deal of free time away from occupation (almost all will be retired) and may no longer be able to take care of themselves and others. Because of the functional losses they have experienced, they may need our help to fill the day with leisure pursuits that increase their quality of life. The professional should keep in mind that:

- Leisure is a state of mind or an attitude.
- Leisure motivates us to recreate.
- Leisure is more the feeling experienced than the activity in which we are involved.

Some elements of leisure are

- Opposite of work
- Pleasant expectations and recollections (reminiscing)
- Minimal social role obligations
- Psychological perception of freedom
- Close relation to values of the culture (cohort factor)

Important factors of leisure for a recreation leader:

- You need to be aware of your own definition of and attitude toward leisure and its significance to quality of life.
- Before you can promote leisure involvement in others, you should look inside and determine your personal motivation.
- Leisure experiences are energizing, relaxing, stress reducing, challenging, playful, and freeing. They promote personal growth.

They can be experienced both in a group and individually.

- The desire to be involved in a leisure pursuit is innate. Leisure itself is learned. So if you are interested in quality of life in your older years, you need to nurture this aspect of your life when you are young. Start today.

Leisure Room[31]

While working as activity professionals, we realized there was a need to have resources more readily available and accessible to the people we serve and the people providing activities.

We felt that the answer was a room containing supplies and resources for a diverse population of individuals. The room would be available during the day and scheduled with supervision. This leisure resource room would provide independence, access, creativity, and learning opportunities both on a one-on-one and a group basis.

The Leisure Resource Room provides a vast variety of tools for reality orientation, sensory stimulation, reminiscing, exercise, and educational growth. There may be musical CDs, equipment, and games. Pets can be brought in for visits and pet care.

The resources and supplies can constantly change as needs change. Newer equipment can be added and new ideas tried. Workstations can be developed and redeveloped. The people we serve and their families will add new ideas and be a good resource for future equipment needs.

In one area of the room, an individual with dementia may be engaged in a sensory stimulation activity, while another individual may be watching a movie while wearing a headset. People may come in to be around others or to see the promotions for the book of the week.

The table space can be used for small sensory awareness groups along with special events such as birthdays, showers, and outside speakers.

[31] by Pat Hubbard, AC, SSD and Elizabeth Best-Martini, MS, CTRS, ACC. Used with permission.

This room is a wonderful space for those with busy therapy schedules during the day who would like to be involved in leisure events after dinner. The hours for this room would depend on individual needs and schedules.

How to Develop this Idea

The first step is a review of your budget. What is the monthly budget for activities? How is it spent? Divide the budget money so you can continue purchasing needed monthly items as well as begin to add new items and supplies for this new area. Each month you should be purchasing educational, musical, and creative equipment that can be used for many reasons and with a variety of individuals. If your budget does not allow for new capital expenditures, seek out donations, discounted merchandise, and items found at garage sales.

Finding a Room

Look around and reassess space usage in your facility. Do you have a large open area that the people you serve spend time in? Are there chairs, a table, a TV? Does the space have potential for this type of resource room? If so, cabinets could be made which can be locked when staff leave for the day.

Many older facilities have a large living area off of the front entrance. Perhaps there is potential in this area. People usually congregate in the front anyway and this would bring the activities to them.

These changes do not have to occur overnight. Begin by building onto what is already there. Add activity supplies and equipment. Have volunteers, family members, and scheduled assistants occupy the room throughout the day, facilitating small groups and assisting independent leisure pursuits.

Ask nursing assistants and other staff to bring individuals to the resource room. A few minutes of encouragement makes a difference.

This room could also be interdisciplinary in nature. The occupational therapist or speech therapist is always looking for a stimulating environment in which to work and the supplies are all accessible for ready use.

Who Uses the Room

All of the people we serve use the room. Now you have an area where all activity equipment is available for use. There will be no more running around to store and retrieve materials.

Think of the possibilities to help meet individual needs and to provide a safe and structured environment for staff to use for all the people they serve. The possibilities are as endless as the imagination in developing activity goals and programs. Of course, you need to let the rest of the staff know about the room. At the end of the section is a suggested flyer to give to other members of the treatment team.

What to Purchase

Since the Resource Room is locked up when activity staff are off duty, you now can purchase valuable equipment that can be accessed for repeated use. Educational books and equipment are no longer kept in boxes or storage only to be brought out on special occasions.

The equipment used in this room should meet the needs of the majority of the people you serve. Is there a larger population of individuals diagnosed with Alzheimer's or other dementias or are there alert individuals who are physically unable to be fully independent? The nature of the population should determine your purchasing needs.

Create a wish list of supplies and keep a file of supply items and ideas for future reference. Below is a list of ideas to start with.

Leisure Room Supplies

Supplies need to be safe, stimulating, purposeful, colorful, age-appropriate, accessible, and used as a resource by all staff. Be aware of what kinds of equipment the people you serve are comfortable using. For example, typewriters may be all that some of the older people want to use, but allow the ones who are more adventurous to learn about computers and other digital devices if they wish. The current set of people entering long-term care will be demanding the latest electronic devices. You will need to be prepared for the information age with all of its communications devices, electronic toys, and gadgets.

Equipment and Supplies

- DVD player and DVDs
- TV
- Computer access
- Pens and paper
- Adult coloring books, art projects
- Poetry books, short stories, books on art, history, health
- Sensory supplies such as soft puzzles, stuffed animals
- Auditory discrimination games, sorting games, mirrors
- Adaptive devices for writing, hearing, and seeing
- Trivia questions
- Etch-A-Sketch
- Mystery box to place hands in and guess object
- Exercise equipment and supplies of all sizes and shapes
- Rhythm sticks
- Tangle game
- Pictures sorted according to objects and themes
- Record player/CD player/tape deck with good speakers, head sets
- Records, tapes, and CDs
- Guitar
- Video game player
- Aquarium
- Homemaking tasks: folding napkins, sorting silverware in a container, counting paper money
- Bird cage
- Large print books, fabric sample books, greeting card books, carpet samples
- Miscellaneous games and large puzzles
- Colorful posters

- Sorting games
- Collection of balls (large and small, various textures)
- Themed sensory boxes
- Magnetic letters and board
- Individualized grooming kits
- Makeup mirror
- Familiar items such as kitchen utensils, hats, gloves, hankies, ties
- Large dominoes, cards, checkers
- Magazines and pictures to sort through and look at
- Large blocks and dice to move and stack
- Sensory apron
- Laundry baskets for storage
- Scarf collection
- Olfactory stimulation kit
- Woodworking ideas: hardware trays, sanding projects, key collections
- Velcro games
- Wii, Xbox, etc.

Leisure Room Notice

The following is an example of a notice that could be posted on the bulletin board outside of the leisure room.

The Leisure Room

The leisure room is designed to provide available leisure activities and supplies to the people we serve with varying levels of needs. The supplies and equipment are accessible for use by all staff to enhance interaction, socialization, and a multi-dimensional sensory stimulation experience.

Because this room is created to encourage active participation at all levels, the supplies are kept in this room and need to be supervised and protected by all staff members. This is a room designed to enhance quality of life for the people we serve. It belongs to all of us and needs to be watched over by all of us.

Supplies will be kept in clear bins, which are marked according to level of cognitive and functional abilities. If a CNA brings an individual into the room and provides him/her with one of these supply items, s/he must return to the room within a short time to reassess how the individual is doing.

The activity staff will schedule times when staff and volunteers will supervise the room. These hours will be posted. When there is no structured supervision, the responsibility lies with the CNA for both supervision and proper management of the materials (i.e. placing supplies within reach, introducing new activities, and putting away supplies in appropriate places).

Any comments, recommendations, and requests in regards to the room and supplies should be discussed with the activity staff.

Person-Centered Activities

The importance of person-centered activities is their focus on individual interests and personalities as well as their focus on abilities rather than limitations. If we can assist an individual in focusing on the strengths s/he still has, his/her limitations seem somehow more manageable. If you are working with an individual who feels that life is over because s/he has lost the ability to write due to a stroke, you can support him/her in therapy goals, encourage trying something new, or find another individual in a similar situation for mutual support. There are many options.

Many times, the importance of therapeutic activities is not measured by the activity itself, but rather in the value of the individual's involvement. Each activity has a purpose and a goal and within that activity each individual has a purpose and a goal.

For all people, the daily pursuit of quality of life and meaning is of profound importance. Sometimes the only way to describe this pursuit is as a struggle. Nevertheless, it is a worthy struggle and one that the professional carries on with dignity, courage, knowledge, and professional expertise.

It is ironic that many professionals in charge of planning the activities of others do not look to their own lives and choices for insights into leisure options and motivations. Ask yourself the following questions:

- What do you do for your leisure?
- Do you enjoy being alone or with others?
- Do your interests vary or do you always seek out the familiar?
- Do you value leisure time as an important component of your own quality of life?
- If you were living in an assisted living community or a long-term care setting, could you still continue your personal leisure interests? What help would you need from other people?
- Could these interests help you in dealing with new situations and problems?
- Could they bring meaning to your life? In what way?

Activity Supplies

Certain equipment is required for running activity programs. Even if you can't put together all of the supplies for a Leisure Room, we recommend that you have the following basic equipment somewhere in your facility to use for activities:

- Slide projector or a computer connected to a large-screen TV
- Large-print books
- Cards
- Bingo games
- Newspaper
- Magazines
- TV and DVD player
- Eraser boards
- Puzzles
- CD player with 4 to 6 headsets and CDs
- Reality-orientation boards
- Exercise balls
- Pens, paints, brushes
- Word games
- Bowling set
- Paper assortment
- Trivia
- Scrabble
- Crossword puzzles
- Pokeno
- Parachute
- Scissors

Keeping track of your supplies is an important part of running activities. The chart on the following page shows one way to keep track of sensory stimulation supplies that are distributed throughout your facility. Whether you use the Leisure Room concept or not, you will still keep some of your supplies in different parts of the facility. This form provides a way to keep track of where they are.

This is the kind of form that needs to be updated often if you are planning to use it to find out where something is. White boards that can be changed as supplies are moved or a computer program that is easy to use are also ways to keep track of your supplies on an ongoing basis. This might be a good project for a volunteer.

If you really don't mind looking for supplies, then a form like this can be filled out every few months to be sure that you still have enough usable supplies where your volunteers, staff, and/or the people you serve can access them easily.

Please note that the numbers of items in the activity supply list below are not recommendations for the number of items you should have in your facility — that decision comes from your analysis of the needs of the people you serve.

Activity Supply List

Date: ____________________________________

Supply Item	Leisure Room	Station One	Station Two	Station Three
Tangle	4	2		
Slinky	3	1		1
Magnetic letters	3 sets			
Frog Tac Toe	1			2
Sing-a-long radio	2	1	1	1
Stacking blocks	2 sets			
CD player	2	1	1	1
CDs	23	12	4	18
Ring toss	1			
Parachute	2			
Dominoes	2		1	
Large print cards	4	1	1	
Flash cards	3	2	2	1
Coaster sets for stacking	3			
Clothespins	1 box		1 box	
Grooming items		2	2	3
Writing materials	3	2	2	1
Trivia games	2			
Velcro catch game	2			
Pat mats		1	1	
Scissors and paper	1	1	2	1
Checkers	2			
Plastic puzzles	3			
Koosh balls	1	2	1	1
Eraser board	2			
Safety locks and bicycle chains	3			
Maps	6	2	2	1

Comments:

Activity Analysis

Therapeutic activities are designed and provided to enhance the individual treatment goals for each person that we serve. When you have determined what the activity treatment goals will be, the next step is to analyze each activity. You can do so by using the form on the next page.

The purpose of this process is to separate the components of the activity and to determine what skills are needed in order to successfully participate and complete the activity.

Analyzing an activity occurs separately from assessing the individual. These are two separate assessment processes. By breaking an activity down into separate components, the professional can recommend specific programs that will enhance interdisciplinary goals and can assist in adapting them to the needs and abilities of the individual.

Use this as a means of walking yourself through an activity experience to determine whom it would be most appropriate for and also to determine what adaptations may be needed in order to offer it to a wider range of individuals.

Each time that you design a new group activity, complete an activity analysis form. This documents your thoroughness and professionalism in designing a meaningful program.

In analyzing activities, you also want to recognize the type of social skills required to participate in the group. As the coordinator, you need to know what the purpose of the group is along with what type of interaction is expected of each individual. Will s/he be interacting with others, needing to work cooperatively, or sitting with others but not required to socialize or share tools?

These are very important questions to ask. If you have an individual whom you have assessed as being in need of stimulation but unable to tolerate other people too close to him/her, you need to closely evaluate and determine what type of setting would meet his/her needs. Perhaps s/he could handle doing an independent project at one table alone while other residents are seated at another table in the same room.

The activity analysis is also a great tool to have available for other staff and volunteers who may be assisting you in leading groups.

Activity Analysis Form

Activity:
Goal:
Equipment and supplies needed:
Precautions and adaptations needed (be specific!):
Physical abilities required:
Social abilities required:
Procedures: This should include set-up and program plan for the activity.
Date:

One-to-One Programming

One-to-one programming is as important and demanding as the general recreation program. To provide appropriate, person-centered activities, much of your time will be spent making sure people who need these kinds of activities receive them. You may provide the activities or you may facilitate the activities being presented by other staff and volunteers. Look for ways to formalize your program to assure quality for all residents. Some of the things to consider include:

- Activity staffing
- How many residents are in need of one-to-one programming?
- Do you have ample supplies for your scheduled visits as well as enough supplies to be left in the rooms for independent activities?
- Do you have volunteers or family members who may be able to help?
- Can you identify family members who would benefit from some program ideas and supplies for their visit times?
- How many residents are in hospice? How closely do you work with hospice staff and volunteers?
- How many short-term residents or rehab residents do not attend group activities? How closely do you work with the therapy team in coordinating therapy goals?
- Do you provide small, sensory stimulation groups at least two to three times per week?
- Is your bedside and attendance documentation up to date?

How to Formalize This Activity Service

Step One

- Identify how many residents are in need of one-to-one activities. Keep this list current.
- Break this list down into categories of need. Some residents are going to need three weekly visits while others may be one or two times per week.

Step Two

- Identify who is going to offer one-to-one activities and schedule it directly onto the calendar. Keep to this schedule.
- Find ways of providing one-to-one activities without having to stay in each room yourself.
- Organize your room supplies in such a way as to provide easy access as well as diversity of programs available for many levels. These need to be activities to go.
- Keep creating new ideas and activities to make it fun and stimulating for you, your staff, volunteers, and the people you serve.
- Post a calendar for bedside auditory stimulation for non-responsive residents. This service may be provided twice a week and you visit on the other days.
- Do you have a good pet visit program? Are you documenting these visits?
- How many volunteers are visiting? Are you documenting these visits?
- How many family members visit? Are you documenting these visits?

An example of a tracking style you could use to document this service and assure that all residents in need of one-to-one programs and interventions are receiving them is shown on the next page.

One-to-One Program Log

Resident	One-to-One Needs	Supplies and adaptations needed	Visitor or Staff	Weekly Schedule
				M T W TH F S S
				M T W TH F S S
				M T W TH F S S
				M T W TH F S S
				M T W TH F S S
				M T W TH F S S
				M T W TH F S S
				M T W TH F S S
				M T W TH F S S
				M T W TH F S S
				M T W TH F S S
				M T W TH F S S
				M T W TH F S S
				M T W TH F S S
				M T W TH F S S
				M T W TH F S S

Multi-Sensory and Multi-Level Theme Activities

Before we look at activities divided into different levels, we want to discuss multi-sensory theme activities. The basic idea behind a theme activity is to create an experience that is appropriate for people with many different levels of functional abilities. Tying many activities to one theme over a period of days or weeks helps facilitate memory, as many activities reinforce one idea. Another benefit of using themes over a specific period of time is that it helps the people you serve measure the passing of time — helping create distinct units of time so that everything doesn't just blend together. An example of a multi-sensory, multi-level theme activity based on a mountain theme is shown below.[32] In reviewing this activity, think about the many ways that you can adapt this theme and continue adding to the sensory components.

Mountain Theme[33]

Trigger Words: trees, streams, pinecones, log cabin, camping

Enhancing the Activity Environment

- Gather bark, pine needles, pine cones, soil, rocks
- Paint trees on butcher paper
- Scent paper with wood musk perfume
- Burn pine-scented incense
- Play environmental CDs of wind blowing, birds singing, thunder
- Hang Christmas lights on ceilings to simulate stars
- Use backpacks to hold supplies
- Set up a parachute and an electric fan to simulate clouds and wind
- Wildflowers
- Potpourri sachet
- Pelts from furrier

Activities

- Create nature trails indoors or out.
- Make a group mural using pine needles for forest floor, tissue paper for leaves or dried leaves. Apply with spray adhesive.
- Make a bird feeder with pinecones and peanut butter, and sprinkle birdseed on the peanut butter. Hang it outside.
- Paint a tree branch on drapery-size fabric and hang it up. Use it for hanging valentines.
- Create a campfire and sing songs.
- Make toasted marshmallows or s'mores.
- Invite SPCA to bring animals who live in the forest — rabbits, owls, birds.
- Flashlight games/tracking.
- Fishing game.
- Storytelling.

Theme Weeks

Here are four mini-themes with ideas that can be used throughout a week. Expand and adapt these activities as desired to have fun![34]

Humor

April Fools' Day Discussion

Origin of April Fools' Day from Charles Panati's *Extraordinary Origins of Everyday Things*.

> There are many theories about the origin of this day, but the most accepted one seems to be that it originated in France in the sixteenth century due to a change in the Gregorian calendar. New Year's Day was observed on March 25, the advent of spring. The celebrations, which included exchanging gifts, ran for a

[32] An excellent resource addressing the issues of themes, special needs, and programming for all levels is *Creative Forecasting*, PO Box 7789, Colorado Springs, CO 80933-7789. Phone: 719-633-3174, fax: 719-632-4721.

[33] From Ann Nathan and Elizabeth Best-Martini, used with permission.

[34] By Mary Anne Clagett, CTRS, ACC. Reprinted with permission from *Creative Forecasting*, A monthly publication for Activity and Recreation Professionals.

week and ended with dinners and parties on April 1. King Charles announced that New Year's Day would be moved to January 1 in 1564. Many Frenchmen who didn't accept or hear about the change had parties and exchanged gifts on April 1 and were called 'April Fools.' People sent foolish gifts and invitations to nonexistent parties to those who celebrated on the old New Year's date. These individuals became known as a poisson d'Avril or 'April fish' because at that time of year the sun was leaving the zodiac sign of Pisces, the fish. It took almost 200 years for the custom of the April Fool jokes to reach England and, later, to America.

Pranks

Read out loud this list of actual April Fools' Day pranks and ask the participants to discuss pranks they have done or heard about.

- Putting salt in the sugar bowl
- Putting pepper in fudge
- Substituting pickle juice for apple juice (in a glass at breakfast)
- Gluing a penny to the pavement
- Stuffing a biscuit with cotton
- Saying, "You have a black mark on your face"
- Taping filing cabinets closed
- Taping down the telephone hook so phone will continue to ring after being answered
- Stapling folders together

Funny Foods

Make the following recipes during a cooking activity.

April Fools' Candy

1 cup milk

1 envelope Knox gelatin

1 cup chocolate chips

In the top of a double boiler pan, pour in milk, and stir in gelatin until dissolved. Place top pan over pan of water and turn heat to medium. Pour in chips and melt them in the milk and gelatin mixture, stirring constantly. Pour mixture into a greased 9"-square pan. Put pan in refrigerator, and the candy will be ready to eat in approximately 10 minutes. Yield: 25 pieces. Per serving: 40 calories, 2 grams fat, < 1 mg cholesterol, 5 grams carbohydrates, <1 gram protein, Exchanges: ½ starch.

Ants on a Log

Celery

Cheddar-cheese spread, cream cheese, or peanut butter

Raisins

Wash and dry celery. Cut into 3"-4" pieces. Stuff cheese or peanut butter. Sprinkle raisins on top.

Funny Charades

Write each action listed below on a slip of paper and place the slips in a basket for participants to draw and act out. This would make an excellent intergenerational activity. The actions may need to be adapted depending on the ages of the children. For younger children, ask each child to imitate an animal for participants to guess.

- Pose like the Statue of Liberty
- Sing a lullaby to a baby
- Pantomime shaving
- Play a harp
- Eat a very spicy food
- Imitate a girl scared by a mouse
- Eat spaghetti
- Roll out cookie dough
- Put on makeup
- Drive a car on a bumpy road
- Paint a portrait
- Fly a glider
- Polish shoes
- Catch and reel in a fish
- Hang a picture on wall
- Play marbles
- Fly a kite

Sensory Stimulation

Here is something for your participants who are in the later stages of dementia. or have similar illnesses to do. Encourage them to touch, hold, and identify pictures of clown (or a visiting clown), unusual hats, comic books, and Sunday comics.

Broadway

Discussion Topic — History

New York City's world-famous Broadway area is the center of professional theater in the United States. Broadway is the theater district in midtown Manhattan. In 1900, it was 1½ miles long; it was less than half that length in 1950 and was six blocks in 1970. In 1900, sixteen of the Broadway theaters were located on Broadway; in 1950, only three were located there; in 1970, two. Most of the houses for legitimate theater are on side streets but are known as Broadway Houses.

From 1900 to World War I, Broadway attracted large audiences of middle class people who were in search of amusement, excitement, and romance. The shows did not seem to depict any relation to art or life. Between the two World Wars, Broadway was bursting with energy and enterprise; the new dramatists and people of the theater were full of hope and fresh ideas and were enthusiastic about new styles of craftsmanship. During those dynamic years, Broadway greatly influenced the theater of the world. During World War II, and even a few years before the war, Broadway began to lose originality and drive. There were fewer dramatists, and there was competition from television and motion pictures.

Brooks Atkinson, Broadway

Topics for Reminiscence

- Ask participants to tell about the Broadway and off-Broadway productions they have seen.
- Ask each participant to tell about the best theater show/play s/he has seen (not necessarily on Broadway).
- Encourage individuals to share experiences of acting on stage at any level (e.g., school, church, professional).

Word Game — Guess the Musical

Ask your participants to complete the names of the popular musicals that appeared on Broadway.

- Annie Get Your _____ GUN
- Bye Bye _____ BIRDIE
- Damn _____ YANKEES
- Fiddler on the _____ ROOF
- Finian's _____ RAINBOW
- Funny _____ GIRL
- Gentlemen Prefer _____ BLONDES
- Guys and _____ DOLLS
- Hello, _____ DOLLY!
- Jesus Christ, _____ SUPERSTAR
- The King and ____ I
- Kiss Me, _____ KATE
- Li'l _____ ABNER
- The Music _____ MAN
- My Fair ____ LADY
- Paint Your _____ WAGON
- Peter _____ PAN
- The Pirates of _____ PENZANCE
- Show _____ BOAT
- The Sound of _____ MUSIC
- South _____ PACIFIC
- A Tree Grows in _____ BROOKLYN
- The Unsinkable _____ _____ MOLLY BROWN
- West Side _____ STORY

One-word musical titles (that could not be included in the word game) include *Brigadoon*, *Cabaret*, *Camelot*, *Carousel*, *Cats*, *Gypsy*, *Hair*, *Kismet*, *Oklahoma*, *Oliver,* and *Rent*.

Lights, Cameras, Action

Form a Drama Club. If some of the participants want to act out a scene from a Broadway play or learn some songs from a musical, this would be an excellent opportunity. Many public, college, and university libraries have scripts that can be checked out. Participants can perform for the club or, on a larger scale, before an audience. Invite a Drama Club from a high school to visit and perform an act of the play they are working on and/or take an outing to see the school's production.

Sensory Stimulation

Here are some items to use with low functioning participants. Encourage them to touch, hold, and identify: top hat, cane, songs from poplar musicals (use list in word game) to listen to, and camcorder.

Ask participants to do some simple pantomimes. These movements are meant to stimulate long-term memories. Suggestions include: play a piano, knead bread dough, stir cookie dough, open a book, type on typewriter, catch and reel in a fish, play a violin, hang clothes on the line, shake wrinkles out of a scarf, nod head yes, shake head no, shrug shoulders.

Rain Showers

Discussion — History of Umbrellas

The umbrella is one of the oldest artifacts in man's history and was a familiar item in many cultures by the time man began to write. The umbrella originated in Mesopotamia (an ancient region of southwest Asia in modern-day Iraq) in 1400 BC. It was an extension of the fan, protecting people from the harsh sun. The word umbrella is derived from the Latin *umbra*, meaning shade. This use of the umbrella continued for centuries. Greek and Roman women used umbrellas or parasols, as they were also called, as sunshields, but the cultures regarded them as effeminate. Roman women began the practice of oiling paper sunshields, to waterproof them. Sun parasols and rain umbrellas were used by women well into the 18th century in Europe and later in America. Men continued to wear hats in the rain and got soaked. It took a British gentleman, Jonas Hanway, more than 30 years to convince other British men that umbrellas were more practical and cheaper than hailing a coach every time it rained. By the mid-1780s, British gentlemen were using umbrellas, also called "Hanways."

"April Showers Bring May Flowers"

Ask the participants to share old wives' tales about how to predict rain. Here are some common weather superstitions to stimulate conversation.

- Rain will come when the north wind shifts to the west and then to the south.
- It will rain when the sky is dark to the west.
- It will rain when there is a ring around the moon.
- If dogs eat grass, there will be rain, maybe a storm.
- If a pig carries straw in its mouth, a storm is on the way.
- When cricket chirps grow long or strong, a storm is coming.

Rainbows

When sunlight is reflected by raindrops (or fog or mist), the water bends the light rays and forms bands of color. The most brightly colored rainbows occur when the raindrops are large. A person can only see a rainbow when his back is to the sun.

The colors of a rainbow always appear in the same order: red, orange, yellow, green, blue, and violet. Red is the brightest band of color, running along the top of the bow. Then come the other colors, each paler than the last. Violet is the hardest to see.

Rainbow Party

Decorate the area with rainbow colors. Place a pot of gold (chocolate coins covered with gold foil or similar treats) at the end of a rainbow on the refreshment table. For an activity, play the word game below.

"Bow" Guessing Game

All answers begin with "bou" or "bow."

- Clear, thin broth BOUILLON
- Something that indicates a border or limit BOUNDARY
- Container used for holding food or liquid BOWL
- Cluster of flowers BOUQUET
- Small, retail shop with specialty goods BOUTIQUE
- Another name for a derby hat BOWLER
- One who pursues a criminal or fugitive for whom a reward is offered BOUNTY HUNTER
- Marked by abundance BOUNTIFUL
- Game played by rolling a ball in an attempt to knock over pins BOWLING
- Knot with large, decorative knots BOW KNOT
- Knot that forms a loop that does not slip BOWLINE
- Type of whiskey BOURBON
- Rubber ball does this when thrown on the ground BOUNCE
- Broad city street, often tree-lined and landscaped BOULEVARD
- Cord attached to both ends of an archer's bow BOWSTRING
- Another word for a match BOUT
- Former name of Hoover Dam BOULDER DAM
- Short necktie BOW TIE
- Held at the end of the college football season BOWL GAMES
- Flower or small bunch of flowers worn in a buttonhole BOUTONNIERE
- Bark of a dog BOW WOW

Before the party, ask a staff or family member to sing "Somewhere over the Rainbow" from the movie *The Wizard of Oz*, to close the party.

Sensory Stimulation

Encourage participants who have sensory limitations to touch, hold, and identify different types of watering cans, umbrella, raincoat, rain gauge, items with rainbows on them, and prisms shining in sunlight.

World of Disney

Discussion — Walt Disney's Life

Source: *The Story of Walt Disney* by Bernice Selden

- 1901 Walter Elias Disney is born on December 5.
- 1918 Walt goes to France to work for the Red Cross Ambulance Corps.
- 1919 Walt gets his first job as an artist and later starts the Laugh-O-Gram Company.
- 1923 Walt creates the *Alice in Cartoonland* series. He moves to Hollywood and forms the Walt Disney Studio.
- 1928 Mickey Mouse is born and stars in *Steamboat Willie*, which opens in New York City.
- 1933 Walt creates *The Three Little Pigs*.
- 1934 Donald Duck makes his debut.
- 1937 Walt creates *Snow White and the Seven Dwarfs*.
- 1940 Walt creates Pinocchio. The Disney Studio moves to Burbank.
- 1941 Walt creates *Dumbo*.
- 1942 Walt creates *Bambi* (Disney's favorite film).
- 1948 Walt produces his first nature film, *Seal Island*.
- 1955 Disneyland opens in Anaheim, CA. The Mickey Mouse Club TV show begins.
- 1964 Walt produces *Mary Poppins*.
- 1966 Walt Disney dies on December 15.
- 1971 Walt Disney World opens in Orlando, FL.
- 1983 Tokyo Disneyland opens in Japan.
- 1986 Walt Disney Productions changes its name to Walt Disney Company.
- 1989 The Disney MGM Studios Theme Park opens at Walt Disney World in Florida.

- 1992 Euro-Disneyland opens near Paris, France.

Topics to Stimulate Conversation:

- First Disney film you saw
- Favorite Disney film
- Favorite Disney character
- Disney's approach to song as story
- In 1937, during the production of his first animated feature, *Snow White and the Seven Dwarfs*, Disney said, "It can still be good music and not follow the same pattern everybody in the country has followed. Really, we should set a pattern — a new way to use music — weave it into the story so somebody doesn't just burst into song."

Disney Movie Music

Ask participants to tell the name of the movie that each song is from.

- *Whistle While You Work* SNOW WHITE AND THE SEVEN DWARFS
- *Chim Chim Cher-ee* MARY POPPINS
- *Once Upon a Dream* SLEEPING BEAUTY
- *Zip-A-Dee-Doo-Dah* SONG OF THE SOUTH
- *You Can Fly! You Can Fly! You Can Fly!* PETER PAN
- *Who's Afraid of the Big Bad Wolf?* THREE LITTLE PIGS
- *I've Got No Strings* PINOCCHIO
- *Cruella de Vil* 101 DALMATIANS
- *The Siamese Cat Song* LADY AND THE TRAMP
- *When You Wish Upon a Star* PINOCCHIO
- *Heigh-Ho* SNOW WHITE AND THE SEVEN DWARFS
- *Supercalifragilisticexpialidocious* MARY POPPINS
- *A Whole New World* ALADDIN
- *Under the Sea* THE LITTLE MERMAID
- *I'm Late* ALICE IN WONDERLAND
- *The Bare Necessities* THE JUNGLE BOOK
- *Bibbidi-Bobbidi-Boo* CINDERELLA
- *Be Our Guest* BEAUTY AND THE BEAST
- *Hakuna Matata* THE LION KING
- *Colors of the Wind* POCAHONTAS

Intergenerational Disney Character Party

Involve participants in choosing the theme and planning the party. Choosing a theme will help plan the decorations, activities, and food. Invite a group of children to the party. Activities could include the showing of the movie used for the theme, a Disney fashion show (individuals showing off their Disney clothes), and songs from Disney movies sung by volunteers (planned beforehand so singers can prepare). Ask participants and the children to wear their favorite Disney clothing. If some individuals don't have clothing showing Disney characters, give them mouse-ears headbands, to wear, made out of construction paper.

Sensory Stimulation

Here are some items to use with low-functioning participants. Encourage them to touch, hold, and identify a variety of Disney characters ranging from stuffed animals, pictures, and memorabilia; music and song from early Disney films; videos from early Disney films (e.g., *Snow White and the Seven Dwarfs*, *Pinocchio*, *Bambi*). Show the first 10 minutes of the videos as participants may recall some of the characters.

Intergenerational Programs[35]

"People of all ages can be friends," Daisy answered when I asked her why she, an eight-year-old girl, enjoyed participating in an intergenerational program.

"My own children, even my grandchildren, are grown-ups now. An adult is not nearly as interesting as a bright, young child. I enjoy sharing ideas with them and hearing about their lives," explained Ted, a former college professor, when asked the same question.

[35] *Intergenerational Program* is from Marcia Weldon. Used with permission.

These simple statements contain the components for a successful intergenerational program. These components are acceptance and enjoyment of each other's differences, sharing ideas, and caring. The task is to provide an atmosphere that will allow these characteristics to flourish.

In 1989 we wanted to start a program that would provide a framework where children's and seniors' natural affinity can blossom. There wasn't a lot of information available on the sort of program that we envisioned, so we learned through trial and error. We have had a few disasters and many high points. As our awareness of our strengths and limitations has grown, along with our ability to trust the process, our program has become a happy event for all of us.

Know Your Participants

Don't assume that all seniors will enjoy children and that all children will enjoy seniors.

A new woman in our group was a retired schoolteacher. Because of this we assumed she would be ideal for our intergenerational program. It soon became apparent she felt that children were just one step above slime on the evolutionary ladder. Fortunately we discovered this before she joined the program or her presence would have caused a few tears and nasty comments.

Another woman, Esther, was also a retired schoolteacher. On our visits with the children there were always at least four little girls hovering around her. She was able to hold an audience of 20 seniors and 30 children listening in rapt attention to her stories. (She must have been a fabulous teacher.) The rule we learned from this is to know the seniors in the program and not to push anyone. Don't assume that because a person was a schoolteacher s/he loves children. Conversely, don't assume that a well-worn Merchant Marine won't melt when s/he is around the kids. Children bring out qualities in seniors that will surprise you!

How to Get a Program Started

The ideal situation can occur if you have a school-aged family member or a friend who can introduce you to a teacher. Most teachers are open to having an intergenerational program. If you don't know someone who is a teacher, make an appointment with the principal of the grade school closest to your facility. Discuss your program idea. They will tell you which teacher would likely be interested. (Usually this is a teacher with an interest in history.)

Set up an appointment with this teacher. Ask him/her the level of the children's writing and reading abilities. We've done this program with preschool, second, third, and fourth graders. Our personal preference is the fourth grade. Nine- and ten-year-olds are young enough to be openly creative and harbor fewer preconceived notions than adults while possessing good verbal and writing skills.

Our favorite teacher has the qualities that work best for our program. S/he is flexible and organized. You may have very different needs. What is important is to determine your needs and find someone who will fulfill them.

The Seniors Who Are Involved

Having tried this with both the frail elderly and with those who attend adult day health centers, our preference is for the latter. However, if you have a stable population of high-functioning adults in your assisted living or long-term care facility, this activity could be perfect for them.

If your seniors will forget the children's visits or if you have a largely fluctuating population due to death, your program will be of a different sort than the one described here. The seniors and children will still enjoy each other's company, but they might not experience connections that are as deep or lasting.

The Time Involved

- Weekly group work for 1–1½ hours, reading and responding to children's correspondence.

- One visit every 1½–2 months, alternating between the school and your facility.

Your Facility

Please don't invite children to your facility if you have a lot of people sitting in the halls, people screaming, or strong odors. One of the positive aspects of this program is to familiarize children with the elderly and to people with physical disabilities. Ideally they will take this comfort into their adulthood. Scaring them will have the opposite effect. If your facility sounds like the one above, meet the children in a park or go to their school.

Introduction — A Beginning

After finding a teacher and a classroom, you can begin your program a few weeks after school begins. We start the program by taking photographs of our participating seniors. We mount them on a poster board. When that is completed, we spend an hour asking the seniors in our group to dictate an introductory letter for us to take to the children's classroom. (They might include anecdotes, jokes, their philosophy of life, etc. How they describe themselves as a group is enlightening.) We take the letter to the children's classroom and read it to them.

We leave the poster with our pictures in their classroom and take pictures of the children to hang on the wall of our facility. We use the pictures as a stimulus for the seniors to discuss the activities they'd like to participate in with the children. We make lists.

Remember: You build the frame; let the seniors and children paint the picture. This is their project!

First Visit

Before the first visit we exchange several letters and/or drawings. It usually works best for the group leader to let the seniors dictate what they want to say. Then, using that information, you write one joint letter. This creates a discussion group and the seniors get to learn things about each other they never knew before. Also, it allows participation for everyone, regardless of dexterity with a pen.

The children enjoy sending separate letters and drawings. Resist the temptation to tie specific children and seniors together in a one-on-one pen pal situation. If someone is sick during a visit or drops out of the program, their pen pal will be very disappointed. It's best to let friendships develop naturally.

Halloween is the perfect time for a first visit. If the children come to your facility, ask the teacher if they can wear their Halloween costumes. The seniors can also wear costumes, hats, and/or makeup applied at the facility or at home. Get your staff involved. We made trick-or-treats and created a spook house in a bathroom.

Throughout the school year, every month and holiday will suggest a project. Here are a few ideas we have enjoyed sharing with each other. These are a sampling of the activities our children and seniors have participated in together. You are limited only by your imagination and the excitement of your participants.

- Letters on construction paper leaves: "What I'm Thankful For."
- Christmas letters, e.g., "My Favorite Christmas."
- Making and exchanging Christmas gifts.
- Hopes, fears, and wishes for the New Year.
- "The First President I Remember" (Some seniors remember hearing a president speak in their hometowns when they were children, etc.)
- Making Valentines.
- Making a huge paper quilt (1–2 children and 1 senior per square), collage forms.
- Seniors begin story/poem; child finishes it
- Child or senior tells dream; child or senior illustrates it.
- Trading riddles and jokes.
- EATING LUNCH TOGETHER!
- Overlaid and printed handprints.
- Sock hop.

- Compile a book of all the stories, poems, etc. you've created. Give a copy to all involved and present one to the school library during a visit to the school.
- Time capsule.

Final Visit

Two weeks before school ends, make your final visit to the school. Eat together. With the teacher, plan a closing ritual. This is the best day of the year! Some kids cry, some seniors cry, and even some activity staff members get teary-eyed. Take your camera or, better yet, bring a friend to film for you. You'll want to have pictures for your bulletin board and scrapbook. A video is nice for starting off your program next year.

Everyone Wins

Seniors and children have a natural bond. Both groups of people get tired of being bossed around by middle-aged members of society. Both groups are willing to have fun, relax, and enjoy simple pleasures.

The benefits of an intergenerational program for seniors are numerous. Children are not only willing to listen to their stories, they listen with enthusiasm. The children's attentiveness and genuine respect raises the senior's self-esteem. Sometimes the children bring books and read to seniors on a one-on-one basis. In this activity the seniors are able to provide a real and valuable service to the children. We have seen children read to seniors even though they were unable to read aloud in the classroom.

"The children are so well-mannered, polite, and considerate." We cannot tell you how often we have heard this after our first visit. The program provides the seniors a sense of peace, safety, and satisfaction by letting them know there are good children in the world despite what they hear and read in the media.

Seniors also benefit from an intergenerational program, because when they are with the children they absorb their energy like a sponge. We have seen elders who shuffle around the facility swinging on swings, playing tetherball, and doing the hokey-pokey. Proximity to youth is a powerful medicine!

The children derive a sense of history and continuity from the seniors. The seniors let the children fuss over them and worry about them. This sort of nurturing empowers the children and gives them a positive role model to carry into their adulthood. They lovingly push the elderly who are in wheelchairs. They walk slowly with those who are able to walk, taking their arm. We have seen several classroom "bad boys" surprise their teacher with their tenderness and compassion.

The old adage "You get as much out of something as you put into it" aptly describes an intergenerational program. It takes work and planning, but the rewards are enormous.

Everyone wins. The children gain a feeling of stability; the seniors are given the gifts of energy, meaning, and purposefulness. Both gain a sense of community and fun. During your final visit when the children and seniors are hugging each other, when people are smiling and crying simultaneously, and you have witnessed small miracles of health and communication — you may feel the biggest winner is the group leader. You created a garden where love and understanding could grow. It doesn't get any better than that!

7. Specific Programs for Dementia and NCDs

In order to truly provide person-centered programs and activities, you always start with the individual. Once you know who this person is and what his/her strengths and skills are, you can begin the process of finding the perfect activities that will be meaningful to this person.

We design programs according to levels but any activity may work for someone if you are focused on what strengths they still possess. Look at the person, not at the disease. This is a small part of a large life. If this person is unable to share with you his/her interests and strengths verbally, watch their physical movements and you will get an insight into what may work. If they are moving their hands over the furniture or wrapping their fingers around fabric, use these movements to create an activity that brings them relaxation, tension release, or creative expression.

Dementia-specific programs include more focus on multisensory experiences.

The types of activities included in this chapter are activities that are appropriate for individuals with severe cognitive impairments. We discuss two different levels of programming for individuals who have little to no ability to take care of their most basic needs: Sensory Integration and Sensory Awareness/Sensory Stimulation.

Sensory Integration and Sensory Awareness/Sensory Stimulation

The primary goal of Sensory Integration is for the professional to provide basic stimulation of the individual's senses: eyes (seeing), ears (hearing), proprioceptors (awareness of the position of the body), vestibular system (balance), tactile systems (touch/feel), and olfaction (smell). Individuals who are functioning at this level will not respond to this stimulation in any clear and meaningful way. Individuals in a deep coma, in the later stages of Alzheimer's and other dementias, and individuals with profound mental retardation would fall into this category.

The primary goal of Sensory Awareness/Sensory Stimulation is to provide various types of stimulation with the express purpose of eliciting a response from the individual. The responses given by the individuals may or may not be a logical response to the type of stimulation provided, but the individual's response appears to be related to or because of the stimulation.

Programming Overview

Most of the settings in which you work have individuals with significant cognitive impairments. You need to specialize and adapt activities to meet their highest potential of function both physically and cognitively.

The basic goal of activity programming for individuals who are cognitively impaired, as it is for any activities program, is to stimulate a person's response and to promote the highest level of functioning of which s/he is capable. Specifically, the goal is to continually simplify tasks so they remain within the individual's diminished abilities, thus allowing her/him to retain as much control over his/her life as possible and to maintain a sense of personal dignity.

Although these individuals may have lost the ability to amuse themselves, because that requires memory capacity they no longer possess, they have not lost the ability to be amused or to feel good. Total inactivity is frustrating for anyone. Meaningless activity in which there is no sense of usefulness or challenge is deadly, even for the person who has memory loss.

In addition to memory loss, we are talking about programming for people who may also be experiencing increasing losses in judgment and initiative; and in their abilities to problem-solve, attach meaning to sensory impressions, recognize familiar objects, and express themselves. They may also exhibit disturbing behaviors such as aimless wandering; carelessness about their appearance; disorientation to person, time, and place; irritability; personality and mood changes; and compulsive repetition. Physical changes may include muscular weakness, gait changes, loss of balance, and difficulties in performing Activities of Daily Living (ADLs). Cognitive deficits are often characterized by the decreasing ability to use past experience to solve current problems.

Because wandering (walking) is a common behavior that most staff work with daily, it is important to remember that all behavior is a means of communication by an individual who may not be able to find the words to describe their emotions. Understanding the walking helps you understand the person.

General Activity Goals

These are some of the goals in programming for people with cognitive impairments:

- To prevent or reverse the tendency to withdraw or deteriorate
- To retain or retrain recognition of articles once familiar
- To utilize physical and mental capabilities
- To feel safe in the current environment
- To maintain or stimulate interests and social contacts
- To focus attention on one's human worth and self-value
- To focus concentration away from physical condition
- To alleviate worry and distress
- To provide an outlet for irritation and frustration
- To promote speech and other forms of communication
- To promote controlled fatigue and prevent excessive sleeping during the day

Sensory Integration

Each individual is born with the potential to organize input from their sensory system: proprioception, touch, hearing, taste, smell, and vision. The sensory input needs to be integrated, — otherwise we experience a profound sensory overload on one extreme or deprivation on the other.

If everything that we felt, saw, heard, and tasted at one time were processed in the upper brain simultaneously, we would be bombarded. Sensory integration is "the ability to organize all of the information that we process so as to better manage ourselves within our environment."[36]

As infants, we make motor responses to the world around us. These responses are global as the entire body learns to move in response to the stimuli. With integration of the senses, the motor responses become more coordinated and purposeful. Each component of the sensory system operates separately and also as a part of the whole system.

An experience incorporating all of the senses leaves an indelible mark, much greater than with only one sensory input. It is as though the inner eye captures the experience so that all five senses can bring up the memory. How often do you smell a scent that reminds you of a past experience? The smell stimulated the memory but was not itself the focal point of the real experience.

When the developmental process has been altered in any way, individuals may not have the sensorimotor capacity to respond to their environment. They also may not have attained a

[36] Ayres, A. Jean, 1971, *Sensory integration and learning disorders*, Western Psychological Services, Pages 1–2.

normal cognitive level due to the sensorimotor deficits.

Individuals experiencing sensory losses or cognitive losses can use the rest of the sensory system to respond to their environment and also to rekindle past memories and learned responses. "A sensory integrative approach differs in that it does not *teach* specific skills — rather the goal is to enhance the brain's ability to learn to do these things."[37]

Deficits in Sensory Integration

Any alteration in the developmental pattern of one's growth will impact the integration process and present one or more of the characteristics listed below:

- Poor body posture and balance
- Reduced visual discrimination
- Short attention span
- Irritability
- Physical rigidity
- Tactile defensiveness (lack of integration of the somatosensory system)
- Poor judgment skills
- Limited cognitive function
- Diminished tactile discrimination
- Distractibility

Many of the people you serve will exhibit seven out of the ten deficits listed above. Any individual who exhibits even a few of these will benefit from sensory integration activities because body- and self-awareness are central components for participating in activity groups.

Goals of a Sensory Integration Focus

- Use recreation and leisure to improve, habilitate, or rehabilitate the physical, social, emotional, and cognitive functional abilities of the individual.
- Educate toward quality leisure functioning regardless of level of functioning.
- Increase attention span.
- Build tolerance to physical prompts.
- Practice fine motor and gross motor skills.
- Increase capacity for interactions.
- Increase tolerance to task levels of social and physical interaction.

Basic Introduction to Sensory Integration

As an introduction to sensory integration, we will look at some of the systems involved in an everyday activity. The components that are involved include:

- Eyes (see)
- Ears (hear)
- Proprioceptors (awareness of the position of the body)
- Vestibular system (balance)
- Tactile systems (touch/feel)
- Olfaction (smell)

These sensory nerve impulses are received and coordinated by the brainstem which in turn sends nerve impulses to our eye muscles so we can see; body muscles so we can sit, stand, walk, turn cartwheels, and still maintain a sense of balance. It takes all of the parts of our body working together to successfully interact with things around us.

A Stroll on the Beach

Imagine that you are walking barefoot on the beach. Your feet are being stimulated by their movement through the sand, your auditory system is processing the sounds of the ocean, you can taste the ocean on your lips, and your eyes are guiding the way (along with enjoying the experience). Looking closer, you might ask, "How do my legs know how to maneuver in sand?"

The sensory nerve impulses are responding to stimuli sent to the brainstem to be processed and sent back to the eyes to see, the spine to hold the body upright, and the legs to move in symmetry with the arms for movement. Within each ear you have both your hearing mechanism (cochlea) and your balance center (the vestibular system).

---

[37] Ayres, A. Jean, 1971, *Sensory integration and learning disorders*, Western Psychological Services, Page 2.

The vestibular system enables the organism to detect motion, especially acceleration and deceleration, and the earth's gravitational pull. The system helps the organism to know whether any given sensory input — visual, tactile, or proprioceptive — is associated with movement of the body or is a function of the external environment. For example, it tells the person whether s/he is moving within the room or the room is moving about him/her.[38]

The vestibular system is your organ of adaptability. This process carries over to cognitive functions. Sensory impulses bring about biochemical changes in the brain that are critical to the learning process.

The muscles, joints, ligaments, and receptors associated with bones provide information to the brainstem about your relationship to the world around you. This is the proprioceptive system.

The relationship among the proprioceptive, vestibular, and tactile systems gives you the ability to carry out the seemingly easy task of enjoying a stroll on the beach.

The vestibular system provides information about changes in your head position with respect to gravity. The objects you see around you and the surfaces you touch or stand on may be changing continually. When your head moves, a biochemical reaction occurs in your inner ear. This biochemical reaction enables learning, increases attention span, and increases memory.

Tactile stimulation refers to the use of the nerves directly under the skin to "touch." Through experience you learn to identify textures, temperatures, and hardness. Just like the muscles, all nerves need to be used. Because disability or living situation tends to decrease opportunities to touch and be touched, purposeful tactile stimulation should be planned.

The vestibular/ocular (ear-eye) nerve literally holds the image of what was last seen. For maximum learning, an individual needs sensory stimulation and input into all sensory systems (vestibular, tactile, proprioceptive, hearing, visual, and olfactory).

Sensory Integration Activities

Here are some ideas for sensory integration activities.

- Encourage movement of the head in groups and individual interactions.
- Create activities that encourage use of fingers and hands. (This movement allows brain to open up to new information.)[39]
  - Clapping and rubbing hands
  - Hand puppets
  - String games
  - Taffy pulls
  - Painting
  - Window wiping
  - Hand holding
  - Hand massages
  - Velcro
- Provide tactile discrimination activities (sandpaper, soft, hard, cold, warm).
- Always add scents to activity (scented objects, room sprays, scented pens). Try to avoid scents that are alcohol based. They actually stimulate a different set of olfactory nerves than a pure scent would. You reach more nerves if you use pure scents or oil-based scents instead of alcohol-based ones.
- Create activities which provide body awareness experiences:
  - Facial brushes
  - Vibrators (need physician's approval)
  - Marbles and sand in a shoe box for foot and hand massage
  - Rhythm balls rolled over joints of the body
  - Parachute games
- Use art experiences with paint rollers. This activity moves the left arm across to the right and vice versa, which crosses the mid-line between brain hemispheres. By crossing

[38] Ayres, A. Jean, 1971, *Sensory integration and learning disorders,* Western Psychological Services, Pages 5–6.

[39] Adapted from Marsha Allen Workshop on Sensory Integration.

midline you are helping to strengthen both hemispheres so the individual has a greater repertoire for responsiveness.

- Create activities that encourage and promote body movements (leaning forward or with head leaning back).
- Use flashlight games to increase visual tracking. One game might be flashlight movement to music. Cover the light with colored cellophane to increase interest.[40]
- Play games of toss and catch or hide and seek with glow-in-the-dark balls and other materials.
- Blow Ping-Pong balls or paint across paper with straws. This can be a group or individual activity. You can also use cotton balls or whatever a straw can blow. Good for increasing lung power and speech skills.
- Tear newspaper or colored paper and play freely as if they were autumn leaves. Then recycle into papier-mâché or stuff paper sacks of various sizes and play games of toss and catch or make a collage or seasonal decorations.
- Use paper punches for activity similar to the one above. Increases hand strength and eye-hand coordination.
- Match a pile of shoes or socks or shirts. Teaches sorting and categories.
- Do string painting with paint applied between two pieces of paper.
- Use milk cartons for bowling and building. They are inexpensive and lightweight.

Sensory Integration Activities

Here are some ideas for sensory stimulation:

Shadow Design

Equipment: Slide projector or similar light source.

Activity: Aim projector light at wall, sheet, or large piece of paper.

For: Gross motor development and body awareness, to learn concepts (e.g., large and small, right and left), for increasing imagination/creativity, to have fun.

Examples: Make yourself tall/small, move right or left, up or down, pretend to be a bird or giant rock, move only your arms, for dancing and movement to music.

Hair Dryer Bubble Blow

Equipment: 1960s-style hair dryer or a fan. Bubble soap.

Activity: Empty room of objects and start making lots of bubbles by holding bubble wand in front of blower. Touch the bubbles in free-form movement.

For: Increasing visual tracking skills as measured by following the movement of the bubbles, eye-hand coordination enhancing imagination, for fun.

Cautions: Bubbles make floors slippery. Use carpeted areas.

Free Form Ball Toss

Equipment: A dozen or more balls of soft texture in varying sizes.

Activity: Empty the room of obstacles and throw balls at each other, kick balls to each other, roll them, kick backwards, etc.

For: Increase body awareness through hand, eye, and foot movements. Increase balance.

Free Form Pillow Toss

Activity: Variation on above ball activity but pillows have the advantage of being easier to manipulate for catching and throwing or kicking with feet.

Powder and Facial Scrubber Time

Equipment: As many Clairol Facial Scrubbers as necessary for your group.

[40] The ideas from here through **Tactile Finger Walk** are from Lois Herman Friedlander, RMT, MFCC.

Activity: Put hypoallergenic powder on arms and "erase" it with the scrubber.

For: Utilizing visual tracking skills, eye-hand coordination, enhancing imagination, for fun.

Tactile Finger Walk

Equipment: Peach packing materials from the local grocery or newspapers or Mylar.

Activity: Place materials on table. Have participants manipulate material.

For: Utilize tactile awareness and discrimination, increase gross motor movement.

The Breath Experience

Incorporate breathing exercises into many of your activities. Our breath not only enhances circulation and focuses attention, but also encourages relaxation and a multi-sensory experience of self.

Begin many of your activities with an awareness of body and breath in whatever way is possible.

Activity Ideas

- (A E I O U) vowel repetition by all participants.
- Blow a feather or Ping-Pong ball across the table.
- Party blowers, whistles, kazoos, or pinwheels provide visual and/or auditory stimulation; then incorporate or reinforce the activity with use of one's breath.
- Blow bubbles. Client touches falling bubbles and blows bubbles as they fall close to him/her.
- Play a familiar (or just active) song and encourage humming along with movement to the music.
- Play an environmental CD of the ocean and assist individuals in stretching arms up and breathing.
- As in all groups, let the participants know that the group has ended (closure) with a special song, handshake, hug, clapping, etc.

Sensory Stimulation

Sensory stimulation is the sensation and input that we receive by using one or more of our five senses: auditory, olfactory, tactile, gustatory, and visual. Sensory input is the basis for all learning and development. The earliest sensory memories that we have are our first and strongest memories. That is why we can smell a familiar scent and be brought back in time to our mother's cooking or favorite perfume, or the smell of a freshly mowed lawn. It is the strongest link we have to our world and environment. Disabilities and injuries may impact the normal route of sensory input. If this occurs, our sensory integration system processes incorrect information and misinterprets the environment. For example, if an elderly person has limited sensation in her hands, and touches something hot, she can injure herself because her tactile sensation is not able to give an accurate reading to her nervous system and neurological response system.

Another example is the lack of touch. A newborn child that is not touched and cuddled can experience a "failure to thrive" syndrome. Children can lose their natural instinct to survive, because they are experiencing sensory deprivation. At the other end of the life span, frail elders who are not physically touched and given affection, will also experience a "failure to thrive" situation due to sensory deprivation that can be life threatening.

Sensory stimulation programs are offered at all levels to all age groups. Many elderly clients have sensory deficits. Because of these, they need programs that bring the sensory world to them. The sensory deficits along with cognitive deficits create a greater need to provide stimulation to keep people aware of and interacting with the world around them. In every program offered, the activity staff has to be aware of how to adapt an activity so as to reach people at their individual level of ability and need.

This need and the appropriate level of interaction are determined through the assessment process. One of the keys to success is a focus on ability and strengths. Look closely to see what function is still intact. That is the area of strength still working for this person. Tap into that with your sensory stimulation activities. Stimulation can be sensory, emotional, social, and cognitive. When an individual at any stage in life is unable to reach out for stimulation, it must be provided through activity, environment, and one-on-one interactions. Meeting these stimulation needs is one of the most crucial components that must be addressed when planning an individual's program.

This need should be addressed throughout the comprehensive assessment process. The professional's goal of providing each individual a high quality of life can be furthered when an interdisciplinary approach is used. Notions that may seem abstract, such as culture, individuality, autonomy, and environment, become real and down to earth when seen as opportunities for individual stimulation and growth.

The charts below show the types of stimulation and sources of stimulation that are important for the people we serve.

The goals of sensory awareness and sensory stimulation activities are to:

- Elicit response or increase level of arousal
- Prevent sensory deprivation
- Encourage the individual to use the senses to respond to stimuli

The types of individuals who need these activities include those who show problems with:

Categories of Stimulation

	Sensory	**Emotional**	**Social**	**Cognitive**
Level of Involvement	Basic neurological stimulation — body responds at the basic nerve level	More complex reaction to stimulation — the interpretation and recognition of stimulation from the sensory level, which is then interpreted by past memories		
Types of Stimulation	Touch Proprioceptive Smell Sight Vestibular Taste Hearing	Anger Insecurity Pleasure Desire	Feed me, I'm empty. Desire for others Need for friendship	Memory (long and short-term) Problem solving Sequencing

Sources of Stimulation

Environment	**People**	**Internal**
Natural (uncontrolled) or controlled stimulation in the individual's environment that stimulates the basic senses as well as the higher senses of emotions and cognition.	Separated from environment only because we are so purposeful in the way we try to use ourselves (and tools) to make up for a lack of stimulation in the individual's environment.	Stimulation originating within the individual him/herself. Includes proprioceptors and things like pain (e.g., from gas) or hearing voices.

- Severe disorientation
- Cognitive and sensory deficits
- Lack of ability to respond without sensory inputs
- Self-stimulation
- Deficits in sensory/perceptual integration
- Rigid body and posture
- Avoiding eye contact
- Constant movement in or out of wheelchair

The way you need to lead these activities includes:

- Using touch
- Being consistent
- Being respectful
- Expecting a response (self-fulfilling prophesy)
- Speaking to the individual in an adult manner regardless of the lack of response
- Using direct eye contact
- Repeating, repeating, repeating
- Letting them know you enjoy being with them
- Being yourself
- Using visual and verbal cues
- Analyzing the stimulation level to avoid over-stimulation

Staff Involvement in Sensory Stimulation

In order for a sensory stimulation program to be successful, all staff members need to understand not only its therapeutic value, but also how they can use this type of stimulation in their work with the people we serve. The activity professional should provide in-service training and various tools and forms for staff use. This is especially true with the Tag F679 interpretive guidelines that identify all staff as being accountable for assuring that meaningful activities are provided to all residents regardless of limitations and lack of response. Examples of the forms are shown on the following pages.

Sensory Stimulation Supply List and Assessment Form

This form identifies supplies to be used in this program. Each item should be assessed for *all* possible types of sensory stimulation. As an example, "magnetic letters" would be assessed as a supply item that could be used for tactile and visual stimulation. It could also be a kinesthetic (body in motion) stimulation. If the staff person was requesting that the individual move the letters around and spell a name, this could be a cognitive stimulation tool also. The intent of the form is to be sure that all of the supply items have been assessed as to types of stimulation, safety issues, and appropriate use. The comment section should be used to address safety and specific uses of the supply item.

We recommend that you have the following items available for a sensory stimulation program:

- Tangles
- Slinky (plastic)
- Magnetic letters
- Ring toss
- Parachute
- Dominoes
- Large print cards
- Flash cards
- Coasters to stack
- Hankies to fold
- Clothespins
- Maps
- Grooming items
- Velcro catch game
- Velcro strips
- Koosh balls
- Writing materials
- Eraser board
- Water puzzles
- Texture books
- Scratch and sniff
- Scents
- Pictures to sort
- Photos to look at

- Stuffed animals
- Name cards
- Cooking items
- Busy boards
- Busy aprons
- Gardening items
- Mystery box
- Fabrics and textures
- Musical instruments
- Etch-a-Sketch
- Hardware trays
- Woodworking games
- Pat Mat (plastic pillow filled with water and a sponge)

We also recommend that each facility have at least one Spinoza Bear for use with individuals. A Spinoza Bear is a soft, cuddly, teddy bear which is also a carefully designed and dynamically effective therapeutic tool that provides sensory stimulation. It comes with a library of CDs. You can order a Spinoza Bear from Spinoza. Phone: 1-800-CUB-BEAR.

Sensory Supply Card

Each sensory supply item should have a separate card filled out on its use and goals. These should be available on a ring or in a binder attached to the supply box. We should never assume that everyone understands how to use a specific supply item. A photo of each supply item can be attached to the card describing it. It is a good idea to laminate the card.

Individual Activity Cards

A card should be filled out for each individual who has been assessed to be in need of sensory stimulation. The card lists specific and individualized information about his/her interests, responses, and types of supplies that s/he has responded well to. Also include any activity that seems to decrease anxiety and elicit interest and focus away from an undesired behavior.

Sensory Supply List

Type of Sensory Stimulation Provided

Supply Item	Tactile	Auditory	Olfactory	Gustatory	Visual	Kinesthetic	Cognitive	Comments

Sensory Supply Cards

Name of supply item: ______________________________

How to use it: ______________________________

____

____

Any adaptations needed: ______________________________

____

Goals: ______________________________

____

____

Comments and precautions: ______________________________

____

____

____

Date written: ______________________________

Author: ______________________________

Activity Card

Name of individual: ______________________________

Identified leisure interests: ______________________________

____

____

What does this individual respond well to? Explain:

____

____

____

What specific sensory supply items work best with this individual?

____

____

____

____

Safety precautions and interventions:

____

____

____

____

Additional comments: ______________________________

____

____

____

Date written: ______________________________

Author: ______________________________

Sensory Stimulation Activities[41]

Sensory stimulation activities are used to help the people we serve increase their interactions with the world around them. Beyond stimulating the senses, these activities are intended to elicit a meaningful response to the stimulus.

There are many ways to help the people we serve maintain or enhance their ability to use their senses. Some basic ideas are presented here with some more detailed activities later in the chapter.

Sight/Vision

Contrasting colors are most important to enhance visual stimulation. The colors red and orange are the easiest to see. Large cards and pictures of bright colors work well with individuals who have poor vision. Other ways of using visual stimulation include showing slide pictures or using playing cards with pictures.

Play a game that increases visual experiences by placing a number of objects on a tray and having the participants name the objects. After the participants observe the tray for three minutes remove it and have the participants try to name all the objects on the tray. A variation would be to remove one or two of the objects and have the participants try to remember what was removed. Start with 6–8 objects and increase or decrease appropriately. Some other activities and objects to use for visual stimulation include:

- Hiding activities
- Colorful objects
- Slides
- Tracking activities
- Electronic games
- Maps
- Mirroring/mirrors
- Eyeglasses with lenses of various colors
- Posters
- TV
- Photos
- Flashlights

Other ways to increase visual stimulation include:

- Using a flashlight, move the light slowly in different directions for the individual to focus on and track.
- Turn the light off and on slowly, and then move quickly.
- Shine light on different parts of individual's body.
- Shine light on different people. If they are able to, ask the individuals to identify or acknowledge those people in some way.

Touch/Tactile

The fingers are filled with receptors that are stimulated by shapes and textures. The lips are also very sensitive to touch. The skin is the largest sensory organ of the body and touch is perceived differently in various areas of the skin. The entire surface of the body is capable of receiving sensory stimuli from the environment. Besides touch, the tactile senses also include pressure, temperature, and pain.

Three of the most pleasurable tactile experiences are

- Being lovingly touched by another person, e.g., hug, massage.
- Feeling the warmth of the sun on one's skin.
- Holding an animal, e.g., pet therapy visits or adopting an animal at the agency.

Remember to:

- Use tactile stimulation to arouse as well as to quiet.
- Verbally describe activity or object, feel it, taste it. Ask about sensation received from an individual who is verbal; describe it for an individual who is nonverbal. Ask about preferences and feelings. Describe the properties — soft, hard, rough, firm, warm, cold.
- Introduce gradually. No more than three things at a time. Use each object at least four

[41] This section (through the Paint Bags Activity) was written by Ann Nathan, MS, CTRS, and Elizabeth Best-Martini, MS, CTRS, used with permission.

consecutive sessions before introducing new things. Return when nine have been presented. Repeat set of nine three times before introducing new textures and sensations.

To stimulate an individual's tactile awareness, objects may be placed in old socks, passed behind backs or under the table. Participants may try to determine what the objects are. A variation is to label paper bags with each letter of the alphabet, fill them with one or more items beginning with that letter, and have the participants guess the objects. Keep in mind that putting more than one item in a bag may be confusing to some individuals. Be careful with small items that could be put into the individual's mouth and cause choking. Rubber balloons are especially dangerous in this regard.

Some items that might be included are

- Apple
- Balloon
- Clothespin
- Cotton ball
- Cuff links
- Dice
- Eraser
- Fork
- Golf ball
- Hair brush
- Harmonica
- Ice tray
- Jelly beans
- Key
- Lemon
- Marshmallow
- Nut
- Orange
- Oyster shell
- Pipe
- Pliers
- Quill
- Raisin
- Rubber ball
- Softball
- Spool
- Spoon
- Sticky tape
- Thimble
- Undershirt
- Vegetable
- Velcro
- Wishbone
- Letter X
- Yarn
- Zipper

Another touching exercise is to give the participants a variety of objects to feel one at a time. If they are able to, the participants may be asked to describe one element of what they feel or they may guess the object. Some possible objects include:

- Cork
- Sandpaper
- Shaving cream
- Rope
- Bird feather
- Powder puff
- Corn silk
- Candle
- Makeup brushes
- Leaf
- Styrofoam
- Emery board
- Moss
- Thimble
- Lotions
- Velvet
- Wet sponge
- Half-peeled raw potato,
- Peeled hard boiled egg
- Ice
- Flower
- Flour
- Rubber glove filled with sand

Rubber puzzles that are manufactured commercially provide good tactile stimulation also. You can make your own game by selecting a shape such as a heart, circle, or other geometric shape and cutting the pattern from materials with a variety of textures e.g., velvet, cork, cardboard, burlap, satin, plastic. Each shape is then cut into several pieces and all are put together in a box.

Participants pick out the pieces and match them by their texture. When all pieces have been separated, the puzzles can be put together.

Sensory integration utilizes many of the same modalities. Refer to the previous level, Sensory Integration, for proprioception and vestibular stimulation activities.

Taste

The sense of taste depends on receptors located on the taste buds, which are on the tongue. There are four taste sensations: sweet and salt on the tip, sour along the sides and bitter along the back. After the age of fifty, there is an increase in the threshold of sensation for all four taste qualities. Because of these changes, those who are older need an increased amount of stimulation in order to be aware of a taste sensation.

Any experience with eyes closed increases taste awareness. It is interesting to see how many tastes people can identify with their eyes closed. Some tastes that they might identify:

- Allspice
- Licorice
- Mocha
- Berries
- Chocolate
- Pickles
- Syrup
- Orange
- Vanilla
- Nutmeg
- Lemon
- Honey
- Wintergreen
- Peanut butter
- Cinnamon
- Peppermint
- Root beer

Smell/Olfactory

A sense of smell seems to have an effect on emotions (e.g., pleasant, unpleasant, harmful, etc.). Care should be taken to prevent the individual from tasting some of these items. Use sharp, distinct smelling substances (e.g., perfumes, colognes, soaps, flowers, herbs, food products, etc.). What smells are common to your environment? Refer to other segments of this chapter. A small amount of different substances may be put into jars and participants may guess the contents. Some suggestions include:

- Vinegar
- Nutmeg
- Apple
- Banana
- Vanilla
- Cloves
- Rose
- Almond
- Bay rum
- Coffee
- Sherry
- Tea
- Lavender
- Lemon
- Lilac
- Fresh cut grass

Hearing/Auditory

To stimulate the sense of hearing, a leader or participant may make a series of sounds and may ask for identification and/or direction. The following are some suggestions:

- Pouring water
- Rubbing wood against wood
- Striking wooden matches
- Shaking a wind chime
- Balling up a piece of paper
- Clinking ice in a glass
- Listening to own voice on tape
- Jingling coins together
- Slamming a door
- Balling up dry leaves
- Rubbing two pieces of sandpaper together
- Banging an aluminum pie plate
- Ripping a newspaper, tearing paper
- Thumbing through a book
- Striking a spoon against bottles containing various amounts of water

- Common sounds in your particular environment

Another suggestion to stimulate hearing is to drop different items and let the participants guess what was dropped, for example:

- rubber ball
- marbles
- keys
- book
- coins
- golf ball
- plastic dish
- soft drink can
- basketball
- tennis ball
- Ping-Pong ball
- aluminum pie plate

Participants may produce their own variety of sounds by utilizing their voices and bodies. Many people can make sounds by clapping hands, snapping fingers, stamping feet, and rubbing palms together. Vocally, sounds may include clucking, whistling, blowing air through loosely closed lips, coughing, crying, laughing, humming, and using a variety of pitches and degrees of loudness.

Listening and identifying nature sounds and the everyday environmental sounds are also good hearing experiences. Other ideas:

- indoor recirculating fountains
- chanting
- large bird cage
- roving reporter exercise
- symphony of emotions exercise
- conversation
- CDs — personal ones made by family, friend, therapist
- radio/TV
- singing

Humor

Humor has been defined as "A sense of joy in being alive." Humor should be incorporated in all activities. It creates a sense of playfulness and should be provided on an age-appropriate basis.

Individuals in stress and confusion oftentimes revert back to a happier time. We often see this in individuals who are no longer in touch with reality.

If we can offer a setting that is safe and playful, we may be providing a wonderful gift of not only reality but also reminiscence about a happier time.

Potpourri Sachet

Purpose: Olfactory stimulation

Skills Necessary: Verbal, fine motor coordination, ability to follow directions, moderate cognitive ability

Goals: Utilize motor coordination (gross and fine)
Stimulate sense of smell
Complete a short-term task
Increase self-esteem by successfully completing the project

Objectives: Each participant will make one potpourri sachet.
Each participant will participate in the use of a sachet.

Materials: Cloth (to be cut into 4" to 5" square pieces)
Yarn or thin cloth ribbon
Fragrant dried flower petals (rose, lilac, gardenia, or cedar chips)
Small bottle of fragrance oil

Process:

(Prior to activity pick and dry flower petals and treat with a few drops of fragrance oil — gardenia, rose, floral, etc.)

1. Seat participants around table.
2. Have prepared:
   a. Cloth cut into 4" to 5" squares
   b. Yarn or thin cloth ribbon in 4" to 6" lengths
   c. Rubber bands
   d. Mixed dried petals, enough for each participant.
3. Have each participant smell potpourri.
4. Have each group member:
   a. Lay piece of cloth flat
   b. Place dried petals in the center of the cloth
   c. Fold edges up around the potpourri
   d. Secure at top with a rubber band (may need assistance)
   e. Tie ribbon in a bow around the rubber band.

Optional — add string, yarn or thin cloth ribbon for hanging in room or bathroom or leave plain to freshen up drawers.

Provide closure for group. Thank each participant for attending.

Spice Kitchen

Purpose: Olfactory stimulation

Skills Necessary: Verbal, moderate cognitive functioning

Goals: Promote/utilize stimulation skills
Practice interpersonal skills
Utilize discrimination skills
Access long-term memory
Promote/utilize expression

Objectives: Each participant will smell and identify at least one spice.

Materials: Herbs and spices (cinnamon, anise, pepper, sage, cloves, lemon peel, orange peel, onion, chives, garlic, mint, oregano, horseradish, etc.)

Process:

1. Gather participants around a table.
2. Give each participant an herb or spice (may have to distribute scents individually throughout activity to preserve group structure).
3. Choose starting participant.
4. Allow each group member to smell and identify his/her herb or spice.
5. Repeat process until all participants have had a turn.
6. Summarize participants' reactions related to herbs and spices.
7. Thank each participant for attending.

Potential Problems and Solutions:

- If participant is nonverbal, s/he can identify scent through gestures and facial expressions or by group leader using questions in which responses are yes/no.
- It is important to allow time for reminiscing between smelling of scents to allow "smell" sensors to become neutral.

Adaptation:

Activity can be done on a one-on-one level and have participant identify several "kitchen" scents.

Auditory Discrimination/Sequencing

Skills Necessary: Verbal/nonverbal, functional attention span, moderate auditory functioning, moderate cognitive functioning

Goals: To promote/enhance auditory awareness
To promote/enhance memory recall
To promote/enhance socialization
To maintain/increase sequencing skill
To maintain/increase attention span
To maintain/increase discrimination ability

Objectives: 1. Each participant will differentiate between at least two different sounds played by group leader.
2. At least 50% of group participants will appropriately sequence more than two sounds (e.g., sticks, bell, drum, snap, clap, hand swish).
3. Each participant will verbally identify (or point to flash cards for) two sound producers.

Materials: Variety of sound producing instruments or objects (not more than five per activity). Hide sound producers in a box, under the table, behind chalkboard, etc.

Process:

1. Seat participants around a table.
2. Explain to participants that various sounds (hidden to them visually) will be produced for them to listen to and identify.
3. Begin by having the group identify the individual sounds that you have selected.
4. Choose a starting participant.
   a. Produce a sound and have the participant identify it, turn toward the sound, or respond in any way possible.
   b. Produce a second sound and have participant identify it.
5. Repeat process with each participant.
6. Select a participant.
   a. Produce three successive but different sounds.
   b. Ask participant to identify them in the order that they were produced.

Problems and Solutions:

1. Try to use sounds that are distinctly different. Some sounds may be too similar for participants to differentiate.
2. If a sequence of three sounds is too difficult, encourage the group to help or cut back to two.
3. If three sounds are too easy, add more sounds.
4. Flash cards of each sound can be made to assist those with verbal limitations.

Adaptation:

Sounds could be categorized by certain themes (e.g., air sounds, animal sounds, or sounds in the facility).

Sand Hide 'N' Seek

Skills Necessary: Verbal/nonverbal, minimal fine motor skills, low to moderate cognitive skills

Goals: To promote/enhance memory recall
To promote/enhance visual and tactile stimulation
To maintain/increase fine-motor coordination

Objectives: Each participant will attempt to find an object in the sand at least once.

Materials: Plastic tub, bucket, or box filled with sand and/or cornmeal
Ten small objects of various sizes and shapes (e.g., comb, ball, blocks)

Process:

1. Arrange group around table (if group is large, use two tables and two tubs).
2. Group leader will identify objects being placed in the sand.
3. Place tub next to starting individual.
4. Place five objects in tub and bury in sand.
5. Request participant to put hands or foot in sand to become accustomed to its texture.
6. Request participant to find one object with hand and remove it from the sand.
7. Replace the chosen object with one not yet used, always keeping the same number of objects in the tub. When all ten have been used, repeat process.
8. Thank each participant for attending.

Potential Problems and Solutions:

- Participants who are low functioning may attempt to eat sand. Cornmeal may be used as a substitute.
- For participants who are nonverbal, promote the use of physical gestures (such as head nods, simulation of object use) as responses to questions asked by the group leader.
- If participants are unable to follow directions, use hand-over-hand method.

Adaptations:

- Use shapes and colors rather than actual objects.
- Use large puzzle pieces. Each member pulls one piece from sand and, when all the pieces have been removed, the group attempts to put the puzzle together.
- Place marbles in sand and move hand or foot over them.

Scented Group Mural

Skills Necessary: Verbal/nonverbal, minimal fine motor ability, minimal cognitive functioning

Goals:
To promote/enhance olfactory stimulation
To promote/enhance visual and tactile stimulation
To maintain/increase fine motor skills
To encourage cooperation within a group

Objectives:
Each member of the group will contribute 1–2 pieces of yarn to the picture.
Any group members who are verbal will contribute at least one statement each concerning the scent of the yarn and its relation to the picture.

Materials:
Large cardboard sheet
Various colored yarn (cut in 1" strips)
Scissors
Glue
Oils or perfumes to pre-scent yarn according to the theme
(Could also use fresh fruit juices)

Preparation:

1. Group leader adds scent to the yarn the night before by dabbing yarn with various oils or perfumes of flowers, fruits, etc., according to chosen theme. Allow the yarn to dry.
2. Group leader draws items from theme on cardboard, for example: fruit (apples, watermelon, grapes, etc.).

Process:

1. Gather group participants around table.
2. Group leader explains theme and the project, displaying the cardboard drawing.
3. Give each participant yarn strips.
4. Have group participants choose a strip.
5. Put glue on small area of cardboard and demonstrate putting yarn on the board.
6. Have first participant choose strip of his/her choice, glue the chosen area, and place yarn on area.
7. Repeat procedure for each participant.
8. Discuss finished picture.
9. Thank each participant for attending.

Texture Collage

Skills Necessary: Verbal/nonverbal, minimal fine-motor skills, low to moderate cognitive functioning

Goals:
To promote/enhance tactile and mental stimulation
To promote/enhance socialization and awareness of others
To promote/enhance group cooperation
To promote/enhance self-expression
To increase eye-hand coordination

Objectives: Each participant will place 2–3 objects on the collage.

Materials:
Large paper or cardboard piece
Textured items preferably relating to a theme
Glue

Process:

1. Place participants around table.
2. Discuss already chosen theme (e.g., nature, spring, flowers, sports, games).
3. Spread out items that the group leader brought related to the theme. Have each participant choose at least 2–3 items that s/he will place on collage.
4. Place large cardboard in front of starting individual.
5. Have participant point or express where s/he would like to place his/her item.
6. Assist participant to put glue there.
7. Ask/assist participant to place item on glued area.
8. If able, participant pushes cardboard to next individual.
9. Repeat steps 5–8 until all participants have placed their items on the collage.
10. Discuss finished collage.
11. Thank each participant for attending.

Potential Problems and Solutions:

Some participants may try to eat the items. Hold back stimulation item until time to be used or implement close supervision.

Surprise Bag

Skills Necessary: Verbal/nonverbal, finger sensation to feel objects, moderate cognitive function

Goals: To promote/enhance tactile stimulation
To promote/enhance mental stimulation
To promote/enhance memory recall
To maintain/increase fine motor skills

Objectives: Each participant will touch and may identify (if able) at least one object in the grab bag.

Materials: Bag(s) (preferably cloth)
Ten small objects of various shapes and sizes

Process:

1. Seat participants in a circle.
2. Explain to participants that there is a bag of objects and they are to:
   a. Reach into the bag
   b. Feel for an object that they can identify (if able).
3. Remove the object from the bag to confirm the identification.
4. Choose a starting participant.
5. Repeat process #2 and #3 with each participant.
6. Optional: Reminisce about objects.
7. Thank each participant for attending.

Potential Problems and Solutions:

- The group leader may need to give verbal clues to assist in identification.
- Flash cards of each object could be made in advance for participants who are nonverbal or for easier identification.

Adaptations:

- Objects can be based thematically such as kitchen items, babies, environmental themes, holidays, seasons, vocations, etc.
- Objects can be based on various shapes or colors.

Paint Bags

Skills Necessary: Verbal/nonverbal, minimal fine motor skills, low cognitive skills

Goals: To maintain/increase fine motor dexterity
To maintain/increase direction following
To promote/enhance creativity and self-expression

Objectives Each participant will move finger, hand, foot, etc. along bag creating a design.

Materials: Zip-lock bags
Various colors of tempera paint

Process:

1. Group leader makes bags taking each zip lock bag and filling it with one color of paint (medium consistency). Use just enough paint so that bag is fully covered but can still lie flat.
2. Gather participants around one table, if possible, or two pushed close together.
3. Place a paint bag in front of each and explain (while demonstrating) that it is to be used like a writing tablet.
4. Suggest simple designs, letters, or numbers to be drawn on the paint bag with finger. Allow time for participants to comply — repeating and assisting when needed.
5. Explain and assist participants in smoothing design off bag front.
6. Repeat process 4 and 5 using various suggestions according to group skills.
7. End the activity by having participants sign their names or make a handprint in the paint bag.
8. Thank each participant for attending.

Problems and Solutions:

- Participants who are lower functioning may not be able to independently move fingers or follow directions. Provide assistance while allowing participant to utilize maximum capabilities.
- Suggest more complex designs for participants who are higher functioning or allow them to create pictures of their own choosing.

Adaptations:

- Various liquid mediums could be used (colored vegetable oil, colored sand, etc.) to provide a variety of tactile stimulation.
- More than one primary color can be used for some participants.

Therapeutic Use of the Vibrator[42]

Always request physician approval for vibrator stimulation.

A vibrator is an excellent tool to be used in conjunction with other sensory stimulation experiences.

Values of this tactile experience:

- To assist the participant in body awareness and specific body parts.
- To stimulate sensory receptors and the kinesthetic/proprioceptive sense of self.
- To experience the sense of touch in a safe and relaxed setting; this is especially helpful in work with tactile defensive individuals.
- To encourage a sense of exploration and curiosity of the world around them.
- To facilitate the experience of "feeling rooted" in one's body — even if only for a short time.

Techniques for use of the vibrator:

- Always tell the participant what you will be doing and what s/he will be experiencing. If possible, let the individual touch and feel the vibrator both on and off.
- Approach slowly to determine tolerance to touch and to the vibrator.
- Stop use of the vibrator if you sense the individual is experiencing any pain or discomfort — you want the experience to be pleasurable.
- Begin to touch individual on shoulders, arms, or hands; avoid extremities if you are unfamiliar with the individual's medical condition.
- Vibrator use is most beneficial and successful with drug-free participants; some medications will decrease one's sense of touch and awareness.
- The average amount of time to use a vibrator is 2–3 minutes per participant.
- Literature indicates that 10 seconds on and then 5–10 seconds off may be the most effective way of building sensory receptivity.

[42] Ross, Mildred, OTR and Dona Burdick, CTRS, 1981. *Sensory integration*, p. 72, Slack, Inc., Thorofare, NJ.

The Sensory Box

The sensory box is a concept created to stimulate the professional's imagination in working with individuals who are limited in sensory and cognitive abilities. This can be a box, a tray, an apron, or any other idea that you create to reach out to those most in need.

This box or tray will be designed, used, and adapted as you work with it. Design new changes or additions to meet individual needs. When designing it, design it so that it is easy to clean between sessions with different individuals.

Description

When working with individuals who have regressed, a leisure goal could be to elicit focus, curiosity, response, and involvement in a sensory experience — if possible. This would be through a multi-sensory experience. The response may be movement of the eyes or tracking of an object (visual), reaching to touch a bright object (proprioceptive, tactile), moving to music (auditory), tasting a piece of fruit (gustatory), recognizing or responding to a familiar scent (olfactory).

Curiosity
= Exploration
= Learning
= Recreating

Creating the Sensory Box

The sensory box or tray can be created with almost any safe, non-toxic, non-edible objects. Use a variety of objects to elicit responses to as many of the senses as possible. Determine if the box or tray is for:

An initial sensory curiosity experience in which the individual does not directly touch the objects but receives auditory and visual stimulation

OR

A hands-on sensory experience.

Create a box or tray that can be used as part of your inventory of supplies for special needs. Be sure to include a picture and a written description of your creation.

Sensory Box Ideas

- A gift box with scarves to fold and tie together. Scarves can also be attached to Velcro to attach and remove.
- Musical instruments in a box. Some of the smaller items can be Velcroed onto the box sides. An individual can touch them or pull one out and use it.
- A box of familiar items to rekindle memories. It could be a box of ties, socks, chains, a wallet, a pocket watch, or photos.
- A television tray with magnetic letters and magnets attached, which can be used as a communication board, color sorting, or letter identification experience. (Remember; never place your magnetic letters near a computer or computer disks.)
- A basket of balls of all colors, sizes, and shapes.
- A bed rail cover with Velcroed objects to stimulate an individual on bed rest during a one-on-one visit.
- A plastic shoe bag with twelve pockets. Add gloves of different types and fabrics. They could be gardener gloves, evening gloves, plastic gloves, bicycle gloves, etc. This could be a visual experience or a tactile and sorting experience.
- Different scents and oils on cotton balls. Each cotton ball can be placed in a zip-lock bag with pinholes in it or in a nylon stocking kept in a plastic container.
- Musical gloves. These are commercially purchased in a toy store. They are battery operated and make music when touched on the fingertips. They are also great for teamwork.

Closing a Sensory Stimulation Session

In order to close the Sensory Stimulation Session, any of the following may be used:

- Song
- Poem
- Story with a theme
- Story book with moveable parts for group members to try
- Review of the time spent together in the group sessions.

Always reassure members that it was good to have shared the time together. Offer a handshake or a hug. Holding hands increases attention span. The day and date should be reviewed.

Activities for Individuals with Cognitive Impairments[43]

The chart below shows activities that are appropriate for individuals with cognitive impairments and their goals. These activities may be done in groups or during one-on-one time with staff or volunteers.[44]

Type	Activity	Goal
Art Activities	Filling in silhouettes Copying figures Collage Assembling pre-cut shapes Group murals Paint bag art Edible art	eye-hand coordination, recognition, sensory stimulation, creativity, accomplishment, follow directions, fine motor movement
Physical Activities	Fitness exercises (purposeful) Supervised walks Movement therapy Kick ball Bean bag toss Dice games	use excess energy, retain knowledge of body parts, competition, stimulation, socialization, maintain or increase range of motion, maintain or increase muscle tone, alertness, cardiovascular conditioning
Word and Quiz Games	Unscramble 3 or 4 letter word Hangman Categories Matching pictures Homonyms, synonyms, antonyms Old sayings, proverbs Discussion questions Trivia Spelling bees What's in a Name	improve cognition, sense of accomplishment, pride, socialization, increase memory, communication skills, competition, mental stimulation, problem-solving ability, attention span, increase self-esteem, reading skills, matching skills
Drama Activities	Musical plays Act out themes "Share a Face" Improvise with props Story telling Pantomime/charades	immediate enjoyment, socialization, cognition, communication skills, release of frustration, creative expression, problem solving

[43] ©1991 E. Best-Martini, MS, CTRS and R. N. Cunninghis, MEd, OTR, used with permission.

[44] Two resources to find out more about working with people with dementia are *Wiser Now* (http://www.wisernow.com/about-wiser-now.html) and Cunninghis, Richelle, 1995, *Reality activities: A how to manual for increasing orientation, second edition*, Idyll Arbor, Inc., Ravensdale, WA.

Type	Activity	Goal
Reality Activities	Review of day's activities Sensory stimulation	identity, socialization, improve/maintain memory, recognition, communication
Activities of Daily Living	Tying shoes/fastening buttons Preparing vegetables Gardening Cooking Grooming	retain skills, sense of accomplishment, eye-hand coordination, object identification, memory, following directions, multi-step tasks
Music Activities	Rhythm band Sing along Movement and music Follow the leader Old time dance steps	sensory stimulation, fun, exercise, reminiscence, coordination, following direction, socialization
Group Activities	Discussion groups Reminiscence groups Simple card games Food and culture	decrease anxiety, encourage use of memory, socialization, past knowledge, creative expression, listening skills
Individual Activities	Looking at photos Large puzzles Memory Box	past memories, manual dexterity, accomplishment
Special Areas/ Undirected Activities	Opening/closing containers Opening/closing drawers Leafing through magazines Articles of clothing activity Art projects Tub of water with boats Fabric fold	exercise creativity, use past skills, coordination, use excess energy, meaningful activity, identifying use/purposes of common objects, fine motor skills
Body Imagery	Sensory boxes Tactile experiences (e.g. hugging, touching) Movement exploration Drawing hands and feet Portraits of each other Writing name in the air	sensory stimulation, identification of body parts, cognitive awareness, socialization, increased awareness of tactile stimulation, range of motion, eye-hand coordination, spatial awareness
Sensory Activities	Touching/feeling Taste Smelling Seeing Hearing Proprioception	sensory stimulation, environmental awareness, reminiscence, body imagery, tactile awareness

Orientation Book

The following pages are for an orientation book that you can help create for residents dealing with memory loss. Work with the resident or a family member to type or write the answers in the book. Including pictures adds to the book. The reminder pages can be individualized according to resident need. Create a book that individuals are able to keep with them to tell their story along with reducing any concerning thoughts that they may be experiencing.

MY MEMORIES

By

My name is

My spouse’s name is

My birthday is

My hometown is

My occupation is

Family Stories

I have ______ children.

Their names are

The number of my room is ______.

Lunch is served at

______________________________.

Dinner is served at

______________________________.

Some of my favorite things to do are

I don't have to worry because all of the bills for staying here are taken care of.

Everyone here knows my name and who I am.

I am very safe here with people who care for me.

My purse is in my room.

My family knows where I live so I do not have to worry.

When I smile, I feel better.

8. Programs for Individuals with Mild to Moderate Cognitive Impairments and Dementia

Many of the people we serve will have impairments and disabilities that are significant enough to lower their awareness of themselves and/or of others. They lose some of the past that helped define who they are. Activities that reinforce their past increase their social skills and improve their general interactions with others. The previous chapter addressed individuals who were very impaired and in need of Sensory Integration and Sensory Awareness/Sensory Stimulation. This chapter offers you information about, and activities for, individuals who function at three levels in the moderately impaired range.

Building on the levels in the previous chapter, this chapter covers: Validating activities, Remotivation/Reminiscing, and Resocialization.

Validating activities are for your participants who are very disoriented, whose goals are not focused on orientation but on feelings and emotions.

Remotivation/Reminiscing activities are for your participants who benefit from a stepping-stone to and from sensory awareness. The participant is aware of self and motivated to seek out others.

Resocialization activities are for your participants who have the skills to socialize and would benefit from being with others in a structured group. These groups are geared toward maintaining an awareness of person, time, and place.

Validating Activities

The goal of validating activities is to validate the memories and feelings of individuals who are very disoriented. They do not focus on orientation but rather on the individual's perception of what happened in the past and his/her memory of this at the present time — Correct or incorrect — it doesn't matter. For more on validation see Naomi Feil, *The Validation Breakthrough*, (Baltimore: Health Professions Press, 2012).

Use these activities with residents who have the following characteristics:

- Moderate disorientation
- Time/place confusion
- Unawareness of environment
- Lack of rational thinking
- Locked into fantasy (as if to embrace a safer, happier time)
- Feelings mirrored in body movements
- Distractibility

Some of the things you need to do to make these activities work include:

- Use touch with approval
- Maintain eye contact
- Communicate with clear and repetitive conversation
- Acknowledge feelings
- Mirror movements
- Validate verbally both their feelings and fantasy
- Use active listening. If s/he needs to go home to feed the children:
    - Acknowledge his/her thought
    - Acknowledge his/her experience as a father or mother

- State: "You must have very special children." or "What is your son's name?"
- Use age-appropriate themes
- Unravel the meaning behind the responses you receive in conversation and body language
- Use simple creative/expressive program ideas
- Encourage laughter and humor
- Be yourself

Validation Activities

Some programming ideas that promote the validating process include:

- Name games — to increase identity and sense of self
- Music — can be used as an opening and closing of group for structure
- Movement — body awareness and identification activities
- Hand-eye coordination exercises
- Parachute games
- Hand gesture games
- Ball games
- Trivia, simple matching games
- Pet programs
- Show-and-tell to stimulate feelings
- Visual cues
- Intergenerational programs
- Discussion groups which rekindle fond memories of different themes (kids, work, school, home, pets, food, holidays, travel)

Another program idea is shown on the following pages.

What's in a Name?

Giving someone back the memory of his/her name — *especially if s/he has forgotten it* — is giving the gift of self. Our names not only represent ourselves, but the history of our family and a personal interest story about the people who named us.

Purpose of Activity:

1. To provide reality
2. To introduce each participant by name
3. To stimulate reminiscence of family and self
4. To encourage social contact within the group
5. To learn the history behind different names
6. To provide a discussion-oriented group for participants who can respond successfully to direct questions regarding their names
7. To feel pride in self
8. To be recognized for yourself as the accomplishment
9. To be part of an enjoyable and sometimes humorous experience
10. To respond to the expectations of others
11. To reduce feelings of being disenfranchised

Participants: This group has been successfully offered to both alert and responsive participants as well as a group comprised of participants with cognitive losses.

Duration: 30 to 40 minutes

Supplies Needed: Nametags (optional)
Library resource books: What to Name Your Baby, Origin of Names, Popular Names According to Years
Famous First Names — Quiz
Family stories of names/nicknames
List of nicknames
Pictures of famous people (optional)
Well-known recordings (to name famous singer) (optional)
Who Am I?

Procedure:

1. Place your participants in a circle facing one another.
2. You should be seated with the group, but able to move about and directly assist or respond to any of the participants.
3. Begin the activity with yourself — state your name and give a personal story about your name, family names, nickname, etc.
4. It is recommended that you add humor to your story since this will set a playful mood for the group.
5. After you share the story of your own name, go around the circle to each person.
6. One by one have the participants state their names, ask if they ever had a "special" name that their parents called them, etc.
7. Mention their last name and country of birth.
8. If one of the participants, upon hearing his/her name, becomes anxious and hesitant to respond, reaffirm the name and mention that you find it to be especially pretty or unique. This will help decrease his/her anxiety regarding the need to respond to you.

9. Depending on how well the activity is received, you may begin the Famous First Name quiz. You name a first name and ask the participants to call out a last name that comes to mind.
10. Using all the names of the group members, the leader may also design an art project displaying the names on a mural, a poem, or a picture as a closure to this group or a future group.
11. To close this group the leader could go around the circle stating all the names and have each individual hear his/her name being spoken one last time.
12. Go around the circle and, while stating each name, have the group member write the name in the air as an exercise.
13. End with a round of applause for the group.

Other related program ideas:

- Use this group as a progression towards a "beginning writing" group — where the participants write their signatures as a first exercise.
- When leading adults through any group process, add the element of education and human interest. This piques their interest in the topic and provides a sense of pride and dignity to the participants.
- Once an individual feels respect for you as facilitator, s/he will be more receptive to respond appropriately because *you* have that expectation of him/her.

Remotivating/Reminiscing Activities

Remotivation is a bridge between the time a participant is concerned only about his/her own problems and the time when s/he is ready once again to help others in the community. It is important for each of us to think of ourselves as an important, contributing member of a community. These activities are designed to help the participant see that s/he has contributed by looking at past achievements. The activities also help to point out that even if the participant has lost some level of functioning, s/he is still able to make a contribution.

The goals of remotivation activities are to:

- Start the process of bringing the individual back into the community
- Stimulate thinking about the real world
- Stimulate and revitalize individuals who have shown interest or involvement in the present or future
- Increase a sense of reality
- Begin practicing healthy roles
- Maintain present functional level

Use these activities with participants who have the following characteristics:

- Fearful of decreased cognition
- Short-term memory loss
- Forgetful
- Passive
- Able to follow directions
- Good potential for progress

Some of the things you need to do to make these activities work include:

- Consistency
- Clarity of communication
- Encouragement
- Ability to facilitate responses
- Reinforcement of strengths and abilities
- Reinforcement for individuality and life
- Humor and laughter
- Touch and eye contact
- Giving immediate feedback for involvement and response
- Being yourself

The activities in this section are usually done one-on-one or with small groups, but notice that it is very possible to have both people in the one-on-one session be participants. The activities for remotivating and resocializing work together. A participant who is remotivated and is now working on resocializing can help you with another participant who is ready for remotivation activities.

With the right group of people you can create activities that run themselves with little effort on your part. Just make sure that each of these activities is documented to explain how and why it was beneficial to each of the participants.

Remotivation Groups

Some ideas that are appropriate for remotivation groups include:

- Name game
- Sharing stories of yourself with another participant or a group
- Gardening
- Cooking
- Pet programs
- Familiar themes (family, pets, work, food)
- Creative writing
- Exercise/movement/breathing
- Trivia
- The question book
- Life review

An interesting idea is shown on the following page.

Food and Culture Class — Italy

Description: Food and Culture is a class emphasizing social interaction and reminiscing, utilizing culture and food as a theme.

Materials: Food to be prepared
Music, slides, and visual aids to enhance the cultural theme

Content: Use geography and culture as the basis for the class. Discuss music, dances, geography, memories

Set Up: Have food, music, and decorations set up in the activity or dining room. Also be sure to include participants who are confined to their rooms by taking decorations and food to them. Perhaps participants could have nametags with their names in both English and Italian.

Activity Process:

1. Welcome.
2. Introduction to theme "ITALY."
3. Movement to Italian music.
4. Geography and description of life in this country (slides, maps, photos, costumes, flags, weather, houses, families, customs).
5. Reminiscing/discussion. Discussion topics may include travel, vacations, family heritage, people we know who are Italian, famous people who are Italian.
6. Class participants receive some token to wear which represents the country (flag, paper flower in country colors, nametag, copy of familiar setting in that country).
7. Social exchange with conversation to complement theme.
8. Food preparation or cooking experience (after lunch so as not to decrease appetite). Example: Bring in a pasta machine, explain how it works, and pass out lengths of fresh pasta for tasting.
9. Discuss other Italian food experiences such as prosciutto ham and melon. Slice melon with a hint of ham for taste. Talk about where the melons are grown, etc. This section can be very adventurous and fun.
10. Closure of class. Using a few Italian phrases, thank participants and look forward to next week's class.

Ongoing Classes: Food and Culture classes can be created for any culture in the world .Gloria Hoffner's book *Going Places in Northern Europe* offers food and activity suggestions for 17 countries.

Resocializing Activities

When an individual has participated and met the goals as a member of a remotivation group, s/he will be encouraged to build onto these social skills and continue to successfully interact with others. This is known as resocialization. Resocialization can be considered step two in the process of bringing the individual back into the facility community.

The participants who are able to participate in resocialization activities are also likely to be able to engage in other thoughtful activities. The activities in this section encourage the participant to explore his/her feelings, as well as interact with others in a meaningful way.

The goals of resocializing activities are to:

- Finish the process of bringing the individual back into the community
- Stimulate and revitalize interest in other people
- Practice healthy roles
- Promote a greater level of independence
- Encourage social interaction
- Build social skills
- Increase ease in social encounters with others
- Build relationships with other participants

Use these activities with participants who have the following characteristics:

- Able to follow directions
- Interested in socializing
- Interested in the concerns of other participants
- Good potential for progress

Some of the things you need to do to make these activities work include:

- Consistency
- Clarity of communication
- Encouragement
- Ability to facilitate interactions
- Reinforcement of strengths and abilities
- Reinforcement for individuality and life
- Humor and laughter
- Touch and eye contact
- Being yourself

Resocializing Groups

Some ideas that are appropriate for resocializing groups include:

- Sharing stories of yourself with another participant or a group
- Problem solving groups, "What would happen if ... "
- Resident Council or other decision-making group for participants
- Creative expressive experiences
- Drama/role playing
- Life review
- Creative writing
- Helping others
- "Who Am I?" quiz
- Dear Abby

You will also need to coordinate groups of participants who are willing to work together to help each other regain the ability and desire to socialize with others.

Other ideas follow. Many of these ideas are considered social services groups, often run by social services professionals. There is no requirement about who should be in charge of them. As with all team situations, the person with the time and understanding of the goals and concerns should be responsible for creating and supervising the groups.

One good thing about these groups is that they involve participants who are able to function well enough cognitively to be part of a group. In many cases these groups provide a pleasant change of pace for the leader. In a well-functioning group, you will be able to have fun, as you explore the past and present through the eyes of people with significantly different experiences than your own.

Resocialization Group Design

There are five important aspects to use in the design of a resocialization group:[45]

- **Climate of Acceptance**. Use introductions to create an accepting environment.
- **Bridge to Reality**. Read an article aloud to develop a group theme.
- **Sharing — The World We Live In**. Develop topics through questions and visual aids to encourage responses.
- **Appreciation of the Work of the World**. Think of work in relation to selves.
- **Climate of Appreciation**. Take time to express pleasure with group and plan next meeting.

Let's Talk![46] *Fifty Topics Guaranteed to Get Discussion Started*

Do you want to improve your participants' self-image, decrease their boredom, increase interaction among staff and participants, decrease negative participant behaviors, and reinforce positive ones, plus stimulate verbalization? Group socialization sessions may be the answer. Conducting weekly group sessions just takes a little planning. Limit meetings to 30–45 minutes, have a definite structure, and only include participants who are not disruptive in a group. Begin each meeting by asking participants to give the date. Next have members recite the names of others (to encourage memory and socialization). Then introduce new participants.

Now you're ready to move on to the topic. The session topics listed here are varied and have all been used successfully at a veterans' nursing home. They are designed to stimulate the senses. This is important because the elderly, whether institutionalized or at home, can become progressively nonverbal as the aging process diminishes vision, hearing, and mobility. These 50 topics are general. By personalizing them you can boost your participants' verbalization and feelings of self-worth. Plus, leading a weekly group can be challenging and rewarding for you.

Sensory Sessions

Colors: Have participants name the colors of construction paper as you hold up the sheets. Ask if the color makes them feel hot or cold, sad or happy. Then name objects indoors and outside that are this color.

Puppets: Ask participants to use the puppets to tell stories, express feelings, and portray fears.

Wildlife: Borrow stuffed animals from a museum or arrange for an animal expert to come to talk. Discuss habitats, mating, foods, pets, and nature facts.

Famous Lady for a Day: Distribute wigs, hats, and scarves to female participants and have each devise a costume and talk about whom she is portraying.

Barnyard Visit: Arrange with a local animal shelter or youth group to bring in various animals. Then have the participants discuss proper care for the animals; allow hands-on contact.

Surprise Bag. Give each participant a shopping bag containing a variety of small, common objects. Ask the participants to select an item and discuss how it is used.

Botany: Bring in fresh leaves or flowers. Ask participants to touch and smell them. Then talk about gardens and favorite plants.

Halloween: Let the participants "dress up" pumpkins with paint, glue, and glitter. They can reminisce about dressing up as a child and maybe read aloud Washington Irving's *Legend of Sleepy Hollow.*

Stuffed Animals: Have participants give the animals names and tell where they might be found in nature or fiction. Discuss the toys the participants had as children.

Ladies' Day: Arrange with a cosmetics company to demonstrate products geared for elderly skin care. Discuss how participants used

[45] Robinson, A. M. "Remotivation techniques."

[46] This section is by Harriet Berliner, RN-C, MSN, ARNP, geriatric nursing service at Harborview Medical Center, Seattle, WA.

to dress up when they were young, fashion changes, and different hairstyles.

Fashion Show: Ask a local clothing store or specialty shop for the disabled to put on a fashion show. The participants can act as models and you can discuss fashions from powdered wigs to grunge.

Art Critique: Bring in sculptures and artwork in different media. (These can often be borrowed from a library or museum.) Discuss different art forms, likes and dislikes, and favorite artists and their works. Let the participants touch the artwork and discuss the different textures and effects.

Touch Stimulation: Have each participant reach into a bag, close his or her eyes, and try to match samples of various fabric swatches and sandpaper by touch.

Architecture: Using large sheets of paper and markers, draw simple house types and discuss them.

Music Sessions

Favorite Music: Get music CDs for your CD player or music downloads for your digital music player from different time periods such as the Big Band era. Participants can sing or clap to the music and reminisce about dates and dancing and favorite singers and groups.

Sing Along: Have someone play piano or guitar and then you can all sing "old favorites." Karaoke systems can also be used.

Percussion Jam: Borrow instruments or make them using common items like combs. Let the participants "play along" to piano or recorded music. This is especially fun at holiday times.

Reminiscence Sessions

War Stories: Talk about wartime job changes, hardships, rationing, and loss of loved ones.

Birthdays: Discuss the ages of participants, who's the oldest and who's the youngest. How did they celebrate in the past? How would they like to celebrate now? Ask what age they would like to be again and why. How old would they like to live to be?

Holidays: Each month, discuss holidays and how participants celebrated them.

Memories: Use CDs or DVDs of old radio or television comedies and humorous old commercials. YouTube has many of these programs for free. Have the participants name all of their favorite comedians and programs, tell some old jokes, and discuss vaudeville versus the comedians of today.

Home Cooking: Bring fresh homemade bread. Then talk about the participants' favorite meals, their own best recipes and helpful hints, and their special cooking talents.

Advertising: Borrow old newspapers or magazines from a library and discuss old versus new products. How have things changed? Compare old and current prices.

Home Remedies: What did their mother give them when they were sick? Discuss advances in medicine, country doctors, and home remedies.

Presidents: Have the participants name all of the presidents, and then discuss old campaign slogans and different parties and platforms.

Sports: Show old sports films and talk about the participants' favorite athletes, "superstars," the Olympics, and artificial turf.

School Days: Ask participants about their favorite teachers, schools, types of discipline, grading systems, and best subjects.

Occupations: Discuss careers and jobs and how they've changed over the years, salaries, equal pay, women in the job market. Ask if they would work for a woman boss.

Idols: Have the participants talk about the most influential people in their life. Then ask: Do you think you have emulated them? Whom do you feel you have had an effect upon? Can you name some famous world leaders?

Old Cars: Pass around photos of old automobiles. What was the participant's first car? What part has the auto played in their lives (weddings, rushing to the hospital to give birth)?

General Discussion

Astronomy: Hang up a large poster of the solar system. Then participants can name planets, describe their sizes and compositions, and discuss space travel, astronauts, and inventions. Ask if they would like to be astronauts and where they would go. What will future life in space be like?

Geography: Use a large map of the U.S. or the world. Have participants show where they were born and have lived. Tell travel stories.

Favorite Dinner: Ask participants where they would go. With whom? What would they eat if they could go anywhere in the world?

Let's Make a Meal: Use pictures from diet or nutrition posters. Serve sliced fruit and iced tea or punch during discussion. Talk about proper nutrition, the food pyramid, and plan a full day's menu. Have participants comment on how they feel about the food pyramid versus the four (or seven) food groups.

Love: What does love mean? Should everyone marry? Discuss weddings and families and today's morals versus the past.

At the Movies: Have the participants name all the cowboys, comedians, male and female stars, animal stars, villains, movie monsters, and silent film stars they can.

Plan a Picnic: Plan the menu, date, and time and enlist volunteers to barbecue or arrange for box lunches indoors. Discuss past family picnics.

Ethnic Day: Talk about ethnic souvenirs, photos, and costumes brought by participants or their families. With the help of families and staff, this can be expanded to include ethnic music, food, and decorations.

Politics: Use current events materials like newspapers and magazines. Discuss present world and national events. Talk about different political systems and how they're changing.

Travel: Choose a specific country and use slides, posters, DVDs, or YouTube to start a discussion of dress, customs, foods, products, and travel. Staff can also show vacation videos.

Guest Speakers: Use the local college and hospital speakers' bureaus, which are often free.

Values: Ask the participants what beliefs and values are important to them. If they had their life to live over, what would they do differently?

Shipwrecked: Ask what three things the participants would pack in their suitcase if they knew they were going to be shipwrecked on a desert island.

Literature: Discuss favorite authors and books, story types, and forms of writing the participants like best. Recording their stories to start a "living library" might be a good idea.

Poetry: Choose a poem and read it as a group or have a member read or recite one of his or her favorites. Discuss what it means, other poems remembered, and poems they had to memorize as a child.

Clowns: Put up posters of clowns or circuses. Talk about the types of clowns they remember, their favorites, and circus memories. What makes people laugh?

Life after Death: What are the participants' religious beliefs, concepts of heaven and hell? Do they fear death? Do they believe in reincarnation?

Inventions: Discuss the first inventions made by man, the most significant ones, and the most harmful. What would the participants like to see invented? Is man's life easier or harder today and why?

Pen Pal Club: Contact the local school or Scout troop and ask that they send letters and photos to the participants to be read and answered as a group.

Alphabet Soup: As you say each letter of the alphabet, have participants call out people, places, and things that begin with that letter.

Creating a Living History Group

One of the most difficult tasks for a leader working with people who are frail is to spark interest, generate conversation and discussion, and keep them involved and curious in the events of the day.

Why is Living History Important?

> No one wants to be a footstep planted in the sand near the rushing sea, a footprint to be washed away into eternal waters, a sign seen for an instant and then erased forever. The sense of identity with other loving creatures, a sense of belonging to the human endeavor or being a part of creative movement, a realization that one's life has counted to someone else have to be realized by persons growing older.
>
> *Author unknown*

Realizing that one's life has counted to someone else by having experienced something, shared this with others, and made their lives richer and easier is giving life purpose. This purpose is important at all ages, but especially for people who are in the process of life review.

How to Develop a Living History Group

The most important elements are personal interest, thought-provoking questions, and topics that can be "brought home." An example would be a headline of an air disaster. Instead of referring to this event as frozen in time, personalize the event with other events that some of your group may have experienced. "Do you recall when the Hindenburg blew up in 1937? How about the problems with the Apollo 13 flight to the moon? How did those affect you and your family?"

Then bring the group back to the present event. Now they have shared personal experiences and the facilitator should direct this energy into a discussion of current events. By incorporating the past and present, you are validating the importance of personal experiences and acknowledging that we all play significant roles, not only in our own lives, but in the lives of those around us.

How to Begin a Living History Group

Begin with a small group of approximately seven to eight individuals. It would be ideal to combine some people who are avid newsreaders and television watchers with those less involved but curious. This creates a good mixture.

Start off the class with a few items on the news, in the paper, or in social media. Also mention the dates and weather conditions in your city and the hometowns of group members.

Take the theme that you started the group with, such as, "The unemployment rate is increasing across the United States." Then bring the national issue closer to the group with "What was your first job and how much did you make? How did Roosevelt's CCC program assist those troubled years?"

The group should now be in discussion, remembering years past and connecting them to events taking place today. It is rewarding for someone to feel proud in sharing personal anecdotes, taking pride in his/her citizenship, and feeling that s/he is still involved in his/her world.

Responsibilities of the Living History Instructor

Be aware of your group member's special interests and backgrounds. Refer to this information and to the individual to acknowledge his/her accomplishments or experiences.

Have your materials prepared with at least three topics to work around. Avoid reading from the newspaper itself. If one topic shows little response, leave it and start another one immediately. Any lapses of interest create distance with your group.

Feel comfortable in directing specific questions to a group member and asking for his/her opinion.

Encourage the group to get involved with voting issues and writing letters to the local Congressional representatives regarding pertinent issues.

Take topics of interest from the group and incorporate these into future classes.

Share personal experiences that are taking place in your life and within the day-to-day confines with your class. Have them get involved with solving dilemmas that you are experiencing. This type of interactive problem solving and discussion among the group creates the ultimate goal of all groups: concern and involvement in a continually changing world.

More Resocializing Activities

The following pages show detailed descriptions of useful resocializing activities.

Pen Pals

Goal: To provide a structured opportunity for participants to write to participants in another facility.

Objectives:

1. Establish a relationship with participants in a similar, yet distant, environment.
2. Compare emotional and physical similarities in lifestyles in the two facilities.
3. Relieve the isolation created by living in a self-contained environment.
4. Reuse social skills (letter writing) not often employed after entrance into an assisted living or long-term care facility.

Participants' needs/problems:

For many participants the world outside seems to fade away as their world becomes more and more centered in the facility. Many also forgo the social skills they had used routinely. Even shopping and churchgoing provided some outlets for these skills. This group will provide an opportunity for the expression of social needs that an enclosed community cannot meet and will, hopefully, stimulate the ability to reach out. It will also be a forum for comparing coping skills with others who are experiencing similar life changes.

Number of participants: 3 to 7
Number of sessions: Variable
Length of sessions: 30–40 minutes
How often: Weekly

Agenda ideas:

1. How do we initiate new friendships?
2. What is it about our everyday lives that we wish to communicate through letters?
3. Can we become interested in someone that we will never see and only know by way of written communication?
4. What can we say that will offer comfort and support to a new friend who is reaching out to us?
5. Do we really have the energy and need to expand our environment?

Using Relaxation to Address Anxiety

Goal: To learn relaxation techniques in response to anxiety produced by living in a community environment and to share relaxation techniques that work for individuals who are participants in the group.

Objectives:

1. Offer a quiet, stress-free environment that will allow maximum participation in this activity.
2. Provide visual and word cues for use as personal focal points to initiate the relaxation process.
3. Exchange personal coping mechanisms with other group members.

Participants' needs/problems:
The group will begin each session with a series of exercises to relax the participants. Individuals will be given attention to ensure that everyone participates. After this portion of the class is completed, there will be group discussion and experimentation with ideas elicited from group members.

Number of participants: 6 to 12
Number of sessions: Variable
Length of sessions: 20–30 minutes
How often: Weekly

Agenda ideas:

1. What visual/auditory images do you use to separate yourself from your surroundings and begin to relax?
2. What are the barriers to relaxation that you currently experience?
3. What is the most effective way to create a stress-free environment in your present situation?
4. Drawing from your past, paint a verbal picture for the group of the most relaxing memory you can think of.
5. What relaxation techniques have you used successfully in the past?

Living in an Institutional Setting

Goal: To provide a special time in the week for participants to express feelings regarding loss of autonomy, to discuss replacements for losses, and to provide a support network for participants by allowing them to share experiences.

Objectives:

1. Stimulate discussion regarding issues of life change.
2. Discuss coping mechanisms that have been adapted to a changing lifestyle.
3. Share feelings of loss and restructuring.
4. Support change as an enabler.

Participants' needs/problems:
The basic group method will be discussion/sharing. Participants will give feedback each week, especially if anyone has tried a new coping skill.

Number of participants: 3 to 8
Number of sessions: Variable
Length of sessions: 20–30 minutes
How often: Weekly

Agenda ideas:

1. List the range of feelings you have experienced since you started living here.
2. What facet of your previous life do you miss the most?
3. What things can be brought from home to give you a feeling that you are living in a place that is more like you want it to be?
4. Has there been any substitute person or thing in your current environment to help you cope with your lost autonomy?
5. Do you find solace in accepting the fact that you are receiving care that you need?

Life and Times in a Long-Term Care Facility

Goal: To provide a structured opportunity for participants to express their feelings and concerns about living in a closed society, i.e. the long-term care facility.

Objectives:

1. Discuss loss of personal freedom: What is the most significant loss for you?
2. Explore choices or options that are available in the long-term care facility.
3. Relate successful and unsuccessful coping skills to others in the group.

Participants' needs/problems:
When living in our own homes, totally independent or with help, we are in control. Options are taken away when hospitalization becomes necessary. Some may never fully adjust to this lack of independence and limited choices. This group may provide a forum for involving participants more fully in their environment and giving them an opportunity to problem-solve some of the obstacles to freedom of choice.

Number of participants: 3 to 7
Number of sessions: Variable
Length of sessions: 30–40 minutes
How often: Weekly

Agenda ideas:

1. What loss has been the most significant for you?
2. What do you do when the facility staff wants one thing and you want another?
3. What coping mechanism do you use to make it okay for you while you're here?
4. How do you assert your right to choice as provided by federal regulations?
5. What gain has been the most significant for you?

The leader may want to modify this activity for individuals in different situations. This modification would require little more than replacing the phrase "long-term care facility" with "assisted living facility" or "adult day program."

About Music and Memories

Goal: To provide a structured opportunity for participants to reminisce about music and the part it has played in their lives.

Objectives:

1. Divide the decades between 1920 and 1970 into segments and focus on the most popular music of each era.
2. Provide historical information that coincides with the music being presented.
3. Identify memory associations of the music and history for each person who is able to express this.
4. Interact within the group to stimulate memory and orientation.

Participants' needs/problems:
This group was formulated as an outgrowth of weekly sing-along sessions which attracted a cross section of participants, probably because of the high energy it provided and also because of the memories it seemed to stimulate. Participants who are not communicative and/or oriented in other areas are often able to sing along with the old songs or even dance. This group is an intellectual extension of that emotional experience.

Number of participants: 5 to 10
Number of sessions: Variable
Length of sessions: 45–60 minutes
How often: Weekly

Agenda ideas:

1. What is it about music that stimulates your emotions?
2. Which music memory has the most significance for you?
3. How does music influence your mood?
4. Is there an era in music that reflects the time in your life when you were happiest?
5. Have you created any music memories since you became a participant here?

Cooking Class — Incredible Edibles

Goals:

1. Provide an opportunity for involvement in a familiar pastime
2. Achieve success in a short-term activity project
3. Encourage socialization and team effort in a group
4. Reminisce
5. Rekindle a past interest
6. Achieve success
7. Provide a time of enjoyment
8. Provide a nutrition-related activity to meet needs of participants and enhance self-care skills

Equipment Needed:

- Recipe
- Handiwipes or wet towels
- Big bowls
- Plates
- Measuring cups and spoons
- Electric skillet, toaster oven, or convection oven
- Potholders and hot pads
- Supply of spices, sugar, flour, etc. (these really enhance the group)
- Blender
- Utensils to serve and eat the finished product
- Some of these supplies may already be available through the dietary department. Be sure to plan these classes with the dietary supervisor to schedule times that work out for both departments.

Length of Activity: 1 hour
Number of Participants: 8 to 12

Precautions and Adaptations:

1. CHECK SPECIAL DIETS BEFORE THE ACTIVITY BEGINS!
2. Be sure to place participants according to equipment proximity and helpful partners (e.g., a participant who is blind should be next to someone who is willing to help him/her).
3. Check the bowl sizes so the participant will be able to reach inside easily.
4. Use utensils that are large and easily manipulated by hands with arthritis.
5. Be careful of all electrical wires, hot pans, and placement of oils, liquids, etc.
6. Create jobs for participants that will be success-oriented, choice-producing, and achievable.
7. Be sure to praise each participant's efforts.
8. As often as possible, have the participants be responsible for making decisions on choices of recipes and procedures.

Procedure:

1. Be sure that all participants have clean hands before beginning.
2. Pass Handiwipes to each participant to clean hands before each session begins.
3. Have the room all ready and prepared to begin. All ingredients, pictures of finished product, and recipes should be on the table.

4. Explain the recipe and procedures to the group. Detail special jobs that you will be delegating.
5. Be sure that the recipe entails jobs for many hands. (If the recipe is made for individual servings, this is not a problem.)
6. Find a recipe that can be completed within an hour's time.
7. If this involves cooking/baking time, have something planned for the interim.
8. Include nutrition and a discussion of the ingredients involved. Cook and make things that are nutritious and a supplement to the diet, if possible.
9. Have the group members share favorite recipes with the cooking group and try to schedule some of these into future classes.
10. When they are experienced enough, have the group make special hors d'oeuvres for a Happy Hour or prepare treats for staff recognition.
11. Don't forget your camera!

Cooking Class Ideas

1. Miniature pizzas (English muffins, cheese, mild sauce)
2. Guacamole and chips
3. Finger sandwiches (bread, cream cheese, olives)
4. Blender fruit drinks (bananas, milk, yogurt, vanilla)
5. Cookies and hot chocolate
6. Melons, their history and differences
7. Cold blender soups (tomato, cucumber)
8. Pita bread with a variety of stuffing (taco style)
9. Pigs in a blanket (small Hormel sausage in white bread or biscuits)
10. Coleslaw
11. Club sandwiches
12. Quiche
13. Stir-fried vegetables

A fun variation is to provide the participants with all of the ingredients that go into chocolate chip cookies but hold back the recipe! Have the group work together to try to remember the recipe for chocolate chip cookies. These cookies take such a short time to bake that the group can try out a couple batches from memory and then vote on the best memory recipe.

Men in a Women's World[47]

Discussion

When a man enters a facility, he may suddenly become aware of an unusual phenomenon. For the most part, he has entered into a world of women, where less than 30% of the population is men. That in itself is unusual, but what is more unusual is the fact that 80% of the staff are women, the majority of visitors appear to be women, and the main group of volunteers are, again, women. It is not that he doesn't like women; it's a problem of being so grossly outnumbered and not represented in his male differences.

Another consideration for the new male participant would be the limited ability of other males to relate to him. More than 1/3 of the 30% of male participants appear to be mentally incapable of communicating or relating because of their medical and/or mental conditions.

It is interesting to note that the number of boys born makes for a greater population of males than females until the age of 18. The shift begins at this age, due to accident, suicide, war, lung cancer, emphysema, and industrial accidents. By the time middle age is reached, the trend is to a greater female population.

For a professional whose responsibility is to meet the needs and interests of each participant and to develop individual activity care plans, it has become an ever-increasing problem to plan successfully for men in long-term care facilities. The majority of activities offered are oriented towards the majority population of women and it is women who attend the predominant number of activities offered.

One experience with a facility planning for a men's activity consisted of an afternoon special event where 15 men were brought into a small dining room. A woman wearing a coat entered the room, set down a tape recorder, removed her coat, and began to belly dance for the men. The dancer was well endowed and wore enough veils to create a suggestive appearance. The veils were slowly removed. For some men, the movement and closeness of the dancer offended their religious beliefs. Others were well entertained. The staff was entertained, too, peeking in to see the men's reactions. After 15 minutes and three dances, the music stopped, the dancer was thanked, beer and chips were served, and the men were taken quietly back to their areas. The belly dancer was the only program offered to the men.

Our planning and scheduling of men's activities has got to involve more depth, consideration, balance, and variety. Here are some basic concepts and recommendations for your consideration in planning activities for the men in your facilities.

The first step is vital and involves assessment of leisure interests. Without an individual assessment of each man's interests, you are not doing justice to their special needs. Review your assessment and activity check sheet and note the types of activities you review with the male participants. Most of the assessments being used have detailed and specific female-oriented activities. An approach to a male-oriented assessment is to include activities where you need to probe for more detail and specifics in discussing both likes and dislikes. For example, following the questions of whether a man enjoys fishing there should be details of what kind, where, when, with whom, and how often. It would be most important in the interviewing and assessment process to concentrate on the individual and his background, rather than the content of your prepared activity program. (Besides, you are not meeting the requirements of the federal laws for nursing homes if you gear your assessment to activities that you offer instead of activities that the participants are interested in.) There will be plenty of time to orient the participant to the existing activity program. Discussing only the existing program

[47] "Men in a women's world" is by Michael Watters, CTRS. Used with permission.

may act as a barrier to his opening up to express his particular interests and background.

The lack of leisure skills or mastery of specific activities in earlier life can cause problems in involvement later. Men are embarrassed to start a new skill with the fear of not being competent or appearing to be unsuccessful. Professionals will need to consider the fear of failure, self-consciousness, or public showing of self with a disability as deterrents to a man's participation. Any one of the above-mentioned situations can be enough to cause withdrawal or resistance to participation. It was also found that, if a person had a positive view of himself earlier in life, it has generally carried over to later life skills. The same is true of a negative view of self and feelings of low self-esteem.

Another interesting fact appears to be that the blue-collar worker engages in fewer leisure activities than those in white-collar jobs and professions. The white-collar worker and professional tended to work outside the home, in the community, and with many different people. Their leisure activities tend to be more diverse and of an active nature. The blue-collar workers tend to engage in more family-centered, home-based activities. Reasons were based on income, educational level, home locations, peer expectations, and access to leisure areas. There appears to be a definite relationship between the man's job role and his use of leisure time. Consideration needs to be given to the elements of technical work, selling, manual labor, the number of hours worked, job isolation, the reading required for a job, the use of tools and specialty tools used, sociability on the job, and overall responsibility which can be useful in developing a creative care plan.

Another major area of concentration and interest appears to be a man's family, especially the children. In a California facility, the activity professional asked a group of men meeting for the second time what they were most proud of and each individual responded with glowing stories about his family. Men appear to talk a great deal about how proud they are of their families and can go into detail of the history of each child and grandchild.

Professionals should begin to make a concerted effort to recruit male volunteers, both group and individual, to provide the meaningful relationships that are otherwise lacking in other areas of the facility.

In one San Francisco facility there was a man who had been a union organizer for the garment industry. After entering the facility, he had reduced his activities to staying in his room and wearing only his bathrobe. Due to his long history as a San Francisco resident, he was asked to make a presentation for a special earthquake survivor party. He arrived, wearing his blue suit with a flower in his lapel, and made a warm and sincere welcome to the gathering. This was the beginning of his continued role as the host and emcee at parties and special events for the facility.

If you search your facility, you will find duties, responsibilities, and roles that give male participants some of those roles that have been lost or re-invest them in duties and activities that they have long since put aside.

For example, the Adopt-a-Grandparent program plays into the role of confidant, friend, and family member, which many have lost as their own family has diminished. Maintenance personnel may become involved by supplying ideas, materials, and leadership for tinkering with projects that many of the men used to enjoy. Adapted setups for tools and workbenches can give back a sense of work and productivity. Barbershop quartets, choirs, sports events, and discussion groups can give some of the camaraderie that has been lost with the reduction of male social contacts.

In summary, although men represent a minority in a world of women, their needs and interests must be given careful consideration, planning, and timely involvement in the overall program. Being left out of the activity program services should not have to be another loss in the series of life's disappointments. Sincere efforts, specific programming ideas, recruitment of volunteers and groups, plus a commitment to involve men in dynamic programming can make a change in the life of a facility.

Programs for Men

Some specific program ideas include:

- Making or repairing toys and children's furniture
- Construction of wooden animals
- Coin collecting
- Animal care and feeding
- Bone and horn polishing and engraving art
- Brass crafts
- Bonsai
- Printing
- Rope tying
- Contests and non-cash gambling
- Storytelling of special events in history
- Cooperation games and events
- Videos of famous men who may have had an effect on the residents' lives
- Sport quizzes, trivia, records and events, personalities
- Men's group singing
- Activities sponsored by men's groups (social clubs, fraternities)
- Debate, Toastmaster speaking groups
- Mime and theater groups
- Walking club — wheelchairs included
- Metal smith work
- Wire work — soft wire sculpture
- Electrical work — tinkering with small appliances
- Soap carving
- Sawdust craft — relief maps
- Monthly breakfast speakers
- Speakers and visits to service equipment: fire station, ambulance, police station, farms, construction sites
- Hardware store owners who show the latest in tools
- Tournaments
- Liar's contest
- Lunch at a local men's club
- Fishing outings
- A day at the races
- Big Brothers sponsorships
- Adopt-a-Grandparent programs
- All male play readings
- Talent show
- Woodworking projects
- Readers for the blind
- Teaching specialized subjects — computers
- Pool and billiards
- Bocce ball
- Bird watching — field identification
- Men's fashion show
- Rock collecting
- Stamp collecting
- Radio equipment
- Gold panning

Men in a Women's World — Activity

Goal: To provide a structured opportunity for men to discuss their lives in a community of women.

Objectives:

1. Compare and contrast life in your facility and life in society as a whole: Who is in control — men or women?
2. Discuss individual adaptations to dependence on women for most care.
3. Interact in a group of mostly men to provide relief from the women's society.

Participants' needs/problems:

The men now in facilities have, for the most part, lived their lives with the assumption that men are dominant in society. It is assumed that they are the decision makers, the ones in control of their life situations. When care becomes necessary due to physical limitations, however, the status of men changes, as does the amount of their perceived control.

What effect does this have on the male ego, this loss of control and this entry into a society dominated and controlled and mostly populated by women? This group explores these issues with men.

Number of participants: 3 to 5
Number of sessions: Variable
Length of sessions: 30–60 minutes
How often: Weekly

Agenda ideas:

1. What is it like to be in a matriarchal society?
2. How do you see your role?
3. How has this changed since you were "out in the world"?
4. What have you learned to do in this environment to enable you to assert yourself as an individual?
5. Is there any way you could have prepared yourself to live in this new "society"?

9. Short-Term Stay: Rehabilitation-Oriented

Many of the individuals you work with will have the potential to regain function. This group will want more than activities meant to keep the skills they have, provide entertainment, and ensure a reasonable quality of life. Individuals who have real potential to improve their function are likely to want to work hard to recover what they can. In many cases an improvement in function will move the individual to a less restrictive setting — and hopefully closer to the ones s/he loves.

Building upon the five levels already discussed in Chapter 7 and Chapter 8, this chapter covers work done with individuals who would benefit from cognitive stimulation, short-term rehabilitation, and community integration.

Cognitive Stimulation/Cognitive Retraining includes techniques used with individuals suffering from trauma to the brain and showing cognitive disorganization. Short-Term Rehabilitation includes programming that enhances personal goals worked on in physical therapy, occupational therapy, recreational therapy, and speech therapy. Community Integration includes individuals who are preparing for discharge; focusing on skills, resources, and independence when back at a previous living situation.

Cognitive Stimulation and Retraining Activities

Cognitive Stimulation is a term coined for techniques used in therapy to stimulate cognitive function and assist in retraining an individual to his/her optimum level of function. These techniques may also provide an individual with memory tools and strategies to compensate for a memory loss s/he has experienced.

There are many excellent resources in this field to draw from. Activity ideas may include concentration games, completion of simple tasks, such as puzzles, color and shape sorting, connecting dot-to-dot puzzles, hand water games that involve sensorimotor skills, analogies, trivia games, problem-solving situations, etc.

Other valuable resources for memory retention and cognitive stimulation activities are the speech therapist, occupational therapist, recreational therapist, and psychologist under contract with your setting. Each of these specialties will offer ideas specific to the immediate needs of the participant.

Memory and cognitive function techniques can also be used with participants who are there for short-term rehabilitation, even though they are generally focused on therapy goals and not interested in most of the other programs that are offered.

Brain Function

The types of cognitive stimulation and retraining activities that are required depend on the diagnosis of the participant. Sometimes there is known damage to some part of the brain (as with a stroke). The chart on the next page provides a brief summary of the functions of different areas of the brain and should help you understand which skills have been lost. In thinking about brain function, it is important to consider how function is tied to person-centered programming. This is a crucial element of *Cognitive Activity Levels*, which was discussed on page 103.

Brain injuries and their effects

The brain controls more than our ability to think. Most of the brain's higher functions are located in the dome-shaped cerebrum, which is divided into four lobes. The cerebellum regulate subconscious activities such as coordination. The brainstem connects the cerebrum with the spinal cord. The diagram below explains what happens when different areas of the brain get injured.

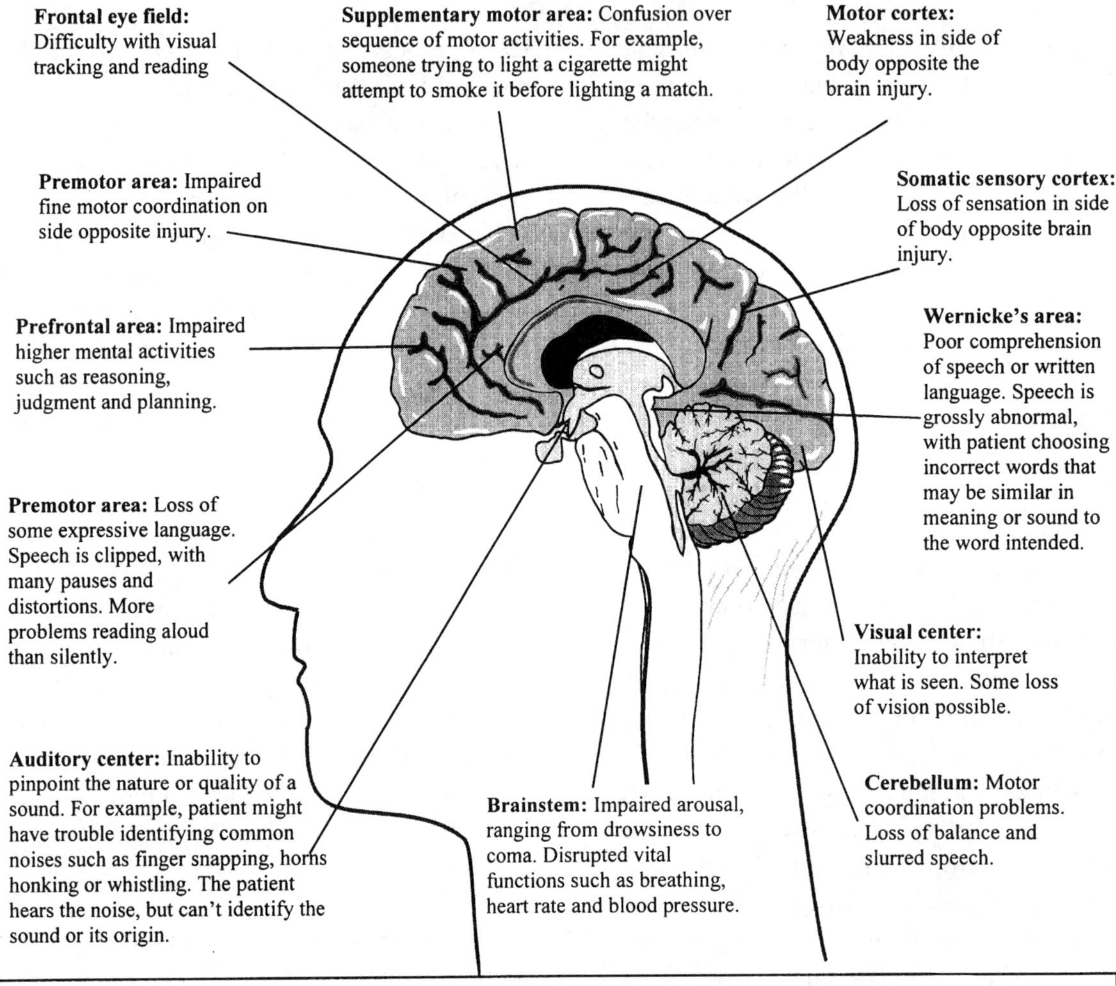
Frontal eye field: Difficulty with visual tracking and reading
Supplementary motor area: Confusion over sequence of motor activities. For example, someone trying to light a cigarette might attempt to smoke it before lighting a match.
Motor cortex: Weakness in side of body opposite the brain injury.
Premotor area: Impaired fine motor coordination on side opposite injury.
Somatic sensory cortex: Loss of sensation in side of body opposite brain injury.
Prefrontal area: Impaired higher mental activities such as reasoning, judgment and planning.
Wernicke's area: Poor comprehension of speech or written language. Speech is grossly abnormal, with patient choosing incorrect words that may be similar in meaning or sound to the word intended.
Premotor area: Loss of some expressive language. Speech is clipped, with many pauses and distortions. More problems reading aloud than silently.
Visual center: Inability to interpret what is seen. Some loss of vision possible.
Auditory center: Inability to pinpoint the nature or quality of a sound. For example, patient might have trouble identifying common noises such as finger snapping, horns honking or whistling. The patient hears the noise, but can't identify the sound or its origin.
Brainstem: Impaired arousal, ranging from drowsiness to coma. Disrupted vital functions such as breathing, heart rate and blood pressure.
Cerebellum: Motor coordination problems. Loss of balance and slurred speech.

The four major lobes

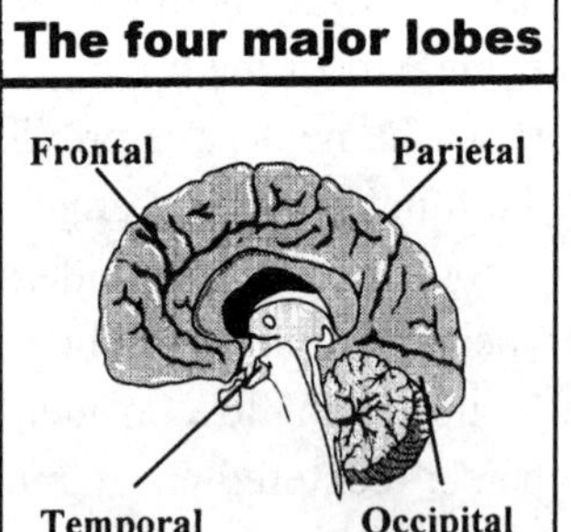
Frontal
Parietal
Temporal
Occipital

General results of lesions in the brain

Frontal: Impaired motor skills, speech, intellectual functions, emotional status. Patient may be apathetic, impulsive, irritable or provocative. Also may have trouble starting, sustaining or ending a specific behavior. For example, a patient sitting in a car might not get up unless told to.

Temporal: Difficulty discriminating and sequencing what is heard. Memory problems. Seizures. Partial loss of vision in upper field of each eye.

Parietal: Loss of sensation in half the body opposite brain lesion. Loss of sense of touch. Patient can have trouble telling what is in hands without looking. Impaired sense of place. Trouble taking things apart and putting them back together. Fifty percent loss of vision in left or right half of visual field.

Occipital: Patient may seem blind since he or she can't identify things by sight alone. Though vision loss is partial, patient needs to touch to identify things.

Used with permission, Dr. William Lynch, Palo Alto Veterans' Administration Medicial Center

Memory

In nearly all of the cognitive stimulation programs offered through activities, memory techniques and interventions will play an integral part.

Memory loss can occur for many reasons. Some of these may be related to depression, nutritional imbalance, medications and changes, emotional losses, and significant transitions. Other reasons for memory loss are more organic such as a head injury, stroke, cerebral tumor, or a progressive degenerative disease such as Parkinson's disease, Alzheimer's disease, and other dementias.

Memory takes place as three separate processes: Memory is quite a miraculous feat and, of course, there are things that can go wrong in all three processes.

Input. From our earliest experiences, we not only explore and learn new things, but, in addition, our brain registers this information.

Storage. The next function of memory is to store this new information in such a way that it relates to the experience.

Retrieval. The final and most important function is the ability to retrieve and use the information experienced and learned before. In the retrieval process, the brain is able to dip into its bank of information and retrieve information specific to the current need.

In addition to the three processes of memory there are also three types of memory:[48]

Sensorimotor Memory. From the physical and sensory experience, we use visual, auditory, tactile, proprioceptive, olfactory, and gustatory senses. An example of this would be a smell that brings back a memory associated with it, such as the proprioceptive experience or whole body experience of walking on sand at the shore. This sensorimotor memory seems to predate all other memory and leaves an imprint on us forever. Sensory stimulation is an intervention to restimulate and remember through this process.

Short-Term Memory. Short-term memory is the ability to experience and replay new information. Short-term memory is exactly as stated, short term. If we read a map and go in that direction, we have processed the new information and applied it to the current task. If we are learning a new card game, we need to understand the rules and process them in order to successfully participate in the game. This is our working memory.

Long-Term Memory. Long-term memory is information that was stored a long time ago. It is our secondary memory. Some participants may not remember who you are or what their own names are, but they will be able to sing all the words of an old song. A similar example would be the ability to recite, word for word, a poem that was learned 60 years ago.

The more that one has memorized in their lives, the stronger the memory. In the early 1900s education was based on memorizing material and reciting it in class. Because of this method, many of the individuals in care settings can successfully recite and engage in activities that focus on long-term memory skills.

Programs we develop need to include all three types and processes of memory. According to the individual's health issues, you can determine what type of memory intervention is most needed.

Treatment for Memory Deficits

The professional will find that s/he is likely to have better results if s/he works on attention span and sensory exercises instead of just working on improving an individual's memory. Zoltan[49] suggests the exercises listed below.

Working with participants who have memory problems can be tough. However, without attention span, memory is not likely to improve, or even stay at the same level of ability. Also, sensory memory and sensory stimulation seem

[48] Atkinson, R. C. and Shiffrin, R. M., 1971, "The control of short-term memory and its control processes," *Scientific American*, 225, 82–90.

[49] Barbara Zoltan (1996). *Vision, perception and cognition, third edition*. Page 140.

to be a more basic activity than verbal memory. There are many different types of memory, including verbal memory, kinesthetic memory, and auditory memory. Work with your participant to see how well his/her short-term memory in all three areas is working.

Visual. The participant is asked to reproduce simple geometric figures, which are presented for 5 to 10 seconds and then covered. Note: if a person's perceptual abilities are impaired, it is likely that this will affect memory for visual material and the ability to use visually based solutions to assist in memory problems.

Kinesthetic. The participant is asked to reproduce a series of hand positions presented to him or her.

Auditory. The participant is asked to reproduce a series of rhythmic taps. Note: if the participant has aphasia, verbal memory and the ability to use verbal memory solutions are likely to be affected.

Some important things for the professional to determine are

- Can the participant continue to learn with practice? Or is the inability to complete a task due to a lack of skill instead of a lack of memory?
- Is the participant's memory loss always a problem, or does there seem to be a pattern to memory loss (e.g., more problems at night)?
- What types of cues help the participant remember better? It is best to give the cue as close as possible to the time the participant needs to remember something.
- Question the participant about what s/he is doing during the activity and wait for a response. If the participant talks about what s/he is doing and gives the activity professional feedback during the activity, the participant will tend to remember more about the activity later.

Some cognitive stimulation and retraining activities are shown of the following pages.

Memory Book

This activity is for an alert participant interested in documenting his/her life for family and friends in a life review process. The use of a memory book is valuable for individuals who remember, recall, and reminisce; and also for individuals who can use these memories and reinforcers to feel safe, enhance long-term memory, reduce anxiety, and promote safe, acceptable social responses.

A memory book highlights the individual and increases a sense of self and self-esteem. This book can be experienced both on a one-on-one basis and in a small group setting. Family and friends are invited to share stories and memories of this individual and perhaps bring in photos to bring the stories to life.

There may be pages with reinforcement statements. Many individuals dealing with memory loss issues become easily agitated and upset with the loss of words and memories. Each person needs his/her own pages of reminders that are individualized to specific needs and concerns.

The book can be filled with art and writings from its owner. This book should always be available and accessible for the individual.

Goal: Opportunities for participant to reminisce about his/her life; to reexamine past experiences, beliefs, values; to recall happier times; to socialize with others.

Equipment Needs: Memory Book — blank book with questions from master list
Photos, drawings, and stories from the participant or his/her family and friends, which can be placed in the memory book
Pen

Length of Activity: 30–45 minutes

Number of Participants: 1–6

Adaptations: Move chair up close to bed; possibly use tray table to write on.

Procedures:

1. Greet the participant; catch up on recent events (briefly).
2. Sit down; ask the participant the next question from the list below or other questions that have been suggested for this participant. (You can briefly review the last session if you like.)
3. Be patient — give the participant plenty of time to answer. Ask helpful questions to stir memory.
4. Do not be too aggressive — this is not a quiz! Be kind, helpful. Keep an open mind — you will hear all kinds of things — funny, heart-warming, aggravating, very sad.
5. Thank participant; read next 1–2 questions for next time.
6. Participant presents completed book to loved one(s).

Questions for a Memory Book about Your Family:

1. From what country or countries did your family ancestors emigrate? When was this and where did they settle?
2. What are your parents' names?
3. When and where were they born?
4. What was your mother's maiden name?
5. What do you remember most about your mother from your childhood?
6. What do you remember most about your father?
7. What work did your parents do?
8. What is your birth date?
9. Where were you born?
10. Was there anything unusual about the circumstances of your birth?
11. Were you born in a hospital or at home?

12. What is your full name and how was it chosen? Does it have a special meaning?
13. Whom in your family do you most look like?
14. How many brothers and sisters did you have? (List them in the order they were born and include children who may have died early in life or at birth.)
15. Where did you fit among them?
16. To whom did you feel closest?
17. How did you spend your time together?
18. Did you ever take trips or vacations with your family? Where did you go? Tell about a favorite one.
19. Was another language besides English spoken in your home? What was it?
20. Did your family attend a church or synagogue? Was religion an important part of your family life?

Map Test

Purpose: To maintain and/or increase the participant's ability to pay attention to task for a short period of time.

Skills Necessary: To scan a document in all directions.
To attend to a task for two minutes.
To distinguish between different symbols.

Goals: To exercise the participant's mental flexibility.
To exercise the participant's attention to task.

Objectives: To attend to the task for two minutes.
To visually distinguish between symbols found on a map.

Materials: Large map with symbols depicting locations on the map. Maps from the parks or cities with large symbols work well. We suggest that you have between four and six maps that measure about three feet by three feet and which are laminated (for infection control). Use an erasable magic marker.

This timed activity requires that the participant search a map for a total of two minutes and circle a particular symbol on the map each time s/he locates one. Some people have the participant use one color marker for the first minute and a second color marker for the second minute. Show the participant the key that contains the symbols that can be found on the map. Indicate which one symbol you want the participant to circle. This helps the professional know how long the participant can attend to a task. Ongoing practice with different maps helps the participant stay "mentally sharp."

Popular Games for Cognitive Stimulation[50]

The following is an alphabetical list of games that are commercially available which could be used in a cognitive stimulation program. This list is by no means comprehensive. The manufacturer of the game is provided after each entry (unless the game is available through several manufacturers) along with a listing by number of the cognitive skills required. The number coding of cognitive skills is as follows:

1. Perceptual accuracy — All games require perceptual (usually visual) accuracy to some extent but some focus on accuracy as a goal.
2. Spatial organization — Games requiring, as a basic focus, organization of material in two or three dimensions are given this designation.
3. Perception-motor functioning — This entails fine-motor functioning or motor speed when it represents a primary component of the game.
4. Verbal skills — Games addressing the generation of words or other verbal material.
5. Math skills — Games in which basic arithmetic plays a central role, including the handling of money.
6. Convergent problem solving — The emphasis here is on piecing together solutions in a step-wise fashion, an essential component to effective strategy.
7. Divergent problem solving — Flexibility in approach is the hallmark. In other words, diverging from step-by-step solutions to generate new strategies.
8. Sequencing — This is often a component of convergent and divergent problem solving but, in some cases, is a goal in itself.
9. Memory — All games require ongoing monitoring and recall as part of the game process but some games focus on memory itself, that is, the ability to retrieve information from long-term storage.

The complexity of the games varies a great deal and is very difficult to rate in a consistent fashion. However, even complex games can be made simpler by altering rules, such as by removing special cards and liberalizing time constraints. For instance, the game Uno (International) can be simplified by removing all special cards, such as Draw Four and Reverse.

Games for Cognitive Stimulation

Aggravation (Lakeside) — 6
Backgammon — 2, 5, 6
Bargain Hunter (Milton Bradley) — 5, 6
Battleship (Milton Bradley) — 2, 6
Bed Bugs (Milton Bradley) — 3
Bingo — 2
Boggle (Parker Brothers) — 4, 7
Checkers — 2, 6
Chess — 2, 6, 7
Clue (Parker Brothers) — 6
Connect Four (Milton Bradley) — 1, 6
Dominoes — 1, 2
Erector Sets — 2, 3, 6
Etch-A-Sketch (Ohio Art) — 2, 3
Foursight (Lakeside) — 2, 7
Gridlock (Ideal) — 1, 2, 6
Lego — 1, 2, 3
Life (Milton Bradley) — 5, 6
Lincoln Logs (Playskool) — 1, 2, 3
Lite-Brite (Hasbro) — 1, 2, 3
Lotto (Edu-Cards)
  Farm Lotto — 1, 6
  Object Lotto — 1, 6
  Go-Together Lotto — 1, 6
  The World about Us Lotto — 1, 6
  Zoo Lotto — 1, 6
Luck Plus (International) — 1, 5
Mastermind (Pressman) — 2, 6
Memory Original (Milton Bradley) — 2, 9
  Animal Families (Milton Bradley) — 2, 9
  Fronts & Backs (Milton Bradley) — 2, 9
  Step by Step (Milton Bradley) — 6, 8
Mhing (Suntex) — 6, 7, 8

[50] Williams, J. M., 1987, "Cognitive stimulation in the home environment," *The Rehabilitation of Cognitive Disabilities*, Center for Applied Psychological Research, Memphis State University, Plenum Press, New York, NY.

Models, plastic replica — 1, 2, 3, 8
Monopoly (Parker Brothers) — 5, 6
Mystery Mansion — 6
Othello — 2, 6
Paint-by-numbers — 1, 2, 3
Parcheesi (Selchow & Righter) — 6
Password (Milton Bradley) — 4, 6, 9
Pay Day (Parker Brothers) — 5, 6
Pente (Parker Brothers) — 2, 6
Perquacky (Lakeside) — 4, 7, 9
Picture Tri-Ominoes (Pressman) — 1
Pic Up Stik (Steven) — 3
Racko (Milton Bradley) — 8
Rage (International) — 6, 8
Risk (Parker Brothers) — 2, 6, 7
Sabotage (Lakeside) — 6, 7
Scotland Yard (Milton Bradley) — 2, 6, 8
Scrabble — 2, 4, 7, 9
Smath (Pressman) — 2, 5, 6
Sorry (Parker Brothers) — 6
Think & Jump (Pressman) — 2, 6
Toss Across (Ideal) — 3
Tri-Ominoes (Pressman) — 1
Tripoley — 1, 8
Uno (International) — 1, 8
Verbatim (Lakeside) — 4, 7, 9
Whodunit (Selchow & Righter) — 6
Word War (Whitman) — 4, 6, 7, 9
Word Yahtzee (Milton Bradley) — 4, 7, 9
Yahtzee (Milton Bradley) — 5, 6

Short-Term Rehab Activities[51]

One of the current issues of professionals is how and what to do with people who are here for short-term or acute rehabilitation who prefer not to get involved in activities and who have very specific and different needs.

This section will look at working with participants who are in your facility for rehabilitation treatment, especially for those admitted to a nursing home. Some of the important questions include:

- What is rehab? What is the team? Who are the players?
- How do you help rehab succeed?
- How do you work with consultants vs. facility employees?
- How do you coordinate care after specialized therapy (PT, OT, RT, Speech Therapy) has occurred and the participant needs to stay in the facility?

The goal of rehab activities is to help the participant get back to the target level of functioning as quickly and easily as possible.

To make these activities work, you need to:

- Understand the differences between the individual admitted for rehabilitation and the individual admitted for long-term care.
- Provide activities that are coordinated with the goals of other members of the rehab team.
- Recognize when the participant is too tired to participate in your activities.

Trends

The profile of the participant in a long-term care facility is as diverse as the services provided. What once was a setting created for individuals who were frail or elderly has evolved into a setting that provides for a profoundly differing participant population. Today a participant may be young or old. S/he may be receiving treatments such as chemotherapy, wound care, IV therapy, or head injury treatment, previously offered only in acute care settings. Along with these specialized treatments, we may see participants needing special care from ventilator dependent services and tracheostomy units. There will also be an increase in the numbers of participants of all ages who are HIV positive.

As the acuity level increases, so does the need to clearly understand medical diagnoses and how professionals play an integral role in quality of care and quality of life issues.

[51] This section is by Lauren Newman, OTR. Used with permission.

The Rehab Team

Working in rehab in a long-term care facility may include working with the following members of the rehab team: doctor, nurses (licensed and aides), physical therapist, occupational therapist, speech pathologist, respiratory therapist, recreational therapist, hospice workers, clergy, dietitian, social services professional, activity professional, psychologist, psychiatrist, and administrator.

Each facility addresses the participant on rehab in a team approach. Facilities hold meetings on a regular basis to design a specific plan for each individual. The content of these meetings may be participant progress, discharge planning, coordination of services, eligibility for current insurance coverage, eligibility for programs, services in the future, planning for family conferences, participant care plan, and sharing of information and techniques that may or may not be working.

It is important to get to know the therapists in your facility and their individual roles as part of the team. Some therapists are consultants under contract and are in the facility specifically to work with an individual participant. They need to be approached directly so that they can understand your role and willingness to help follow through with their treatments. On the other hand, some therapists are full-time employees within the facility. They may be available for additional support for the activity department regarding specific participants and their therapy.

With the new Medicare PPS (Prospective Payment System), the rehab team needs to very closely monitor a participant to ensure they are meeting the criteria to receive specific rehab services according to their diagnosis and rehab potential. Review the PPS guidelines in Chapter 12.

The Role of Professionals

When the Resident is Actively Involved in Therapy

When a participant is newly admitted to a long-term care setting and is receiving therapy on a daily basis, his/her primary goal is to regain strength and independence and be discharged. Because the focus is short-term and centers on returning home, this individual is usually not interested in activities that are offered. For some, the experience of socializing with participants who are confused and disoriented is a hard and constant reminder that they may also need to remain long-term and possibly begin to experience further declines in function. Because of this, their choice is often to go to therapy and then spend the majority of the day in their rooms. Some participants in rehab will seek out other participants in rehab programs for support and contact because of their common challenges and goals.

The professional needs to listen closely at the rehab meetings so that s/he understands clearly what the therapy goals are and how the participant is progressing with them. At this stage, you should discuss with the therapists how activity staff can reinforce and align themselves with the current therapy goals. If the therapist encourages the participant to work with you, there is a greater chance for either involving the participant in a group or in working with them on a one-on-one basis. Therefore, it is important to make agreements with the therapists regarding the non-therapy time the participants may have.

When Assisting with the Therapist's Treatment Goals

The following set of goals show examples of ways that activities can help participants make progress toward their therapy goals:

Increase endurance of walking. When the therapist has given approval for independent ambulation, the activity professional can assist with increasing endurance of walking. This can be done with the help of a walker or other device. Activities such as mail delivery and assistance with participant transportation to and from activities may be appropriate.

Increase endurance in time out of bed in wheelchair from 1 to 2 hours per day. The activity professional can find activities that will not only challenge but also engage the participant in meaningful activity, which can at the same time be enjoyable.

Increase strength in upper extremity. This could be incorporated into an exercise group, beanbag toss, balloon volleyball, parachute game, and movement to music.

Increase endurance and accuracy in upper extremity. This could involve stacking and sorting activities, sewing or weaving, bingo, checkers, puzzles, and many other activities.

Improve visual scanning skills. This could be done through bingo and flashlight tag.

Improve conversational skills: auditory comprehension, intelligibility of speech, word finding. This could be done in discussion groups or as part of an activity where conversation goes on between the participants.

Improve reading and writing skills. This could be done using current events groups, through discussions of literature, or by writing down life histories.

Improve skills in ADLs: grooming and dressing. This could be helped with various grooming activities (including fixing nails or hair) and activities involving period clothes.

When the Participant Stays on after Formal Therapy Has Ended

When participants are discharged from formal therapy services and need to stay in the facility for additional convalescence or long-term stay, the need for activity involvement becomes crucial. Many participants feel a sense of failure and loss when they have not been able to achieve their therapy goals. They often develop close and significant relationships with the therapist. This therapist plays a pivotal position in refocusing the participant's goals and establishing a new framework. By encouraging work with the professionals with goals similar to the ones previously established, the therapist provides the participant with a better chance of not giving up and continuing his/her work towards a higher functional level.

In determining the best and most realistic discharge plan for a participant, the interdisciplinary team works closely with the physician to assess the participant's level of independence. The activity professional can help assess this level of independence and orientation by including the participant in a "helper" or a volunteer role and closely observing him/her in group settings and projects. Things such as mail delivery or requesting the participant's assistance with special projects and events help not only to assess abilities, but also to give him/her a sense of usefulness and self-esteem, which are paramount to continued progress.

When the Participant is in Need of Long-Term Stay

The activity professionals may be among the most helpful staff members facilitating the transition to long-term care and daily routine. After acute rehab is completed, there is usually a room change for the participant. This means new roommates, new orientation to the area of the facility, and, sometimes, different staff members attending to his/her needs. The activity staff may be *the* point of stability for these participants.

When the Participant is in Need of Recreational Therapy Services

The types of rehabilitation treatment provided by a recreational therapist are different from the types of interventions offered by the activity professional (even if the activity professional is a recreational therapist). So the question is: what types of special treatments or procedures fall within the scope of recreational therapy practice which are not already considered to be part of expected and required activities listed under Tag F679? (Tag F679 is the section of the U.S. OBRA '87 nursing home law which outlines the type of services required by the professional — recreational therapist, activity professional, occupational therapist-certified, or occupational therapy assistant — who is in charge of ensuring that each resident's needs related to activities are being met.)

To understand what falls outside of the expected and required activities, it is best to understand what types of activities are expected and required. These can be found at Tag F679 under both the regulation and the guidelines for surveyors. Tag F679 states:

Tag F679 (Regulation) The facility must provide, based on the comprehensive assessment and care plan and the preferences of each resident, an ongoing program to support residents in their choice of activities, both facility-sponsored group and individual activities and independent activities, designed to meet the interests of and support the physical, mental and psychosocial well-being of each resident, encouraging both independence and interaction in the community.

(Guideline) Because the activities program should occur within the context of each resident's comprehensive assessment and care plan, it should be multi-faceted and reflect each individual resident's needs. Therefore, the activities program should provide stimulation or solace, promote physical, cognitive, and/or emotional health; enhance, to the extent practicable, each resident's physical and mental status; and promote each resident's self-respect by providing, for example, activities that support self-expression and choice. Activities can occur at any time and are not limited to formal activities being provided by activity staff. Others involved may be any facility staff, volunteers, and visitors.

(Probes to Surveyors) Observe individual group and bedside activities. Are residents who are confined or choose to remain in their rooms provided with in room activities in keeping with life-long interests (e.g., music, reading, visits with individuals who share their interests or reasonable attempts to connect the resident with such individuals) and in-room projects they can work on independently? Do any facility staff members assist the resident with activities he or she can pursue independently? If residents sit for long periods of time with no apparently meaningful activities, is the cause: resident choice; failure of any staff or volunteers either to inform residents when activities are occurring or to encourage resident involvement in activities; lack of assistance with ambulation; lack of sufficient supplies and/or staff to facilitate attendance and participation in the activity programs; or program design that fails to reflect the interests or ability levels of residents, such as activities that are too complex?

Some of the key words and phrases found under expected and required activities are

- Interests and well-being of each resident
- Provide stimulation/solace
- Promote health
- Enhance status
- Promote self-respect

For the recreational therapist it is often very difficult to determine if the treatment is enhancing and providing well-being and health or if it is a treatment intervention that goes beyond that.

Most of the treatment that allows the resident to maintain his/her status (or to slow decline) and which allows the resident to engage in leisure/free time activities is considered to be part of the required and expected services. Required and expected activities would include reality orientation; exercise group; almost all adaptation of supplies and activities to allow the resident to engage in activity; modifying activities; providing activities which are culturally, age, or gender appropriate; cognitive stimulation; reminiscing; remotivation; resocializing; solace; generalized relaxation techniques; most in-room activities; range of motion through activity; activities to increase self-esteem and self-respect; teaching new leisure skills; and providing structure to modify behavior.

Other activities, generally outside what is traditionally thought of as the activity professional's job, relate to general resident safety and well-being. These activities would include infection control; ensuring that residents have adequate skin protection including pressure releases, changing positions, and appropriate padding; maintaining a safe environment; and ensuring a respectful environment.

Most of the work that a recreational therapist does in a long-term care setting that is different from the work of an activity director relates to community integration, improved function through the use of aquatic therapy, increased independence through adaptive computer equipment, and cognitive exercise through cognitive retraining/cognitive therapy. Greater detail can be found in Chapter 3 under the section Recreational Therapy Services.

Community Integration Activities

At times it may be vital, prior to discharge from our services, for the participant to be escorted into the community on short outings. Not all participants can adjust immediately to a new (usually lower) health status. They may need the professional to venture into the community with them, helping to solve problems along the way. Such help from the professional (and the rest of the team) involves preparatory activities, which take place both inside and outside of the facility.

Some of the activities involve the use of standardized integration programs such as the *Community Integration Program (CIP)*[52]. Others involve the use of activities in the facility for the development of skills such as working, communicating, and the basic ADLs. One important element of community integration activities is to never let the community get too far away from the participant's day-to-day life.

Professionals work with the interdisciplinary team's goal of discharging participants to their next level of care. Some of the ways that professionals can assist in this process are

- Identify and list community resources for leisure activities in the community.
- Assist participant in contacting support groups or recreational groups s/he has expressed interest in joining.
- Create a map of the community including names and addresses for reference.
- Offer participant the name of an individual or staff person to call if s/he has any questions or needs to talk after discharge and during integration into the community.
- Identify transportation systems which participant may need to contact in community.
- Touch base with family briefly by phone or during discharge to offer them support in and after discharge.

As a step toward a return to the community, you can establish programs such as the Intergenerational Program (see Chapter 6) to reconnect your participants with the community outside the facility. Even if the participants need to stay in a long-term care facility for medical reasons, they can still be an integral part of the community outside.

Recreational Therapy Services in Community Integration Programming

Using a pre-established set of community integration treatment protocols such as the *Community Integration Program (CIP)* (Armstrong and Lauzen, 1994) helps the therapist ensure that the treatment provided is likely to have positive outcomes based on the participant's actual level of ability. An example of one of the *CIP's* treatment protocols is the *Module 1A: Environmental Safety* protocol. The purpose of the protocol is to first determine how safe the participant will be in the community

[52] Armstrong, Missy, and Sarah Lauzen, 1994, *Community integration program, 2nd edition*, Idyll Arbor, Inc., Ravensdale, WA.

and, second, to provide training in the community safety areas that will limit the participant's safe use of the community after discharge. This is important information for the entire treatment team to know as they plan the participant's discharge.

The therapist takes a 3" x 5" card with instructions written on one side of the card. The instructions take the participant from one of the doors of the facility and use five turns along sidewalks, driveways, and other areas to have the participant get to a spot where s/he can no longer see the door from which s/he started. At this point the therapist asks for the card back and then instructs the participant to return to the door from which s/he started. *Module 1A* provides the therapist with a series of questions related to participant knowledge, endurance, safety of ambulation/locomotion, speed of both gross motor and cognitive actions, problem solving, personal safety, awareness of his/her own needs for assistance, appropriateness of grooming and clothing for situation, and ability to tolerate stimulation in the environment.

It is a common practice for the recreational therapist to use a standardized program for community integration interventions. There are many other commercially available programs that help teach advanced activities of daily living. The therapist should have a variety and use the ones appropriate for a particular participant.

10. Documentation

What is a health record? Why are health records kept? Who owns the health record? Are there rules to follow when making an entry in a health record? Are there mandated forms and content to the health record? These questions and more will be answered in this chapter. While the specifics found in this chapter apply to nursing homes, the general principles apply to all settings.

First, an introduction to the basic requirements of clinical record keeping as defined in the federal regulations (483.751 1–5, Tag F842 Clinical Records). The health record is owned by the long-term care facility and kept for the benefit of the resident (or his/her legal guardian) and the health care team. The record is used for primary resident care, continuity of care, quality assurance, proof of care given, research, and reimbursement or billing. The health record must be protected from loss, destruction, or unauthorized use. The record must be kept for the period of time required by state law or five years from the date of discharge if there is no requirement in state law; for a minor, three years after the resident reaches legal age under state law.

All information in the health record must be kept confidential. No information may be released without authorization from the resident except when it is required by law. The resident's records may not be released without prior, written consent even to his/her insurance company or to a facility to which s/he is being transferred. The facility must permit the resident to inspect his/her records within 24 hours of request and must provide copies no later than two working days after notice from the resident. All records are kept in accordance with accepted professional standards and practices. Records must be complete, accurately documented, readily accessible, and systematically organized. These are the minimum requirements for record keeping.

Every state may have additional requirements and facility and corporate policy may also require additional record keeping practices. The wise practitioner will be familiar with all regulations and policies. If copies of the federal and state regulations are not readily available in the facility, they may be reviewed at the local county law library or the Internet. (To find the federal health care regulations on the Internet go to <http://www.cms.gov/> or use a search engine like *Google* and search for "State Operations Manual.")

Let's look again at the purposes of the health record.

- *Primary Care.* The record gives the information the health care team needs to deliver direct care — orders for medications, treatments, diet, and nursing care as specified in the treatment plan.
- *Continuity of Care.* The record provides a means of communication among members of the health care team and gives a report of assessments, interventions, evaluations of the individual's progress, and response to the treatment plan.
- *Quality Assurance/Proof of Care.* The record documents care and services provided. The record can be examined by outside reviewers for evidence of appropriate care and intervention. The record is a legal document and can be used as evidence in defense of claims of providing inadequate care and intervention. (If a treatment *isn't* documented in the health record, the legal assumption is that it *wasn't* given.)

- *Research.* The record can be used by health care professionals for research in many fields.
- *Billing/Reimbursement.* The record is reviewed by third party payers for proof that services, supplies, and equipment were provided as claimed.

Because there are so many purposes for the record, including its use as evidence in legal proceedings, standard documentation principles have been established. Following these principles assures that the record can be used for all of the purposes listed above. Failure to follow the principles may render the record useless.

Documentation Principles

Entries into the record must be permanent, legible, timely, accurate, and authenticated. Let's examine each of these principles.

- *Permanent.* Electronic records must be kept for the legal time requirement. They may not be edited, revised, or removed once they have been entered into the electronic record system. Paper entries must be made with an indelible ink pen. Do not use pencil, erasable pen, or a felt tip pen, which may run when wet. Your entry should not be erasable or alterable once in the record. Pages of the record should never be destroyed before the legal time requirement nor should the record be modified by crossing over or using correction fluid.
- *Legible.* Do not use short hand or other personal abbreviations. (A list of generally recognized abbreviations can found in Appendix A.) For paper records, write clearly. If your penmanship is poor, try printing. You and others must be able to easily interpret what you write. Use a pen dark enough that the entry is capable of being photocopied or faxed. Black ballpoint pen is best.
- *Timely.* Document as events occur noting the complete date: month, day, year, and time. Don't rely on your memory and don't document actions in advance. Never backdate, tamper with, or add to notes previously written. It should never appear that the record has been altered with the intent to mislead. For paper records never write between lines or squeeze in words after the fact.
- *Accurate.* Entries should be factual and describe only events that you know to be true through direct observation. Entries should be objective, describing what you can see, hear, smell, or touch. Subjective entries — hearsay, statements from others, opinions, or feelings — should not be used unless they are documented in the form of a direct quote from a resident or family member.

Another part of accuracy is that the entries are within the scope of your education, training and, if applicable, your professional credential. Entries should be specific to your discipline and appropriately express your clinical opinion. Use only words that you understand. Don't attempt to diagnose or assess an individual's psychological or physical condition unless you have the appropriate training. Never speculate about possible causes or interpret behavior unless it is your legal responsibility as a credentialed therapist or social worker to do so. For an example, weeping may be caused by many factors, both internal and external. Unless you are trained to assess the causes with assessment tools or observation, you must wait for the individual to tell you what is causing the weeping before you state a reason. Even then the reason should be documented as a quote from the individual.

Document only what you do. Do not document actions of other members of the health care team. Do not document actions or interventions that you aren't legally allowed to perform (and don't perform them in the first place!).

- *Authenticated.* Sign all entries with your name and title. First initial and full last name with title is acceptable. Example: M. Smith, AC. In signing with your title, you let the other members of the health care team know your background and training. If your facility is using electronic health records (EHR) you may sign with an authenticated signature key.

All of this may make the documentation process look intimidating. You may be saying to yourself, "But I'm only human! Humans make mistakes!" You're right. Because you are only human, there are methods for correcting honest mistakes. It is important that corrections look like corrections and not deliberate attempts to mislead or defraud. In paper records simple errors in charting, the wrong word, date, or name, may be corrected by drawing one line through the error, dating, and initialing it. The time is sometimes recommended.

Example:

The first part of an entry was correct but then ~~the words that were here originally were not correct.~~ error PW 1/16/18

Electronic systems will have similar functionality for making a correction, but the way it is done depends on your system. Be sure you know how to make corrections so they are tied to the entry that is being corrected.

Omissions in charting, forgetting to record an event, may be made as late entries to the record. The current date and time is entered, then the phrase "late entry for ______" entering the date and time for the missed event. Some electronic record systems will have a specific tab for late entries.

Example:

1/5/18 2:00 PM Late entry for 1/4/18 10:00 AM

Late entries should not be made long after the event and are generally recommended to be made no longer than 48 hours after the missed event. Some states will allow late entries only if they are made in 24 hours or less. Check with your medical records professional or legal counsel. If a late entry is not allowed and the information is felt to be important to the record of resident care, an addendum may be made. This is done on a separate page of the record. The current date and time is entered, then the phrase "Addendum to the record for _____" entering the date and time for the missed event.

Both late entries and addenda to the record should be used sparingly. The impression created (and it is an accurate impression) is one of inaccuracy and lack of timeliness in record keeping. Late entries and addenda cast doubt on the reliability of the entire health record. In all documentation, remember that many people, including the person we serve and his/her family, may look at the record.

Claims for slander and defamation of character may be avoided by describing events factually, by avoiding blaming and finger pointing, and by avoiding personal opinions. Do not document an observation in the record that you would not support in public. Entries into the record should be objective as stated above. Instead of describing a resident as a "nasty old man," the description could be a "99-year-old male dissatisfied with facility routine."

Be aware of the individual's rights when documenting and remember that the individual and the family should be a part of the decision-making process. Statements of problems and concern about the individual and family behavior should be discussed openly and should not be discovered by the individual or family only upon reviewing the record.

Introduction to Required Documentation

Non-medical/non-nursing professionals are responsible for five types of documentation about the resident. Each one must be written carefully to be sure that it reflects the actual state of the resident and meets all federal and state regulations. The documents include the initial assessment, the care plan, the discharge plan, ongoing monitoring, and reassessment and updates.

Initial Assessment

Each department is responsible for completing an initial assessment of the individual who is newly admitted. Although state law and facility policy will determine the time frame for completion, it should be completed prior to completion of the *Minimum Data Set* (MDS). The MDS is the name given to the assessment tool mandated for use by every nursing home in the United States that accepts federal or state reimbursement. All of the different professionals who work with residents in nursing homes are expected to participate in the assessment process.

The initial assessment is the first step in getting to know the individual. There is no mandated format for the assessment. It is up to each facility or activity professional to determine which format will best meet their needs.

The activity assessment includes identification of past and present interests, previous lifestyles, and functional limitations and sensory deficits that need to be accommodated. The assessment will also identify individualized programming plans.

The recreational therapy assessment includes information about the individual's functional ability as it relates to advanced activities of daily living:

- Basic environmental/community safety skills
- Community mobility skills
- Consumer skills
- Community resource identification
- Advanced dressing skills
- Time management skills
- Social interaction skills.

The scope of the assessment is often determined by the physician's order for recreational therapy services.

Resident Assessment Instrument (RAI)

Completion of the Resident Assessment Instrument is required for all residents residing for 14 days or longer in a nursing home that accepts federal or state reimbursement. The RAI is a comprehensive assessment that includes the Minimum Data Set (MDS) and the Care Area Assessments (CAAs) and is the first step towards care plan development. Care Area Assessments (CAAs) is the name for a set of decision-making tools that help team members know if a specific, standardized intervention should be used. The CAAs do not cover all interventions, just the most common ones. The MDS identifies real or potential problem areas, which are then further assessed by using the CAAs. This in-depth assessment determines whether or not identified problems need to be addressed in the care plan.

The RAI establishes a baseline functional status for each resident, which is reassessed quarterly with an abbreviated MDS. Improvements or declines in status are tracked through this process to maintain the residents at their optimal level of functioning. The RAI process is completed at least yearly, more often if a resident experiences a significant change of condition.

The RAI's main purpose is to improve the quality of care and quality of life for each resident. It is also used for reimbursement and monitoring of care issues by state and federal regulatory agencies.

Care Plan

A comprehensive care plan is required for all residents residing in a nursing facility. As of November 28, 2017, each facility is required to complete an interdisciplinary baseline care plan for each new resident. The baseline care plan is started on admission to manage the resident's immediate needs. The comprehensive care plan, including all of the resident's identified needs, is completed within 21 days of admission. Both the RAI and the initial assessments are used to develop the comprehensive care plan.

The purpose of the care plan is to provide a "road map" to resident care. The care plan identifies a resident's needs and strengths and establishes goals to maintain a resident at the optimal level of functioning through aggressive staff interventions.

Care plans are developed with the resident's and family's participation. Resident rights require that the resident or his representative is "afforded the right to participate in care planning and is consulted about care and treatment changes." The resident is given the "opportunity to select from alternative treatments" and to refuse treatment. The social services professional needs to be very proactive in promoting the resident's participation in the care planning process and act as an advocate when the resident cannot represent himself/herself.

Discharge Planning

Most residents and families say that their goal is discharge back home or to the prior placement, such as an adult family home or assisted living. While sometimes this is not realistic, it is important to proceed as though it will happen. This is why discharge planning begins at the time of admission. There are some instances when this is not true, but each person who is admitted to the facility must be treated as if there is a potential for discharge until it is proven otherwise.

There are five steps in discharge planning, starting with admission and ending with a final discharge plan. We will look at them here.

Admission

The social services professional's first assessment, the Social History and Psychosocial Assessment, needs to document the potential for discharge based on the facts presented at the time of admission. Review the history and physical and hospital notes prior to beginning the initial interview.

The discharge assessment and documentation respond to the following issues:

- Describe the "crisis" that necessitated placement at this facility. This will usually be the primary diagnosis on the health and physical.
- Describe the resident's prior living situation. S/he may have lived alone or with a spouse. It could have been a community setting such as board and care or assisted living. Note the resident's prior level of functioning, any supplemental care, including the frequency and nature of the care. Finally, describe the support system of children, neighbors, etc. that the resident currently has.
- Describe the resident's functional goal for discharge and the family's goal for discharge. At the time of the initial assessment, it does not matter whether or not the facility staff share this goal. It is only important to get a sense of the resident's and family's commitment to discharge planning. Describe the barriers to reaching the functional goal or the problems that need to be solved in order for the resident to reach that goal.
- Describe desired placement following discharge. Usually the choices for discharge include independent living at home, at home with support, assisted living, board and care, or a skilled nursing facility.
- Assess the support system that will be available after the discharge. Assess whether it will be enough to meet the projected follow-up support necessary for a safe discharge. Some things to consider are increased home care, durable medical equipment, transportation, Meals on Wheels, and Lifeline. List any other support issues found during the assessment

Patient Care Plan

This is the next step in the discharge planning process. The resident's care plan should describe a short-term placement that resolves discharge issues with the goal of discharging the resident to the desired placement once the resident's functional goals have been met.

From Admission to Discharge

There are instances when the discharge plan is clear-cut and the resident seems to breeze from admission through therapy to discharge. This is most likely to happen if the resident was relatively independent before admission, if he has generally intact cognitive/problem solving skills, and has a support system that is involved.

However, when one or more of these factors is missing, the social services professional has a major role in problem-solving placement issues. The best venue for this is a patient care conference with resident, his support system, rehab staff, the interdisciplinary team, and the social services professional in attendance. The issues to be addressed include:

- Resident's abilities and how they have changed
- Necessary resources to assure a safe discharge
- Resident and family ability to provide these resources (financial, personal)
- Community resources that might act as support for a safe discharge.

There may be a question of the resident's cognitive abilities, especially his/her problem solving skills for independent living. The Saint Louis University Mental Status Examination is a test which can detect early cognitive loss. Early cognitive loss impacts problem-solving skills and may be a predictor of discharge success.

The occupational therapist may help in this process as her work with the resident often contains executive problem solving, which is necessary for independence with ADLs.

Additionally, the social services professional might ask someone from a placement agency to come to the facility to assess the resident for appropriate placement if there is a question of the safest environment for discharge. Knowing what is expected of a person in the lesser level of care can be compared with the resident's ability in the current facility. A conclusion can be drawn as to the best possible placement.

The social services professional is the major support person during this process. S/he interfaces with the rehab department and communicates progress or lack of progress to the resident and family. The goal of this communication is to bring the discharge plan to a logical conclusion. This may or may not coincide with the goal as written in the initial assessment but remember that the goal of discharge is placement in the safest possible environment.

Social Service Charting

The social services professional's charting reflects the decision making involved in the discharge plan. From beginning to end, the social services professional will be charting the steps to the final resolution.

Think of the notes as the story and capture your interactions with the resident, the family, and rehab in relation to the plan. The notes should indicate progress (or not) and the supportive counseling given to the resident and family along the way.

The charting regarding discharge will end with a summary of the solution giving the rationale or justification for the decision. Five examples are shown here.

Resident will stay in long-term care, as he has not progressed with therapy to the point of independence or even less supervised care. There is not enough support from family or community to insure a safe discharge.

Resident has not returned to his prior, independent level of function but will be able to maintain some independence, with support, at the board and care level.

Resident has reached his functional goals and will be returning home with follow-up home care per MD orders and suggested durable medical equipment.

The resident and/or family have been asked for their preference for Home Health Agency and have chosen __________ from among the options offered.

Resident wishes to return to the Home Health Agency which he has used in the past. Social services professional to follow up with phone call and MD orders.

Final Charting

The last step in discharge planning is the final charting. In addition to the discharge plan of care which many members of the interdisciplinary team participate in, we recommended a final, comprehensive note in the social services section of the medical record. Examples of the kind of information that should be in the note include:

Resident has been informed that his projected discharge date is on or about _______. At that time, discharge issues were discussed as follows.

HOME CARE has been ordered by the MD. It will consist of PT, OT, nursing and social work. The agency that will follow is

name, phone number

OR

No follow-up home care indicated

Durable medical equipment will include: walker (Medicare to be billed), commode (Medicare to be billed), and tub chair (private expense)

OR

Resident has all necessary equipment

Transportation: Family to pick up resident

OR

Van has been arranged

Approximate discharge time is ______

Address for discharge is ________

A follow-up appointment has been made with your primary care physician on day, month, and time at address

At the time of discharge, nursing will instruct resident and/or family about the medications that will go home with the resident and treatments (e.g., fingersticks) that will be necessary follow-up.

The resident has said that he is excited to be returning home and is "anxious to be reunited with his cat"

OR

"I am in better shape now than I was before I broke my hip"

OR

"I am scared but have great family support so will make it through this."

Monitoring

As part of ongoing documentation, the resident's progress and response to care interventions are monitored. The activity professional documents daily participation in activities to track the effectiveness of the individualized activity program and the care plan. The daily attendance log will also track refusals to participate in the activity plan. This can be used to modify the plan to meet resident's interests. It can also be used as proof that activities are offered to residents when surveyors question why a resident appears not to be involved in activities or when residents state that no activities are offered.

For some residents a bedside log will be maintained. This should document the type, frequency, length of visit, and resident response to the visit. Again, this serves as proof that the care plan interventions are being carried out.

The recreational therapist maintains documentation for each treatment session. This would include the treatment offered, the individual's response to the treatment offered, and plans for the next treatment session.

Reassessment and Updates

At a minimum, the resident is reassessed on a quarterly basis when either the quarterly or the annual MDS is due. At this time, the professionals review the resident's progress over the last three months. The monitoring logs are reviewed; staff, resident, and family are interviewed; and the chart is reviewed.

After the MDS is completed, a quarterly progress note is written summarizing the resident's progress, identifying any new or unresolved problems and establishing goals for the next quarter. The care plan is then reviewed and updated as necessary.

The discharge plan is updated at this time if required by state regulation or facility policy.

During the resident's stay slight changes in functioning may occur. These may be transitory and resolve with immediate staff interventions. In some cases, the changes may be major and more permanent. These will require review by the interdisciplinary team to determine the need for a new MDS and revision of the care plan. Professionals should document their assessment of the change in condition in the progress notes. The note should include an assessment of the impact of the change on the resident's psychosocial well-being, activity participation, and functional ability.

More detailed information about each of these types of documentation will be found in the following chapter. A summary of documentation, in flow chart form, is shown on the next three pages.

Activity Documentation

1. Initial Assessment Form
Assessment of the newly admitted resident. The activity assessment identifies needs, strengths, and lifestyle. Leads to development of an individualized activity program. Completed prior to the MDS.

2. Resident Assessment Instrument (RAI) = MDS + CAAs
Comprehensive interdisciplinary assessment of the newly admitted resident by day 14 of admission. Activity professional is responsible for completion of MDS 3.0 Section F and, if triggered, the Activity CAA and the information on the CAA Summary Form. Quarterly MDS completed every 90 days thereafter and a full MDS annually and on significant change in condition. Additional MDSs may be required for billing purposes.

3. Care Plan
Started on admission to address immediate needs. The guidelines require activities to participate in the baseline care plan completed within 48 hours of admission to begin the process. Then the comprehensive, interdisciplinary care plan based on assessments and the RAI completed within 21 days of admission. Sets goals for resident to measure progress each quarter.

4. Attendance
Daily documentation of activity attendance. Proof that activities were offered to each resident. Bedside log to be used for room-bound residents reflecting type, frequency, length of visits, and response to visit. Resident refusals to be documented with each occurrence.

5. Quarterly Progress Note
Completed with the MDS review. Documents overall progress and response to programming for the previous quarter. Addresses any changes in coding on the MDS and the need to revise the activity care plan interventions in response to these changes. The rationale for the decision to revise or not revise the care plan is documented in the progress note.

6. Change in Condition Progress Note
Completed with a change in level of activity participation or ability to participate. Changes may be temporary, due to an illness like the flu, or may be permanent. Progress note addresses the need for a revised activity plan and the care plan is updated. Permanent changes due to a decline in physical, mental, or psychosocial functioning are assessed by the interdisciplinary team for the need for a new MDS.

Social Services Documentation

1. Initial Assessment Form: Assessment of the newly admitted resident. Identifies psychosocial needs, concrete needs, interests, strengths, and lifestyle. Leads to development of the resident care plan. Completed prior to the MDS.

2. Resident Assessment Instrument (RAI) = MDS + CAAs: Comprehensive interdisciplinary assessment of the newly admitted resident by day 14 of admission. Usually responsible for completion of Sections D, E, and, if triggered, the related CAAs and the information on the Summary form. Quarterly MDS completed every 90 days thereafter and a full MDS annually and on significant change in condition. Additional MDSs may be required for billing purposes.

3. Care Plan: Started on admission to address immediate needs. The federal guidelines require social services to participate in the baseline care plan completed within 48 hours of admission to begin the process. Comprehensive interdisciplinary care plan based on assessment and the RAI completed within 21 days of admission. Identifies mood, behavior, or psychosocial problems that need resolution or management. Sets goals to measure effectiveness of interventions.

4. Social Services Log: Ongoing documentation of services and counseling provided to the resident. May be documented in a separate log or in the resident's health record. Follow up note is required to document resolution or outcome of the interventions.

5. Quarterly Progress Note: Completed with the MDS review. Documents overall progress for the previous quarter. Assesses the resident for any unmet needs. Addresses any changes in coding on the MDS and the need to revise the care plan interventions in response to these changes. The rationale for the decision to revise or not revise the care plan is documented in the progress note.

6. Change in Condition Progress Note: Completed with any changes in mood or behavior problems, including starting or stopping use of a psychotropic drug or a physical restraint. Changes may be temporary, due to an illness or changes in environment, or may be permanent. Progress note addresses the need for a revised interventions and the care plan is updated. Permanent changes due to a decline in physical, mental, or psychosocial functioning are assessed by the interdisciplinary team for the need for a new MDS.

7. Discharge Plan and Progress Note: Started on admission to assess potential for discharge. A care plan is initiated for the resident with a potential for discharge to a lesser level of care. Periodic progress notes track the progress of discharge planning. A final note must show that sufficient preparation and orientation have been provided to assure a smooth transfer. The note summarizes the outcome of the plan and post-discharge planning. Resident/family training, resident counseling, and post-discharge referrals are documented.

Recreational Therapy Documentation

1. Initial Assessment Form
Assessment of resident after receiving prescription for recreational therapy services from resident's physician. Identifies needs and strengths within the scope of the prescription.

2. Resident Assessment Instrument (RAI) = MDS + CAAs
Comprehensive interdisciplinary assessment of the resident by day 14. Recreational therapist (CTRS) is responsible for completion of MDS 3.0 Section O concerning RT services. Subsequent MDSs completed depending on length of prescription received from physician and/or significant change in resident status.

3. Care Plan
Started when prescription for recreational therapy services is received from physician. Set goals for resident to measure progress for duration of prescription or quarterly time period, whichever is shorter.

4. Chart Note for Each Treatment Session
Recreational therapy to document resident's performance and feelings after each treatment session.

5. Progress Note
Complete weekly or quarterly note. Quarterly notes are completed with the MDS review. Documents overall progress and response to programming for the previous quarter. Addresses any changes in coding on the MDS and the need to revise the recreational therapy care plan interventions in response to these changes. The rationale for the decision to revise or not revise the care plan is documented in the progress note.

6. Change in Condition Progress Note
Completed if there is a change in level of function within the scope of the prescription. Changes may be temporary, due to an illness like the flu, or may be permanent. Progress note addresses the need for a revised treatment plan and the care plan is updated. Permanent changes due to a decline in physical, mental, or psychosocial functioning are assessed by the interdisciplinary team to determine the need for a new MDS.

11. Assessments

This chapter will look at the assessments used to evaluate a resident and what is required in the discharge summary. The next chapter will look at using the RAI to create a care plan.

Initial Assessment

The first step in an individual's care is to assess the person. Assessment is the process of discovering who the person you will be serving is and what his/her physical and psychosocial needs are in terms of optimum care and functional status. You use that information to create the care plan.

The assessment process begins with the first information that you receive about the individual. During the first few days after admission, you should introduce yourself to this individual in an informal visit. At this time you will be making observations in areas such as appearance; understanding and comprehension; orientation to person, time, and place; understanding of diagnoses; and any personal possessions or items in his/her room that give information on past lifestyle and interests. You may or may not have had a chance to review this person's medical chart before meeting him/her the first time. With the information gathered from this initial visit, you proceed to the medical chart for more information specific to past social and medical history, primary and secondary diagnoses, rehabilitation issues and goals, etc.

There are some basic concepts to remember as you move through the assessment process. First, people do not perceive themselves as their chronological age. The spirit of adventure and the child within is always much younger. Find the key to this real age of the person to open an understanding of who they really are. Look less at age and more at the individual. Help identify potential. Regardless of limitations, there are many strengths, abilities, and talents to discover about this person. Additionally, consider:

- Individual leisure interests and hobbies
- Customary routine — what is or was an average day like?
- Educational background
- Community involvement and volunteer work
- Family, children, grandchildren
- Previous travels
- Hopes and goals/aspirations
- Leadership experiences
- Spiritual/religious affiliations, needs, and interests
- Special talents and strengths
- History of physical activity and current level of fitness
- Mobility issues
- Adaptive equipment needs and sensory aids
- Functional abilities/independence in activities of daily living
- Special requests for programs or resources

As you get to know the individual better, you will make updates to your assessment. The original assessment and the updates provide important information for making program plans. Planning programs for individuals requires making plans based on what the person is like now and making adaptations when the individual has a change in ability or situation. That is what the ongoing care plan process is designed to let you do.

Assessing a New Individual

The assessment process employs a variety of techniques to reveal as complete a picture as possible of an individual's situation and condition. On the following pages are forms for gathering information on a new admission.

Usually there is an initial assessment or screening form. The information you gather using this form will be used to fill out the MDS and the CAAs. Some states require an assessment in seven days and others allow up to fourteen days. Whatever your state mandate is, use the maximum amount of time to assess the person. This will give the individual time to more fully present to you a picture of who s/he is. Initially there is pain, disorientation, often depression, and sometimes delirium — all of which will color your assessment.

The assessment of new individuals is the key to individualizing and understanding individual needs. Meet with him/her informally to introduce yourself. Offer support and welcome him/her without too many questions during this first visit. Make your visit short unless s/he asks you to stay longer.

During the first informal visit, you are in the first stage of the assessment process. Keep your eyes open and listen carefully to the conversation. There is some factual information that you need to find out during the initial assessment process. Some you will be able to get from talking to the individual and his/her family. Other information will come from the medical chart. The information includes:

- Date of birth
- Lifestyle
- Level of alertness
- Marital status
- Leisure interests
- Orientation
- Children
- Hobbies
- Hearing
- Religion
- Talents
- Vision
- Occupation
- Political interests
- Adaptive devices
- Physical history
- Social history
- Compensatory skills
- Language(s) spoken
- Voter registration
- Communication skills and deficits
- Discharge plan
- Allergies
- Emotional health
- Attention deficits
- Special diets
- Dependency issues
- Grooming issues
- Mental attitude
- Short-term memory loss
- Long-term memory loss
- Diagnoses
- Prognosis

But what is more important to creating an appropriate care plan is understanding the individual as a person, not as a set of facts. When you complete this part of the assessment form, do it away from the individual so the person will not feel anxious about the answers that s/he gives you.

- Discover who this person is — the goal is to provide a "person-centered" plan.
- Be aware of cognitive and functional levels.
- Be aware of sensory deficits.
- Be aware of ability to communicate needs and interests.
- Be aware of personal possessions in the room.
- Be aware of previous lifestyle issues and interests.

We have included forms that you can use to gather information about new individuals. The forms, as they are presented, include information that we feel is most important, but you may need to modify them to meet the needs of your facility. Following the forms are some additional tools and techniques to help you gather information for the initial assessment.

Barbara's Story

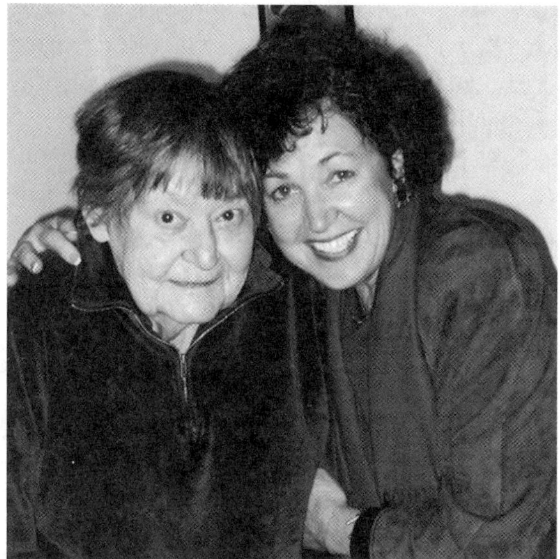

To show you why it is important to put your best effort into understanding each person your serve, we will tell the story of Barbara. Barbara Best was Betsy Best-Martini's aunt. Her personal story and experience brings alive the journey that we each take with family and friends through the long-term care experience. It is important to personalize this experience both as a staff member and as an individual so that the entire staff can participate in creating culture change and quality of life for each member of the community. The following is Betsy's story about her relationship with Barbara.

As a geriatric recreational therapist working in long-term care settings for many years, I have had the privilege of working with unforgettable residents who have left an imprint on my life and work. These people and clinical experiences made it possible for me to be a better family member, daughter, and niece, when it was my time to play the role of family member and responsible party to my own family. My perspective, as a family member with two relatives who were both in assisted living and convalescent care, has heightened my personal and professional focus on the importance of culture change and what that magical thing we all look for in creating a "meaningful and quality" life really is. Recreation, Leisure, Family and Friends are significant components of this puzzle.

Throughout this edition of *Long-Term Care*, you will get acquainted with Barbara Best. Her story, life history, case history, and documentation will help you understand how to "find the key" to who someone is, identify strengths and limitations, create a treatment plan, and follow it through the changes that life and age create.

As you get to know Barbara, use the skills that you have learned to better understand and provide services to other residents with rich lives and special needs.

A Life History

Barbara was born in Coronado, California, on December 2, 1921. She was the youngest of a family of four. She had two brothers, Charles, Isaac Shelby (my father), and one sister, Louise. Being from a Navy family, she lived in many places as a child, including China. These early memories shaped a strong curiosity and interest in people and places that would be a part of her life, work, and continued travels.

She attended the University of Southern California on a full scholarship and graduated from the School of Journalism in 1943. Upon graduation, she was recruited by 20th Century Fox and for six years she was the youngest unit publicist, and the rare woman, in the motion picture industry. This position led to other administrative positions, newspaper reporter, and her own TV show. She then went into business for herself as a publicist and worked with many famous and wonderful entertainment personalities. In addition to her professional career, she volunteered many hours a week to assist non-profit organizations and groups in business. She was a co-founder and former chairperson for the Vikki Carr Scholarship Foundation, which awarded more than 100 college scholarships to students from Mexico who never could have imagined attending college in the U.S. She was a president of the Publicist Federal Credit Union and was listed in *Who's Who of American Women* starting in 1974.

Barbara was a strong and active member of the Hollywood Women's Club and assisted in planning the Golden Globe Awards for many years.

In addition to work, Barbara had many leisure interests. She traveled and cruised all over the world and brought her nieces on trips with her so they could get the travel bug, too. She was a very independent and proud, self-made woman who took pride in her home, garden, many pets, and numerous home improvement projects. She could be found laying brick in her yard late into her 70s.

Technology always fascinated her, and she needed to be the first with the newest high tech gadgets, including her first computer in the late 1970s. She loved her family and made a point of keeping in touch with all of them with visits, phone calls, and then e-mails. She taught herself how to use a computer and then taught this author how to use one, too.

A Case History

Barbara was very physically active her entire life. She had been a heavy smoker for over fifty years, which caused her to take more breaks during the day, but did not slow her down too much until she began experiencing breathing difficulties in her 60s and was diagnosed with COPD (Chronic Obstructive Pulmonary Disease).

She first started experiencing memory loss in her late 70s. She was still in business and started to spend more time at the office and at the computer so that those around her would not be able to detect her early struggle with finding the right words and forgetting appointments. Her office colleague was the first person to express concern about the changes that she was seeing. As the memory loss continued and her ability to balance the books became more challenging, she decided to retire. This was in 1998/1999. She asked for help from her nieces to organize and move out of her office. Spending time together organizing in her office was when it became very apparent that the ordinarily simple tasks of sorting and filing and moving were becoming more than she could handle. She became irritable and short-tempered with those around her and had difficulty experiencing the everyday joys that had been such a part of her life.

She went to her doctor to discuss the memory loss and other concerns. He ordered an array of tests to rule out any other disorders. After extensive tests were completed with a colleague geriatrician, her primary physician discussed his findings with her — that she had dementia due to Alzheimer's disease.

He recommended a caregiver at home. She then had someone with her at home twenty-four hours a day and continued to work in the garden, read the paper, and enjoy caring for her animals with assistance. One evening at home she fell unconscious and was hospitalized. She was diagnosed with sick sinus syndrome and had a pacemaker implanted.

In 2000, Barbara and her cat named Sam moved to Northern California to be closer to her nieces. She lived in a small residential care setting for two years. She started to need more care and supervision and moved to a specialized assisted living setting for individuals dealing with dementias. She continued to enjoy one-to-one short visits and spending most of the day walking, eating favorite foods, and sleeping. She responded to verbal conversation, but was non-verbal herself except for repetitive verbalizations that were expressed with great concern. Always having been an excellent communicator, she was trying to express herself and her concerns with all those around her.

At the same time she was also beginning to experience frequent falls. One of these falls brought her to the emergency room with lacerations over one eye. It was determined at this time that she needed a higher level of care. She was then admitted to a skilled nursing facility, in 2003. She lived in this setting for another four years. She became total care for all ADLs, but was walked daily with two-person assist. She seemed to come alive and be more aware of her surroundings when up on two feet, as she had always been such an active person. She was brought to some group activities, but became upset and verbally agitated, as the stimulation was too overwhelming for her. She spent the majority of her time in her room with two other residents with similar levels of cognitive function. She would smile for familiar staff for a short period and then spend the rest of the day asleep or with her eyes closed.

She responded to the sound of my voice and would open her eyes during our many visits. Upon making eye contact with me, she would begin to speak in her new private language but with great emphasis. Barbara always had music playing in her home. So, each visit, we would listen to Broadway favorites and sit together holding hands. She responded the same way to visits with her other niece, my sister who is named Barbara (after her aunt).

My Aunt Barbara died in February 2007. Her cause of death was heart failure. The heart failure was due to pneumonia, COPD, and an advanced dementia with dysphagia. As we go through the book we will spend more time looking at Barbara's story

Activity Assessment

The activity assessment form in this section is designed for the activity professional completing the initial activity assessment. This is an example of an intake assessment form. There are many variations and styles. The form will be completed before the MDS and used in conjunction with the MDS assessment process. This intake form may be used in a variety of settings.

Background Information

Background information, such as the person's name, date of birth, educational background, etc., can be found in the medical chart. It might be a good idea for the activity professional to fill this part of the form out (as much as possible) *before* interviewing the new participant. This allows the professional to check the individual's answers to these questions against what is in the medical chart. (Remember, a "wrong" answer by the person you are interviewing could be a mistake in the medical chart and not problems with dementia!)

Voting status is an important part of the background information. Is the individual registered to vote? Is s/he interested in voting? Does s/he have an absentee ballot? This question is not asking for political party preference but whether an individual is interested in registering or completing a change of address form.

Diagnosis

Include a brief description of the individual's diagnosis, especially related to activities.

Ability to Do Activities

This area addresses areas that affect the individual's ability to participate in activities. It includes the types of medication, mobility issues, adaptive devices, behaviors that might be a problem during activities, issues with pain management, language barriers, and sensory deficits. This information is important in addressing how functional and independent an individual may be and how much you will need to individualize your program to meet his/her needs.

Previous Leisure Interests and Information Related to Previous Lifestyle and Customary Routine

In order to better understand a new person, it is important to know his/her previous interests. They give you clues as to what you might attempt to offer him/her in terms of one-on-one interventions or programs. What did a typical day in his/her life look like? How can we assist in maintaining the normalcy of routine and interests?

Levels of Programming

When you reach this part of the assessment, you have not only reviewed the medical record, but also interviewed and possibly observed the person on a one-on-one basis or in a group activity. This is your assessment of what level of activity programming s/he needs. Check the types of programs from the list. If you need to add to the list, be sure to do so. Remember: for each level checked, you must document involvement and response to this type of program. So, when you check two areas, you must also document on these two areas in the progress notes.

Independent Interests

If the individual has independent interests, be sure to document it. This is important in explaining why the individual is not participating in group programs in the facility.

Observations, Comments, and Plan

This section should be used to record any other areas that you feel need to be addressed. Be specific about the treatment plan and goal.

Remember — the individual has the right to know about and agree with all aspects of his/her care before it is written into the care plan.

Person-Centered Activity Assessment Form

Admit Date: ______________________ **Date of Birth:** ______________
Former Occupation: ______________________ **Marital Status:** ______________
Religion: ______________________ **Voting Status:** ______________
Diagnosis:

____

Medications: ☐ Antidepressants ☐ Antipsychotics ☐ Antianxiety ☐ Sedatives
Mobility information:
Adaptive devices and supplies needed:
Identified behaviors needing activity interventions:

____

Pain issues and management through activity interventions:

____

Language barrier:
Sensory deficits:
Previous leisure interests and information related to previous lifestyle:

____

According to this activity assessment and in addition to the MDS, the following level of programming is identified as appropriate for this resident's leisure needs and interests:

- ☐ Bedside Music
- ☐ Creative Expressive
- ☐ Group Activities
- ☐ Group Games and Projects
- ☐ Community Outings
- ☐ Intellectually Stimulating Activities
- ☐ Music
- ☐ One-to-One
- ☐ Outdoor Activities
- ☐ Pain Management/Intervention
- ☐ Physical Activities
- ☐ Pet Visits
- ☐ Reading/ Writing
- ☐ Rehab-Oriented Activities
- ☐ Relaxation
- ☐ Religious
- ☐ Resident Council
- ☐ Sensory Stimulation
- ☐ Solace Activities
- ☐ Spirituality
- ☐ Other (describe below)

For Residents with Independent Leisure Interests:

- ☐ *Involved with previous leisure interests and customary routine*
- ☐ *Expresses interest in new leisure activities*
- ☐ *Prefers not to attend group activities*
- ☐ *Prefers change in routine*
- ☐ *Involved in individual leisure interests independent of activity program offerings*

Assessment Observations, Comments, and Plan:

____

Activity Coordinator: ______________________ **Date:** ______________

Resident Name: ______________________ **Room:** ______________

Assessment Box: Assessing the Less Responsive Individual

There are many reasons why an individual may not be responsive to some facets of the assessment processes. The assessment box is a therapeutic tool to assist the individual in taking a more active role — to participate more fully in the initial assessment process. The box should include both familiar and unusual items. Some of these items should be leisure related. Some should be orientation objects. Others should be unique and unexpected in order to stimulate the senses.

Some items found in an Assessment Box could be

- Paint brush and paints
- Wallet
- Potpourri
- Small balls of various types
- Deck of cards
- Newspaper
- Sandpaper
- Sports equipment
- Mirror, lotion, makeup
- Camera, view finder
- Binoculars
- Gardening tools
- Whistle
- Egg beater
- Scarves, gloves, ties
- Pictures of familiar things
- Maps
- Coins
- Keys
- Sheet music
- Music box, CDs and player
- Silverware

Assessment Procedures:

- Eliminate as many distractions as possible.
- Sit across from the individual at a distance where there is close eye contact and s/he does not need to strain to hear you.
- Place the objects either on the table in front of the individual or leave them in the box and place the box on the table.

At this stage of the assessment, the goal is to create curiosity about the objects and then to assess the individual's response to the objects. The goal is for the individual to identify items that appear familiar to him/her. This tells you what is familiar to the individual from his/her long-term memory. These may become leisure activities or games created for this individual because of *his/her* response to them.

There are a multitude of observations you can make. You are most often looking for response of either familiarity or interest. For example, if there is positive and immediate response to a picture of a dog, this could indicate a past and also present interest and affection. If further indications confirm this observation, animal-related programming would be a good idea. Puzzles with more than one shape that require the individual to place a piece in the correct outline, could indicate that s/he recognizes and processes the steps necessary to engage in this leisure pursuit.

Some individuals have experienced cognitive and sensory losses. Visual cues may assist them in participating more fully in the assessment process. Regardless of the functional level, you should strive to make the assessment experience an empowering one and the Assessment Box is an ally in this effort.

Some specific questions you may seek to answer through observation include:

- Does the individual seem most interested in bright objects? small objects?
- Does s/he appear to recognize the object presented?
- Does s/he use the objects as intended (e.g., does not try to eat the photograph)?
- Can s/he repeat the name of the object or acknowledge recognition with a yes/no or a nod?
- Is there any differentiation between positive or negative responses?

- Does s/he look for an object that has been removed?
- Is s/he unwilling to return an object to you?
- Does s/he refuse to respond to this entire experience?
- Is s/he able to use small motor/fine motor movements to pick up and examine objects?

Focus on task and successful involvement can be nurtured and expanded with information gained through this assessment activity. Curiosity can initiate involvement and growth.

Social Services Assessment

The social history of the individuals: who they are and were, where they lived, whom they lived with, their occupations, and the kinds of community support they received prior to joining your facility describe the patterns of previous lives. These patterns help you tailor treatment plans to match each individual's unique needs.

Typically, gathering this information for the rest of the team is the responsibility of the social services professional. That person should ensure that an accurate picture of the individual's social history is presented as inaccuracies could lead to inappropriate treatment goals. Ideally you will create a biography of the resident: begin at the beginning and make logical progress through his/her life. However, do not limit yourself to facts; assess also what you see. Mood is often worn on one's face, in one's affect. It takes more than words to assess mood. Use your skills of observation for a complete picture of the individual. When you are finished, you may have the data for a social history. If you are unable to obtain biographical information (because the individual is unable to give it and there is no one else to act as historian), you will need to "see" the individual to produce a psychosocial assessment. Hopefully, you will have access to both forms of information.

Two methods of obtaining the information are presented. The next two pages have a set of questions you can ask to help you write a narrative social history. The two pages after that show a more structured form for gathering much of the same information. Adapt the forms as required to meet your particular needs.

A note of caution: do not allow yourself to be constrained by these intake forms. These forms are simply tools to provide a skeleton of selections to be used during the assessment process. Also, some corporations have specific policies related to the forms you must use. Check this out before you begin.

If you are inclined to write a narrative note, take a blank progress note and develop your statement based on what you have seen and what you have heard about the individual. This kind of note will allow you to focus freely on the personality of the individual: describe actions and reactions and important relationships. Use anecdotes the individual and his/her family tell you.

Narrative notes are fun to write and interesting for the staff to read (isn't that our goal?). You will develop your own story-telling style and can more fully depict the individual. Remember that you must use your skills every day. No one's assessment is ever finished; even the most ill individual continues to evolve within the boundaries of the facility.

Identify changes because change is what we must be alert for. It drives our care interventions. Do not stop with the identification of change. Chart it. Make sure that the rest of the care team also knows about the change. Be assertive; be proactive; do not wait to react. Act on behalf of the individual every day by assessing, documenting, and keeping all information current.

Social Services Assessments for New Admissions

1. Reason for Admission to a Long-Term Care Facility at this Time

- Where was individual living previously/now?
- What were precipitating factors for this change?
- How was admission decision made? Was the individual involved in the decision?
- Were family or friends involved in the decision? Did they help with the moving or the transition?
- Who is primary contact person for the individual?

2. Social History

- Where did the individual live?
- Where was the individual born?
- What was his/her occupation?
- Why did s/he stop working?
- Was s/he married? Length and quality?
- Did s/he have children?
- What other important relationships did s/he have in the past or present?
- What were the most significant life events and/or losses? How did s/he react to these events?
- How does s/he feel about them now?
- What is the ethnic, cultural, and religious background? How important were they to the individual?
- Has s/he seen a psychiatrist or other similar professional? Why? How long?
- What are his/her current relationships with family or friends like?
- Who provided this information?

3. Current Psychosocial Functioning

- Does the individual have the capacity to make decisions regarding individual needs and wishes?
- How does the individual present herself/himself to other people?
- Is s/he well groomed? Is there anything striking about his/her appearance?
- Does s/he have any idiosyncratic mannerisms?
- What is his/her general behavior like (e.g., nervous, clingy, sad, quiet, content, etc.)?
- What is his/her cognitive functioning like? Is s/he oriented to person, place, and time?
- Is s/he forgetful of recent or remote events?
- What does s/he talk about most of the time?
- What are his/her fears?
- How does s/he cope with physical and emotional losses?
- What is his/her sense of humor like?
- What achievements is s/he proud of?

4. Psychosocial Care Plan Recommendations

- What difficulties is this individual likely to experience in adjusting to the program?
- What can be done to ease his/her adjustment?
- How can specific departments in the facility be of help?
- Will family members also need assistance? What kinds?
- Will family members participate in the individual's care? How?
- Should this individual be encouraged to attend group activities or be left alone?
- Should this individual be referred for social work assessment?

5. Discharge Planning Assessment

- What was the "crisis" for admission?
- What was prior function (how independent, or dependent was the resident in ADL terms)?
- Where did the resident reside? With whom?
- What supports were necessary: care givers, transportation, banking, cooking, etc.?
- What equipment was used?
- What is the resident's functional goal for discharge?
- What is the family's functional goal for the resident at discharge?
- Where is the desired discharge placement?
- What supports might be necessary: extra care, Meals on Wheels, walker, wheelchair, etc.?
- Why is this level of care required?
- Under what conditions will this individual be able to go to a less structured environment?
- What social or environmental supports would be required?
- What is the projected timetable?
- Does the individual agree with discharge plan?
- Does family agree with discharge plan?
- What difficulties can be anticipated in implementing this plan?

Social Services Assessment

Medical Record # ____________________ Admission Date ____________________

Room # ____________________ Admitted From ____________________

Readmit Yes _______ No ______ Date of Birth ____________________

I. Identifying Information

Name: ____________________ Age: ________ Sex: M ____ F ____

Religion: ____________________ Contact: ____________________

Diagnosis: ____________________

Marital status: Never Married _____ M _____ W _____ D _____ Sep. _____

Financial Resources: Medicaid _____ Medicare _____ Private _____ Other _____

Responsible Party or Conservator: ____________________ Relationship: ____________________

II. Mental Status

	Yes	No	At Times
1. Oriented to:			
Person	_____	_____	_____
Place (Facility/Room)	_____	_____	_____
Season	_____	_____	_____
Staff	_____	_____	_____
2. Long-Term Memory Problem	_____	_____	_____
Short-Term Memory Problem	_____	_____	_____
3. Problem Behavior:			
Wandering	_____	_____	_____
Verbally Abusive	_____	_____	_____
Physically Abusive	_____	_____	_____
Socially Inappropriate	_____	_____	_____
Indication of Delirium	_____	_____	_____
4. Quality of Life:			
Makes Own Decisions	_____	_____	_____
Uses Telephone	_____	_____	_____
Manages Own Money	_____	_____	_____
Takes Own Medication	_____	_____	_____
Sets Own Goals	_____	_____	_____
5. Has Verbal Expression of Distress	_____	_____	_____
6. Has Observable Signs of Mental Distress	_____	_____	_____
7. Receives Psychoactive Medication	_____	_____	_____

	Yes	No	At Times
8. Emotional Status:			
Moods Interfere With Daily Activity	_____	_____	_____
Aware of Diagnosis	_____	_____	_____
Participates in Care Plan	_____	_____	_____
Accepts Facility Placement	_____	_____	_____
Upset over Lost Roles/Status	_____	_____	_____
Unsettled Relationships:			
Family Member	_____	_____	_____
Other Residents	_____	_____	_____
Staff	_____	_____	_____

III. Personal Data:

A. Family Relationships/Emotionally Supportive Persons:

Name	How Related	Phone
______________________________	____________	_________________
______________________________	____________	_________________
______________________________	____________	_________________
______________________________	____________	_________________
______________________________	____________	_________________
______________________________	____________	_________________
______________________________	____________	_________________

B. Birthplace ______________________ Education ____________________________
Lifetime Occupation(s) ____

C. Cultural Background ____
Interests/Hobbies ____

D. Adaptive Aids Used/Needed:
Hearing Aid ______ Glasses ______ Dentures ______
Clothing ______________________ Special Eating Equipment __________________
Ambulation Equipment ____

E. Information Received From ____
____

IV. Identified Psychosocial Problems/Needs/Concerns:
Areas include: psychosocial, family, financial, and social

____
____
____
____

Date Plan Reviewed with Resident: ____
Discharge Plan: ____
____

Social Services Professional ___________________________ Date of Assessment ________

Recreational Therapy Assessment

The recreational therapy assessment in a nursing home setting is limited in scope and must reflect measurement of the specific areas prescribed by the physician. The prescription from the physician (along with a physician's signature) should indicate the frequency, scope, and duration for treatment of the functional skill area to be addressed.

If the physician wants the recreational therapist to test the patient's use of public transportation to reach his/her outpatient appointments, then the recreational therapist will need to assess the patient's skills related to public transportation and not leisure interests. The recreational therapist will use a standardized assessment such as *Module 4B (Taxi/Taxi Vans)* or *Module 4E (City Bus)* from the *Community Integration Program* (Armstrong & Lauzen, 1994). For patients with less physical impairment but large deficits in executive function the *Bus Utilization Skills Assessment* (BUS) (burlingame, 1989) may be more appropriate.

If the physician wants to increase muscle strength and to increase range of motion for a patient who is so weak that hydrotherapy is the best choice, then the therapist may want to use the *Oxford Scale for Muscle Power Modified for Water* (Skinner and Thomson, 1983). The Oxford Scale is a modification of the standard 0 (zero) through 5 scores given for muscle strength on land. When the patient is able to increase his/her Oxford Scale up to 4 or 5, s/he may be ready to work on muscle strengthening exercises on land.

As our communities and population become more computer literate, information technology will greatly enhance the independence of our patients. A recreational therapist might get a prescription to help an older patient "get on line" so that the patient can be more independent and return home. The therapist can increase the technology's usability by understanding the needs and characteristics of individuals who are older. As an example, age-related changes in visual functioning include a "reduction in light sensitivity, color perceptions, resistance to glare, dynamic and static acuity, contrast sensitivity, visual search, and pattern recognition." (Kosnik et al., 1988)[53] Make sure that the patient has a computer system that will work for him/her, such as a large screen monitor that allows high contrast. The patient will also need to be taught how to use the various web pages to shop on line, communicate with others via e-mail, access social media, and keep up with daily events through the Internet.

Standardized Scales and Assessment Tools

One of the standards of practice for almost every health care profession is the standard to measure the individual's functional (skill) level before any type of intervention or activity is taken to modify that function. This standard requires that some kind of measurement be taken that measures the individual's ability and can be understood by the other members of the health care team. For this reason health care professions have developed "standardized" testing tools and scales.

A *scale* is a type of measurement that goes from the least to the most, usually using numbers (e.g., 1 to 5). An *assessment* is a tool to gather information that may or may not use scales to record the information gathered. Because the measurements are standardized, they can be taught to students all over the world, developing a common language. This section provides you with an introduction to a few of the standardized scales and tools. The next chapter covers one specific standardized tool, the Resident Assessment Instrument that is used in every nursing home in the United States that accepts federal funding and other countries throughout the world.

---

[53] Kosnik, W, Winslow, L, Kline, D. (1988). Visual changes in daily life though adulthood. *Journal of Gerontology: Psychological Sciences, 43,* 63–70.

There are two primary scales used by the professionals who work with the people we serve. These are the Functional Independence Measure (FIM®) and the Manual Muscle Evaluation. Other scales frequently seen by the professional include the vital signs (blood pressure, pulse, and respiratory rate).

Some professionals may use a standardized testing tool in addition to scales to obtain more information about an individual. Some assessment tools have been written using ideas and information obtained from rigorous research. An example, the *Checklist for Nonverbal Pain Indicators*, is shown below.

The FIM® Scale

The Functional Independence Measure, or FIM® scale is a standardized, seven-point scale that measures the degree of independence an individual is able to demonstrate for any type of task. The professional may take any skill attempted by the individual s/he is assessing and use the FIM® scale to show how independent the individual was in completing the task. The FIM® Scale is shown below.

Manual Muscle Evaluation

One important measurement to be aware of is muscle strength. By knowing how much strength the individual has, the professional should also be able to understand how far the individual can walk, how long s/he can physically engage in activity, and what modifications to equipment (that might be too heavy) will be required. While the activity and recreational therapy professionals do not usually measure strength, it is important that they understand the meanings of the numbers used in the manual muscle strength evaluation. The table on the next page shows the five levels of the manual muscle strength evaluation.

FIM® Instrument

Independent — Another person is not required for the activity (No Helper).

7 **Complete Independence** All of the tasks described as making up the activity are typically performed safely without modification, assistive devices, or aids, and within reasonable time.

6 **Modified Independence** Activity requires any one or more than one of the following: an assistive device, more than reasonable time, or there are safety (risk) considerations.

Dependent — Another person is required for either supervision or physical assistance in order for the activity to be performed or it is not performed (Requires Helper).

Modified Dependence The subject expends half (50%) or more of the effort. The levels of assistance required are

5 **Supervision or Setup** Subject requires no more help than standby, cueing, or coaxing, without physical contact. Or, helper sets up needed items or applies orthoses.

4 **Minimal Contact Assistance** With physical contact the subject requires no more help than touching and subject expends 75% or more of the effort.

3 **Moderate Assistance** Subject requires more help than touching or expends half (50%) or more (up to 75%) of the effort.

Complete Dependence — The subject expends less than half (less than 50%) of the effort. Maximal or total assistance is required or the activity is not performed. The levels of assistance required are

2 **Maximal Assistance** Subject expends less than 50% of the effort, but at least 25%.

1 **Total Assistance** Subject expends less than 25% of the effort.

Manual Muscle Evaluation — Strength

100%	5	N	Normal	Complete range of motion against gravity with full resistance
75%	4	G	Good	Complete range of motion against gravity with some resistance
50%	3	F	Fair	Complete range of motion against gravity
25%	2	P	Poor	Complete range of motion with gravity eliminated
10%	1	T	Trace	Evidence of contractility
0%	0	0	Zero	No evidence of contractility
S			Spasm	If spasm or contracture exists, place S or C after the grade of a movement incomplete for this reason.
C			Contracture	

Pain Indicators

The most common scales used to measure pain show faces indicating the degree of pain. The resident indicates his/her current level of pain by choosing one of the faces. There are many scales to measure the severity of pain felt by a client. JCAHO provides a few examples including the *Wong-Baker FACES Pain Rating Scale* (Figure 1).

The *Wong-Baker FACES Pain Rating Scale* was originally developed for use with children at the Hillcrest Medical Center, Tulsa, Oklahoma, to help the staff measure the severity of a child's pain. While many of the other scales that measure pain used a metric scale of ten choices, the original authors, Donna Wong and Connie Morain Baker, felt that a six level scale (no pain plus five levels of pain) would be better understood by children. A modification to this six-point scale for use in nursing homes is the conversion of the scale to a 0–10-point scale using the numbers 0, 2, 4, 6, 8, and 10.

Figure 1: Wong-Baker FACES Pain Rating Scale (Wong, et al, 2001)

Wong-Baker FACES Pain Rating Scale	0	1	2	3	4	5
	No Hurt	Hurts Little Bit	Hurts Little More	Hurts Even More	Hurts Whole Lot	Hurts Worst
Alternative Coding	**0**	**2**	**4**	**6**	**8**	**10**

Brief word instructions: Point to each face using the words to describe the pain intensity. Ask the child to choose face that best describes own pain and record the appropriate number.

Original Instructions: Explain to the person that each face is for a person who feels happy because he has no pain (hurt) or sad because he has some or a lot of pain. **Face 0** is very happy because he doesn't hurt at all. **Face 1** hurts just a little bit. **Face 2** hurts a little more. **Face 3** hurts even more. **Face 4** hurts a whole lot. **Face 5** hurts as much as you can imagine, although you don't have to be crying to feel this bad. Ask the person to choose the face that best describes how he is feeling.

Rating scale is recommended for persons age 3 years and older.

From Hockenberry, M. J., Wilson, D, Winkelstein, M. L. *Wong's Essentials of Pediatric Nursing, ed. 7*, St. Louis, 2005, p. 1259.

Checklist of Nonverbal Pain Indicators

Date: ____________ **Patient Name:** ____________

Write a "0" (zero) if the behavior is not observed, and a "1" (one) if the behavior occurred even briefly during activity or rest.

	With Movement	Rest
1. **Vocal Complaints: Nonverbal** (Expression of pain, not in words, moans, groans, grunts, cries, gasps, sighs)		
2. **Facial Grimaces/Winces** (Furrowed brow, narrowed eyes, tightened lips, dropped jaw, clinched teeth, distorted expression)		
3. **Bracing** (clutching or holding onto side rails, bed, tray table, or affected area during movement)		
4. **Restlessness** (Constant or intermittent shifting of position, rocking, intermittent or constant hand motions, inability to keep still)		
5. **Rubbing** (Massaging affected areas, in addition, record verbal complaints)		
6. **Vocal Complaints: Verbal** (Words expressing discomfort or pain — "ouch," "that hurts" occurring during movement, or exclamations of protest — "stop," "that's enough")		
Subtotal Scores		
Total Score (Movement + Rest)		

Checklist of Nonverbal Pain Indicators

Measuring pain in residents with cognitive impairments is a challenge. They are not able to select a level of pain, even with pictures. Because of this difficulty with measurement, residents with cognitive impairment are significantly more likely to be undermedicated for pain than clients who exhibit little or no cognitive impairment (Geriatric Video Productions, 1998). Feldt (2000) developed a tool to measure pain in residents with cognitive impairment called the *Checklist of Nonverbal Pain Indicators* (*CNPI*) shown above. The *CNPI* is best used when the resident is moving about and engaging in activity, so this test is very appropriate for the activity professional to use.

Other Assessments

Two books that provide greater information on the subject are *Assessment Tools for Recreational Therapy and Related Fields, 4th Edition* by burlingame and Blaschko, 2010 and *Assessing Older Persons: Measures, Meaning, and Practical Applications* by Kane and Kane, 2004. A widely used assessment, the *Therapeutic Recreation Activity Assessment* (*TRAA*), measures fine motor skills, gross motor skills, social behavior, expressive communication, receptive communication, and cognitive skills. The *TRAA* may be used with individuals who range from very impaired and on bed rest to individuals who have only slight impairments. Another standardized testing tool is the *Leisure Assessment Inventory* (2002), which measures the leisure behaviors of adults using laminated color photographs. The *LAI* has four subscales: 1. the Leisure Activity Participation Index, reflecting the person's leisure participation, 2. the Leisure Preference Index, measuring activities in which the individual would like to increase participation, 3. the Leisure Interest Index, measuring the degree of unmet leisure involvement, and 4. the Leisure Constraints Index, assessing the degree of internal and external constraints that inhibit participation.

Discharge from the Nursing Home

The process of planning for discharge begins at the time of admission to the nursing home. At that time the treatment team will use the medical database and the resident/family goals to begin the process of discharge planning. This includes an assessment of the change in medical status that has necessitated admission, an assessment of the home situation (from resident/family interview), and discussion with the rehabilitation staff concerning the possibility of improvement.

Then progress must be monitored. To do so, it is essential to attend weekly rehab meetings. In terms of any successful determination of discharge potential, this may be the most important meeting of the week. At this session, you will have available to you all of the resources which are acting in either a rehabilitative or a supportive role with the resident. You will be able to examine his/her daily pattern from every aspect: dietary to therapy to activity level to nursing. From this comprehensive overview, you will be able to note progress (if any) and to inform the resident and the family of the consensus opinion, thus neither becomes unnecessarily discouraged nor encouraged and they can begin to plan and prepare the home environment if this seems feasible.

Many residents and families regard admission to the long-term care facility as final, but it is actually possible for many residents to return to a lesser level of care, either as a result of rehabilitative service or a change of condition toward — not away from — wellness.

Although some residents may not be able to go home due to the constraints of care needs or lack of support, other options exist in most communities and you can explore the choices with the resident while s/he is in the facility.

When home is the best answer, the family should enlist the assistance of the occupational therapist for a home visit to assess the safety and accessibility of the home. S/he can make valuable recommendations about removing hazardous rugs and other obstacles, and suggest ramps and safety bar placement (especially in bathrooms). The responsible party should be able to follow up on these suggestions, using parts that can be found in most hardware stores, to improve the safety of the home.

Once the environment has been made safe, follow-up care can be arranged. Home care agencies, some hospital-based, some private, are a rich source of assistance. They can provide physical therapists, occupational therapists, recreational therapists, skilled nurses, and home health aids.

If there is a Meals on Wheels program in the community, which can bring at least one hot meal a day, check to see if the resident would like to have the service. We like to recommend it for the first two weeks at home. It must be ordered by the doctor.

If the resident wants a homelike setting, but does not want all of the responsibilities that entails, there may be assisted living complexes in the community.

There are several variations on this theme. Some include well care, supervised care, and skilled nursing. Some have only the first two options. Some are only for those who are independent. Research the possibilities to find the best match for the resident.

Assisted living facilities will allow the individual to have all the possible amenities in his/her apartment, including his/her own furnishings and kitchen facilities. S/he will be able to use congregate dining facilities and planned activities within the complex, too. This is often a good transitional environment from total independence to the beginnings of supervised care. It is an excellent option if the individual is still able to be independent and manage his/her own personal and health care needs.

The next step toward supervised care is a board and care facility. Most board and care facilities pride themselves on being homey, but the sizes vary considerably and it is important to visit them to find the one that will best suit the resident's needs. Look for the availability of supervised care: medication administration and personal needs such as bathing and dressing. Then consider the match between the facility and the personal style of the resident:

- Does s/he prefer social settings or quiet and privacy?
- Are there grounds for strolling (and does the resident care)?
- Are there animals?

Board and care facilities will allow the resident to bring personal possessions such as a favorite chair. This will help the move seem more like a return home rather than like being a guest in someone else's home.

For both assisted living and board and care facilities, home care agencies will follow residents who have a doctor's order for follow up. Take advantage of these resources since they provide an excellent bridge between long-term care facility dependence and the next level of independence.

As exciting as the prospect of a discharge might seem to the health care workers, do not forget that the time leading up to the long-term care facility placement may have been extremely traumatic for the resident and the family. They may be reluctant to accept a discharge plan, seeing it as another opportunity for failure. It is important to assure them that a support system (usually home care) will be built into any discharge plan and that they, as the major components of the plan, must be honest and forthcoming with their input and their anxieties. Involving them at all levels of planning and organizing the discharge will give the discharge the best chance of success.

In anticipation of the discharge, the interdisciplinary team must complete an interdisciplinary discharge summary. In this way, resident and family will be given some of the tools needed to insure a successful return "home."

Writing the Discharge Summary[54]

A discharge summary is a report that the professional writes when s/he will no longer be treating the patient. This report may be seen by another health care professional the same day that the report is written or it may be reviewed by a health care professional years later. To help make the discharge summary useful and easy to understand, it is recommend that:

- Whenever possible, refer to the specific instead of the general; be concrete instead of abstract.
- Take care with what you say and how you say it. Avoid fancy or obscure words, abbreviations, or words that overstate. Avoid qualifiers such as "rather, very, little, pretty."
- When you write, be clear, document sequentially; be brief but do not take short cuts that might leave out key information.
- Whenever possible, write your statements in the positive, e.g., "patient was able to ambulate 45 feet between stores before needing to rest" versus "patient was not able to ambulate between stores before needing to rest." The second sentence leaves the reader wondering if the patient had no functional ambulation skills or if the patient could go 50 feet before needing a rest — two very different cases. While being positive, do not be reluctant to provide realistic or negative findings.
- If the treatment was as a result of a referral, make sure that all issues addressed in the referral are answered in the discharge summary.
- It will not be helpful to future readers of the discharge summary if you include just raw data from your assessments. Include a concise interpretation of all data presented.
- Whenever you make a recommendation, make sure that the justification for that recommendation can be found in your discharge summary.

[54] This section is used with permission from *Idyll Arbor's Therapy Dictionary* (2001). Idyll Arbor, Inc.

- Without being long-winded, include an alternative recommendation or an alternative course of action, if it is appropriate for the situation.
- Make your recommendations realistic for the patient, his/her cultural, social, and economic background, and for his/her discharge destination.
- Remember that the discharge summary is just that, a summary. All of the information presented should be brought together in a way that presents the entire picture of all the pertinent information. (Armstrong & Lauzen, 1994 and Zuckerman, 1994)

The MDS 3.0 amended Section Q to include question Q0500 asking the Resident (or family or significant other if resident is unable to respond): "Do you want to talk to someone about the possibility of returning to the community?"

A positive response requires contact with the Local Contact Agency. The Local Contact Agency may have different names for different states including Aging Disability Resource Center (ADRC), Center for Independent Living (CIL), Area Office on Aging (AoA), Area Agency on Aging (AAA), Relocation contractor, Dept. of Medicaid, MFP program, managed care organizations, etc. A state-by-state list is available from the national Department of Health and Human Services https://www.dhhs.nh.gov/dcbcs/beas/nhpct/documents/statecontacts.pdf

These agencies are given the responsibility of assessing and, when necessary, assisting with appropriate placement and supports for a disabled person in a skilled nursing facility who wishes to pursue other housing options. When speaking with a resident about this possibility, it is essential to stress that leaving the facility does not necessarily mean going to his/her own home. This might alter a person's desire to leave the nursing facility.

In 1999, the Olmstead v. L.C. decision by the Supreme Court ruled that people with disabilities do not need to remain in nursing facilities if they have the desire and potential to live in the community. It is important to know that it is not up to the skilled nursing facility to determine feasibility of community placement. The social services professional initiates contact with the Local Contact Agency which determines feasibility after interviewing the resident and family.

The county ombudsman's office should be able to provide the name of your Local Contact Agency.

A resident must have been living in a skilled nursing facility for 90 days on Medicaid in order to initiate the process of discharge through the Local Contact Agency.

When completing Q0600, there are two NO responses: For normal discharge planning purposes, check 0. When a person is likely to be long-term care, check 1. 2/yes, is in response to an actual referral to the Local Contact Agency based on the response to question Q0500.

12. Resident Assessment Instrument: MDS + CAAs

Every facility in the United States accepting Medicare and Medicaid funds is required to complete a comprehensive assessment using the Resident Assessment Instrument (RAI). Each state must use a standardized form that is approved by the Centers for Medicare and Medicaid Services (CMS). It must cover required core items and may include additional approved items individualized to each state. It is a functionally based assessment tool designed to establish a baseline for each resident. It is then used to track changes in a resident's psychosocial and functional status throughout his/her stay. The RAI provides a holistic view of each resident by assessing both quality of life and quality of care issues.

There are three components of the RAI: the Minimum Data Set (MDS), the Care Area Assessment (CAA) process, and the RAI utilization guidelines. The comprehensive care plan is the end result of the assessment process and may be thought of as the fourth component.

The Utilization Guidelines are found in the *RAI User Guide*, which is published by the Center for Medicare and Medicaid Services (CMS). It is a public document available online at www.cms.hhs.gov/manuals/Downloads/som107ap_pp_guidelines_ltcf.pdf or through various publishing houses. The *User Guide* explains each of the above components in great detail, and has numerous examples and case studies to make the instructions for MDS, CAA, and care planning completion very clear. Every professional should have a copy of this manual for his/her department and refer to it often when learning the RAI process.

A copy of the full MDS form can be found in Appendix B. Referring to the form while you read the various sections of this chapter will help you better understand the RAI assessment process.

Planning an individual's care is a five-step process. It starts with the initial assessments that you and the rest of the treatment team complete. After all of the assessments have been done, the team meets with the individual or his/her representatives to create a care plan that is designed to meet the needs of the individual, the goals you will be working on for the next quarter, and the progress you expect to see. The third step is implementing the care plan and monitoring the progress the individual is making. The fourth step is updating the care plan based on your observations of the individual or because the individual's condition changes. The final step, which may not be appropriate for all of the people you serve, is discharge planning. The discharge plan summarizes the current condition of the person, the care s/he has received, and the continuing care that will be needed.

Purposes of the RAI

The primary purpose of the RAI is to improve the quality of life and care for the nursing home resident. It facilitates assessment, decision making, and care planning as well as the implementation and evaluation of care.

There are several secondary purposes for the data gathered from the MDS form itself. The data is first transmitted electronically to a state repository. Once encoded, the data can be used for statistical purposes, for reimbursement, to monitor the quality of care in an individual nursing facility, to compare nursing home performance within the state and across the nation, and to provide information for consumers when choosing a nursing home.

These purposes and their corresponding data sets — Prospective Payment System (PPS), Resource Utilization Groups (RUG), the Quality Measure/Quality Indicator Report (QM/QI), the Quality Measures (QM), the Quality Indicator Survey (QIS), and the Nursing Home Compare web site will be discussed in more detail later in the chapter.

Overview of the RAI Process

The RAI provides a standardized structure for identifying and managing an individual resident's strengths and functional needs. It provides a smooth flow from problem identification to evaluation of the treatment plan.

Think of the RAI as a series of screens, going from a large screen to a finer screen. The MDS provides the first screen, which lets the Care Area Triggers (CATs) through, the CAAs provide the second screen, which lets actual and potential problems through, and the care plan is the last screen, which develops an action plan to address the problems and allows for ongoing assessment and screening out of unmet goals or resolved problems.

MDS — core data

CATs — areas for further in-depth review

CAAs — suggested problems/strengths for care planning (actual or potential high-risk problems/strengths)

Care Plan

Ongoing Review and Revision

Standardized Assessment

CMS mandates the core items in the assessment, the sequencing, and the definitions. States may add additional items at the end of the forms. There are three types of MDS forms:

- A full or comprehensive MDS, which is used for the initial, annual, and significant change assessments.
- A quarterly MDS, which is a subset of the full MDS.
- An MPAF MDS, which may be used for the Medicare PPS assessments.

A further standardization includes the requirements for completing the RAI and timing of ongoing assessments.

Timing of Assessments

The RAI completion date schedule that follows explains the completion requirements for each type of MDS. Please note that the day of admission is always counted as Day 1.

A typical resident will have a full assessment completed within 14 days of admission, three quarterly MDSs, and an annual full assessment. This cycle will continue while the resident remains in the facility. Additional assessments will be completed if the resident experiences a significant change in condition or if the resident is receiving Medicare Part A benefits.

Admission → Quarterly → Quarterly → Quarterly → Annual

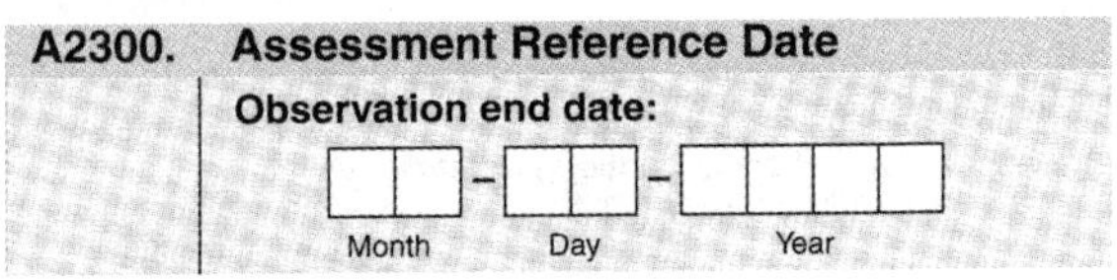
A2300. Assessment Reference Date
Observation end date:
Month Day Year

MDS Section A2300

The due date of the next assessment is calculated by using the Assessment Reference Date (ARD) of the previous assessment. This date is found in section A2300 of the MDS. For example, an annual assessment is due on the ARD of the last full assessment + 366 days. And a quarterly MDS is due on the ARD of the last assessment + 92 days. The MDS may be completed earlier than these dates but no later.

When completing the assessment, it is important that all persons involved use the same observation period. This is accomplished by setting an assessment reference date (ARD). This establishes the last day of the observation period. Commonly referred to as the "look-back date," this date is recorded in Section A2300 above. For example: if the look-back date is March 7th, all disciplines completing the MDS "look back" at the period between March 1 12:00 AM and March 7 11:59 PM. Only observations for this time period are used on the MDS. The exceptions are those questions that have a longer look-back period. The time frames for the look-back are specified in the RAI Guide and on the MDS forms. The majority of the look back periods are seven days.

When completed, the comprehensive MDS is electronically transmitted within 14 days of the Care Plan Completion date (V0200C2). A quarterly MDS is transmitted within 14 days of the MDS Completion Date (Z0500B). Failure to transmit on a timely basis can result in federally mandated sanctions. The list of completion day schedules is shown below.

RAI Completion Date Schedule

Assessment Type	Requirement	Assessment Reference Date (A2300)	Grace Day Period	Completion Date (V0200C2)	Payment Dates For Medicare
Medicare 5 day	PPS billing	Days 1–5 of admission	6–8	No later than day 14	Days 1–14
Admission assessment*	Regulatory compliance	Days 1–14	not applicable	No later than day 14	not applicable
Medicare 14 day	PPS billing	Days 11–14	15–19 unless used as admission assessment	No later than day 14 or 14 days from A2300 date	Days 15–30
Medicare 30 day	PPS billing	Days 21–29	30–34	14 days from A2300 date	Days 31–60
Medicare 60 day	PPS billing	Days 50–59	60–64	14 days from A2300 date	Days 61–90
Medicare 90 day	PPS billing	Days 80–89	90–94	14 days from A2300 date	Days 91–100
Quarterly	Regulatory compliance	No later than 92 days from V0200C2 date	not applicable	No later than 92 days from V0200C2 date	not applicable
Significant change* PPS	Follow definitions for significant change**	Within 14 days of noted change	not applicable	14 days from A2300 date	pays days from A2300 date to next assessment
Significant change*	Follow definitions for significant change**	Within 14 days of noted change	not applicable	No later than 14 days from the noted change	not applicable
Annual review*	Regulatory compliance	No later than 366 days from V0200C2 date	not applicable	No later than 366 days from V0200C2 date	not applicable

RAI Completion Date Schedule (continued)

Assessment Type	Requirement	Assessment Reference Date (A2300)	Grace Day Period	Completion Date (V0200C2)	Payment Dates For Medicare
Other Medicare required assessment (OMRA)	When all therapies are discontinued and no significant change in condition	8–10 days from discontinuation of the CAAs	not applicable	14 days from A2300 date	pays days from A2300 date to next assessment
Significant correction of prior assessment	follow definitions for significant correction	not applicable	not applicable	not applicable	adjusted prospectively from A2300 date

* requires completion of the CAAs and the care plan

** refer to the *RAI User Guide* for definitions of significant change

Completion of the MDS

The most accurate completion of the MDS is best accomplished by an interdisciplinary team (IDT), the resident, resident's family, and the direct caregivers. The coordination of the RAI completion is assigned to an RN, known as the Resident Assessment Coordinator (RAC). The RAC is responsible for assuring that all sections of the MDS and the CAAs are completed on a timely basis.

Often certain sections are assigned to an individual discipline for completion. If this is the case, the MDS should be reviewed as a group after each discipline has completed its sections. This allows the interdisciplinary team to get a holistic view of the resident before proceeding to care planning.

MDS Section		Designated Discipline
Section A.	Identification Information	Admitting, Social Services
Section B.	Hearing, Speech, and Vision	Nursing, Social Services, Speech Therapy
Section C.	Cognitive Patterns	Nursing, Social Services, Speech Therapy
Section D.	Mood	Social Services
Section E.	Behavior	Social Services
Section F.	Preferences for Customary Routine and Activities	Activities, Social Services
Section G.	Functional Status	Nursing, Therapies
Section H.	Bladder and Bowel	Nursing, Therapies
Section I.	Active Disease Diagnoses	Medical Records and Nursing
Section J.	Health Conditions	Nursing
Section K.	Swallowing/Nutritional Status	Dietary, Speech Therapy
Section L.	Oral/Dental Status	Nursing, Dietary
Section M.	Skin Conditions	Nursing
Section N.	Medications	Nursing
Section O.	Special Treatments and Procedures	Nursing, Therapies
Section P.	Restraints	Nursing
Section Q.	Participation in Assessment and Goal Setting	Social Services, Nursing
Section V.	CAA Summary	All
Section X.	Correction Request	RAC
Section Z.	Assessment Administration	All completing the form

For a detailed explanation of completion requirements including the assessment reference date and signature requirements, see Chapter 2 of the *RAI User Guide*.

Suggested responsibility for completion of each section is shown above. Note that these are suggestions only. Every facility will assign responsibilities according to staff strengths.

Conducting the Interview

The MDS 3.0 revision increased the resident's voice in the assessment process by introducing several resident interview items. All attempts should be made to have the resident be the primary source of information regarding their choices over aspects of their lives. The manual emphasizes the need to interview all residents capable of *any* communication. This includes residents with moderate to severe cognitive impairment who may be able to answer some simple questions.

If a resident cannot participate in the process, the family and/or significant other should be interviewed. If there is no family and/or significant other available, the staff completes the assessment.

Review of *Appendix D — Interviewing to Increase Residents' Voice in MDS Assessments* in the RAI user guide gives an idea of basic approaches that can be used to make the interviews effective. These include tips such as offering assistive hearing devices, using cue cards, and breaking questions apart so that a confused resident can better respond. Another reference provided for improving interview techniques is an instructional video titled *Interviewing Vulnerable Elders*. The video can be ordered directly from the Center for Medicare Services (CMS website https://www.cms.gov/Medicare/Quality-Initiatives-Patient-Assessment-Instruments/NursingHomeQualityInits/NHQIMDS30TrainingMaterials.html or from pioneernetwork.net.

Testing Tools

MDS 3.0 includes several standardized testing tools. The Brief Interview for Mental Status (BIMS) which identifies cognitive impairment, the Confusion Assessment Method (CAM) which assesses presence of delirium, and the Patient Health Questionnaire (PHQ-9(c)) which assesses for presence and frequency of depressive disorder.

These are conducted for all residents that can be interviewed. The results of these tests, found in Section C and D, should be reviewed prior to conducting the interview in Section F.

Section D: Mood

The information in this section looks at the most significant indicators of mood problems related to depression. Mood problems usually need to be addressed as an important part of the care plan.

Interview Questions

The instructions for conducting the interview are found in the Chapter 3 of the RAI user guide. These should be thoroughly read and understood prior to completing any interviews. There are nine questions regarding how the resident is feeling. The resident indicates if s/he has been feeling this way. For positive responses, the resident is asked how much of the time (or how often) s/he has had these feelings.

D0200 Interview Questions — Resident Mood

"Over the last 2 weeks, have you been bothered by any of these problems?"

A. Little interest or pleasure in doing things
B. Feeling down, depressed, or hopeless
C. Trouble falling or staying asleep, or sleeping too much
D. Feeling tired or having little energy
E. Poor appetite or overeating
F. Feeling bad about yourself — or that you are a failure or have let yourself or your family down
G. Trouble concentrating on things, such as reading the newspaper or watching television
H. Moving or speaking so slowly that other people could have noticed. Or the opposite — being so fidgety or restless that you have been moving a lot more than usual
I. Thoughts that you would be better off dead or of hurting yourself in some way

Response Coding
There are two answers coded on the score sheet: symptom presence and symptom frequency. The frequencies should be on a cue card that can be used to assist the resident, family member, or significant other. (See the sample cue card below.)

The response choices for symptom presence are
0: No
1: Yes
9: No response or non-responsive

The response codes for frequency (based on a 14-day look back period) are
0: Never or 1 Day
1: 2–6 Days (several days)
2: 7–11 Days (half or more of the days)
3: 12–14 Days (nearly every day)

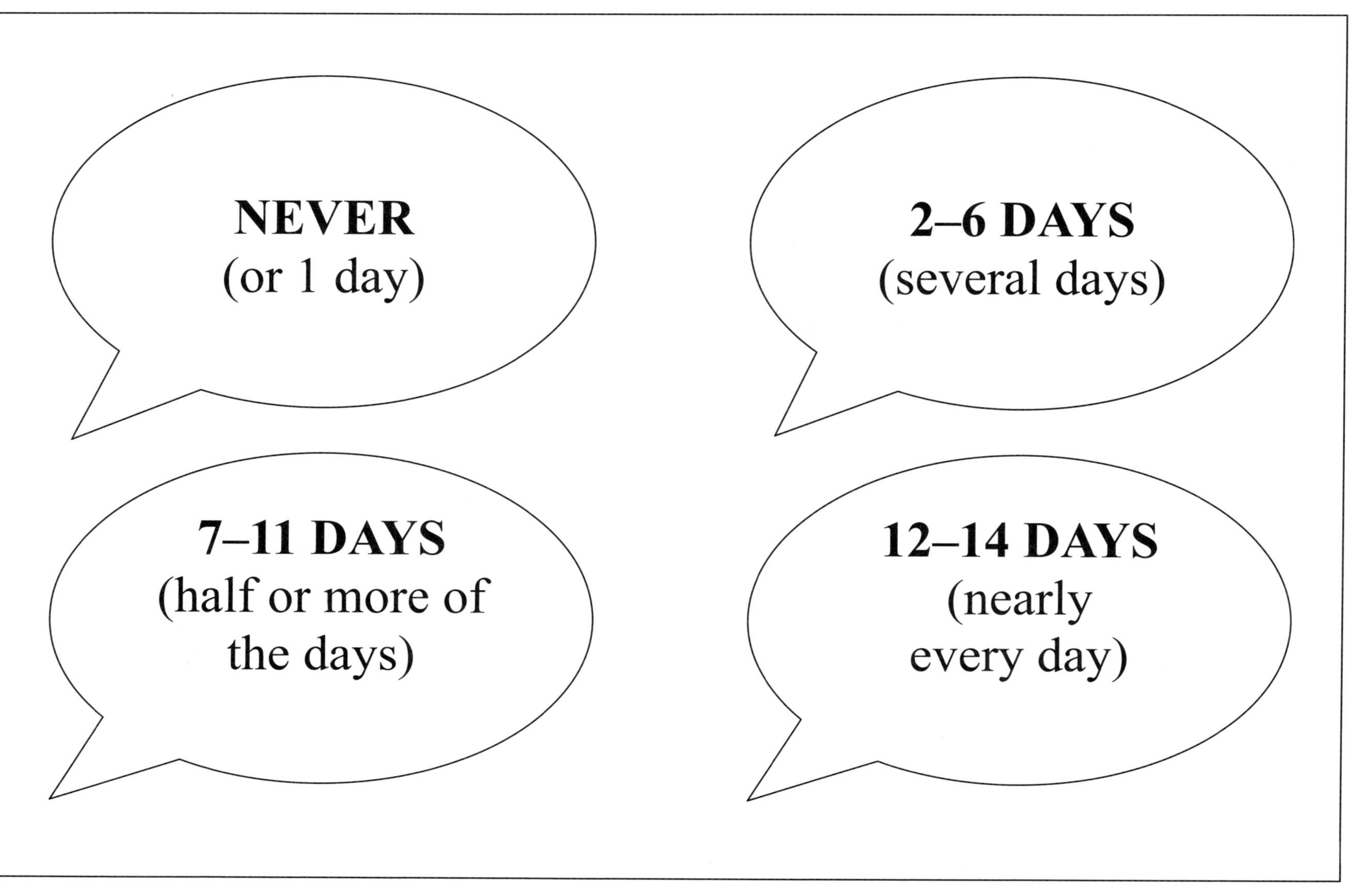

Figure 1: Sample response card for mood symptom frequency.

Section F: Preferences for Customary Routine and Activities

The information obtained from this section allows the resident to state what things are important for his/her ability to maintain a distinct lifestyle. It allows the resident's voice to be used in developing the care plan. As mentioned above, interviews should be attempted for *any* resident with the ability to communicate verbally, by pointing to their answers on the cue card, or by writing out their answers.

Residents exempted are those who are rarely/never understood (coded in section B0700 of the MDS) who need an interpreter but one is not available, and who do not have a family member or significant other available for the interview. In this case, the instructions state to skip to F0800, (Staff Assessment of Daily and Activity Preferences). The assessment is then completed using staff observations across all shifts and departments. Staff assessments should be needed for only a small percentage of your residents.

Interview Questions

The instructions for conducting the interview are found in the Chapter 3 of the RAI user guide. These should be thoroughly read and understood prior to completing any interviews. There are eight questions regarding preferences for individualized daily care and eight questions regarding what activities are meaningful and enjoyable for the resident.

F0400 Interview Questions — Daily Care
"While in this facility…"

A. how important is it to you to choose what clothes to wear?
B. how important is it to you to take care of your personal belongings or things?
C. how important is it to you to choose between a tub bath, shower, bed bath, or sponge bath?
D. how important is it to you to have snacks available between meals?
E. how important is it to you to choose your own bedtime?
F. how important is it to you to have your family or a close friend involved in discussions about your care?
G. how important is it to you to use the phone in private?
H. how important is it to you to have a place to lock your things to keep them safe?

F0500 Interview Questions — Activities
"While in this facility…"

A. how important is it to you to have books, newspapers, and magazines to read?
B. how important is it to you to listen to music you like?
C. how important is it to you to be around animals such as pets?
D. how important is it to you to keep up with the news?
E. how important is it to you to do things with groups of people?
F. how important is it to you to do your favorite activities?
G. how important is it to you to go outside to get fresh air when the weather is good?
H. how important is it to you to participate in religious services or practices?

Response Coding

There are five options for responding to the interview questions. These should be on a cue card that can be used to assist the resident, family member, or significant other. The code corresponding to the response is entered on the MDS.

The response choices are

Code 1: Very important

Code 2: Somewhat important

Code 3: Not very important

Code 4: Not important at all

Code 5: Important, but can't do or no choice

This choice reflects something that is important to the resident but can't be done due to health reasons, because it is not available in the facility, or because there is no choice due to scheduling. For example, the resident would like to stay up late but needs to be up early for physical therapy.

Code 9: No response or non-responsive

This code is used when the resident, family member, or significant other refuses to or can't answer the question. It is also used when the resident cannot formulate an answer or gives an incoherent or nonsensical answer.

A good resource for activity coordinators and other staff wanting some ideas and examples for interviewing and completing MDS 3.0 is *MDS 3.0 Interview Guidebook Section F Preference for Customary Routine and Activities.* Michele M. Nolta, CTRS, ACC. www.rec-therapy.com 858-546-9007.

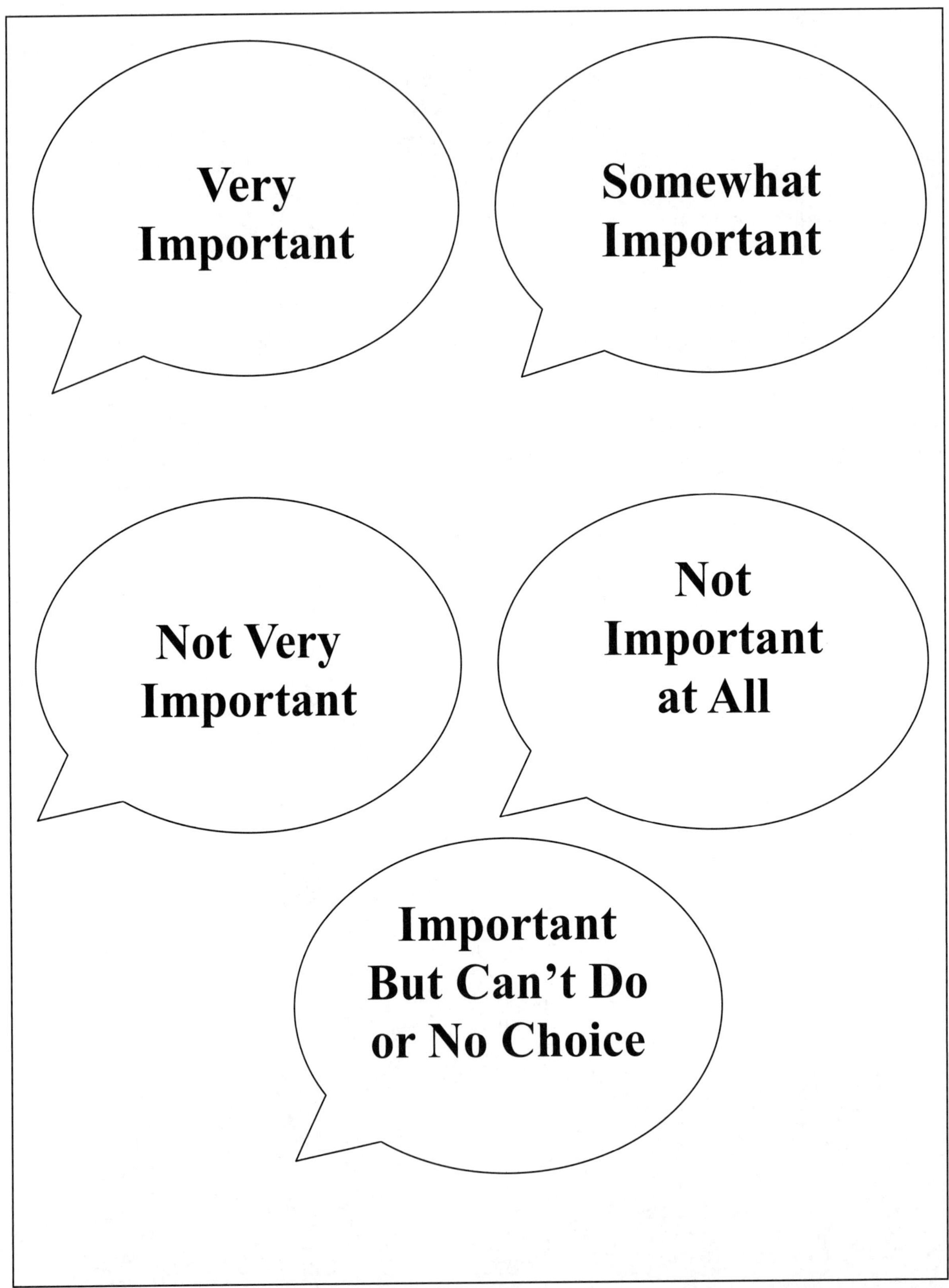

Figure 2: Sample response card for Section F questions.

The Care Area Triggers (CAT)

When the MDS is completed it provides a foundation for a more thorough assessment. Completion of a comprehensive MDS will trigger the Care Area Assessment (CAA) requiring further review. These are identified by responses to items coded on the MDS.

The items that "trigger" the CAAs can be found in each CAA. Review the Activity CAA in Appendix C of this book. Note that this CAA is triggered by items coded in Section D and Section F. Note also that other related CAAs that were triggered are also identified.

The first step in completing the CAA should be to understand why it triggered. This will help focus the further assessment on the potential problems, needs, or strengths identified.

Care Area Assessments

There are 20 Care Area Assessments:

1. Delirium
2. Cognitive Loss/Dementia
3. Visual Function
4. Communication
5. ADL Functional/ Rehabilitation Potential
6. Urinary Incontinence and Indwelling Catheter
7. Psychosocial Well-Being
8. Mood State
9. Behavioral Symptoms
10. Activities
11. Falls
12. Nutritional Status
13. Feeding Tubes
14. Dehydration/Fluid Maintenance
15. Dental Care
16. Pressure Ulcer
17. Psychotropic Medication Use
18. Physical Restraints
19. Pain
20. Return to Community Referral

Reviewing the triggered CAAs is the first step in developing a comprehensive care plan. The CAAs provide further assessment of "triggered areas" from the MDS. Just as the MDS provides broad screening for real or potential problems, the CAAs provide finer screening to determine actual needs and possible interventions. It helps to remember that the CAAs are the second screening process to determine whether or not a triggered area requires further follow-up through care planning.

Some triggered CAAs do not require care planning. The main determination of whether care planning is warranted or not is whether or not a realistic and achievable goal can be established for the suggested problem. In some cases it may be due to the resident's refusal to accept the IDT's suggested interventions. This should be documented and alternatives should be offered to the resident.

CAAs are required for the full MDS only. Completion of the CAAs is not required for the quarterly MDS or for PPS assessments.

CAAs for Activities

Although the activity department may be responsible for completing only one of the CAAs, it is necessary to review the entire MDS and all triggered CAAs prior to developing the activity department's person-centered plan. This is usually done in care conference; but if not, the activity department must take the responsibility to complete a thorough review of each section of the MDS and take note of which CAAs have triggered.

The MDS coding, especially in Cognition, ADL, Incontinence, and Mood and Behavior, will give more in-depth assessment information, and possibly more current information, than was gathered on admission. Many of the CAAs require or suggest interventions by the activity professionals in conjunction with the other interdisciplinary team

The following table lists the CAAs and suggested interventions to be considered by activities when developing the resident care plan.

CAAs Requiring Activity Intervention

Delirium	• Caused by recent relocation: Orientation program to provide calm, gentle approach with reminders and structure to help resident settle in. • Caused by diagnosis: Activity program to help prevent further cognitive decline and improve quality of life while problem is being treated.
Cognitive Loss or Dementia	• Provide positive experiences (e.g., enjoyable activities) for the resident that do not involve overly demanding tasks and stress. • Design programs to enhance resident's quality of life. • Provide opportunities for independent activity and participating more in decisions about daily life. • Segment tasks to make them easier to accomplish. • Provide small group programs. • Create special environmental stimuli (e.g., markers, special lighting).
Communication	• Provide opportunities to communicate, e.g., availability of partners. • Provide tactile approaches to communication. • Participate in restorative communication treatment program.
ADL	• Provide a program that supports rehabilitative goals for the resident.
Psychosocial Well-Being	• Provide social relationships. • Alter environment to allow access to others or routine activities. • Provide activities to address cognitive/communication deficits that may cause a lack of interest in activities or interactions with others. • Focus on a daily schedule that resembles the resident's prior lifestyle.
Mood State	• Passive residents with distressed mood may be overlooked. • Evaluate those with no involvement in activities (alone or with others) or little initiative.
Behavior Problems	• Participate in support programs that focus on managing behaviors. • Participate in activities where coping skills, relaxation, and anger management techniques are taught.
Activities	• Focus on residents who have indicated a desire for additional activity choices; cognitively intact, distressed residents who may benefit from an enriched activity program; cognitively deficient, distressed residents whose activity levels should be evaluated; and highly involved residents whose health may be in jeopardy because of their failure to slow down.
Restraints	• Participate in the restraint reduction program by providing activity programming to distract the resident with diversional activities or to relieve boredom. • Participate in exercise and strengthening programs to promote maximum functional independence.
Psychotropic Drug Use	• Participate in development of behavioral programming to support ongoing plans for drug reduction.
Pain	• Participate in interventions to reduce pain levels.
Return to Community Referral	• Support the resident's plans to return to a lower level of care.

CAAs Requiring Social Services Intervention

Delirium	Assess and intervene if caused by: • Isolation, • Recent loss of family/friend, • Depression/sad anxious mood, • Recent relocation, and/or • Sensory losses.
Cognitive Loss or Dementia	• Develop strategies to assist staff. • Teach staff and resident how to deal with behavioral manifestations of cognitive loss. • Develop a behavior control program. • Assess if problem could be remedied through improved staff education, referral to OT/RT for training, or an innovative counseling program. • Assess if emotional, social, excess disability, and/or environmental factors play a role in cognitive decline.
Visual Function	• Referral to optometrist/ophthalmologist if necessary. • Evaluate for appropriate use of visual appliances: glasses clean, labeled, reading glasses not used for walking. • Evaluate for effect of sad or anxious mood on visual dysfunction. • Provide appropriate devices for level of vision: large print calendar, clock, high wattage light, large print signs. • Refer to activities if necessary.
ADL	• Evaluate the effect of mood or behavior problems on ADL performance and motivation. • Develop a behavior control program to improve functioning.
Incontinence	• Evaluate the effect of incontinence on psychosocial well-being and social interactions and assist resident with coping with the dysfunction.
Psychosocial Well-Being	• Evaluate the effect of mood and behavior problems on feelings about self and social relationships. • Develop treatment program to focus on mood and behavior problems. • Develop corrective strategies to address distressing relationships and concern about loss of status.
Mood State	• Evaluate the need for new or altered care strategy when mood state problem are present: sad mood; feelings of emptiness, anxiety, or unease; loss of weight; tearfulness; agitation; aches and pains; bodily complaints and dysfunction.
Behavior Problem	• Develop alternate interventions and treatments to address behavior problems. • Identify the various factors involved in the manifestation of problem to identify behaviors that could be resolved and eliminate the problem.
Psychoactive Drug Use	• Develop monitors and care plan to address possible decline or impairment of cognitive and behavior status.
Physical Restraints	• Evaluate conditions associated with problem behaviors and physical restraint use: delirium impairment, cognition impairment, unmet communication needs, psychosocial needs, sad or anxious mood, resistance to treatment, medication, nourishment, motor agitation, confusion, gait disturbance. • Evaluate resident's response to restraint use. • Evaluate the philosophy, values, attitudes, and wishes of the resident regarding restraint use. • Develop monitors and care plan to address possible negative outcomes from restraint use.

How to Complete a CAA

The Interdisciplinary Team can complete CAAs as a group effort or CAAs can be assigned to certain disciplines. Usually the social services professional completes the Mood State, Behavioral Symptoms, and Psychosocial Well-Being CAAs. The activities professional is usually responsible for completing the Activities CAA. All triggered CAAs must be addressed.

The CAAs function as decision facilitators. They provide the basis for developing a problem list and formulating the resident's plan of care. After the MDS and CAAs are completed, the interdisciplinary team will be able to decide if:

- The resident has a cognition deficit that warrants intervention and addressing this problem is a necessary condition for other functional problems to be successfully addressed.
- Improvement of the resident's functioning in one or more areas is possible.
- Improvement is not likely, but the present level of functioning should be preserved as long as possible with rates of decline minimized over time.
- The resident is at risk of decline and efforts should emphasize slowing or minimizing decline and avoiding functional complications (e.g., contractures, pain).
- The central issues of care revolve around symptom relief and other palliative measures during the last months of life.

The most important requirement for CAA documentation is that you show the thought process in working the CAA. There are no mandated formats or forms for the process. A separate form can be used for CAA documentation or the CAA review can be included when completing the disciplines assessment form or the progress note. Four areas should be addressed when completing a CAA review:

- Nature of the condition
- Complications and risk factors that affect the staff's decision to proceed to care planning
- Factors that must be considered in developing individualized care plan interventions
- Need for referrals or further evaluation by appropriate health professionals

To complete the CAA review, use the following steps: *(Go through the CAA found in Appendix C for examples of how the steps are done in practice.)*

1. Determine Why the CAA is Triggered

This is an essential step in working the CAA. A CAA cannot be properly reviewed unless the reason for triggering is understood. A CAA is triggered by the MDS coding. Most computerized MDS programs will print a list of the triggered items for review. If not, a manual review of the MDS will be necessary.

2. Interpret the Significance of the Triggered Areas

There are no tools mandated for completing the further assessment of the triggered areas. The facility is instructed to use sound clinical problem solving and decision making. What is important is the facility uses tools that are current and based on current clinical practice guidelines. Appendix C of the RAI manual provides specific and general resources that the facility may use. The resources chosen for use must be available for surveyor review.

The key here is to determine if this is a real problem for the resident and, if so, why? For example, a resident may trigger the Activities CAA because he states it is not important at all to participate in religious practice. If the resident has been a life-long atheist, then this would not indicate a problem in need of care planning.

3. Problem-Solve

Determine what the nature of the problem is and why it is a problem for this resident. Don't stop at the condition but keep asking why until a root cause is identified. For instance, the resident triggers the Activity CAA because he states it is not at all important to do things with groups of people. Why is it not important? Is it because the resident is intimidated by large groups? Is it because of an image problem? Is it because of a hearing or vision problem? If it is because of a hearing problem — why? Is it due to a lost hearing aid, earwax, need for amplifier set? Keep asking questions until the underlying problems have been identified.

4. Complications and Risk Factors

The next step is to determine what complications or risk factors are associated with this problem. What other areas might need care planning to avoid associated declines? A resident with a hearing problem will have complications with communication. Associated risks might be a decline in cognition, mood, increase in behavior problems, and increase in safety needs.

5. Document the Rationale for Proceeding or Not Proceeding to the Care Plan

The MDS manual suggests the following process to decide whether to proceed or not.

How to Decide to Proceed or Not Proceed

- **Proceed** when a triggered condition affects a resident's functioning or well-being and the cause is resolvable, the problem can be minimized, or declines can be avoided. In this case, a realistic and achievable goal should be evident.
- **Do not proceed** if the triggered condition does not affect a resident's functioning or well-being. In this case there would be no problem to resolve, no goal to be met. If the resident does not want to pursue a problem, e.g. an overweight resident does not want to lose weight, even though it may affect her health, a care plan is not warranted. A goal cannot be met without the resident's participation.

The clinical decision-making process should be very clear in the documentation. A lengthy statement is not needed, but enough information should be given to clearly identify the rationale for proceeding to the care plan. Or if the decision is made not to address the problem in the care plan, you must make it clear why you determined that the triggered condition is not a problem for the resident.

This may appear anywhere in the record. It could be a narrative note, an assessment, a flow sheet, or the CAA summary sheet provided in the MDS manual. (See Appendix B.)

The resources or tools used for decision-making should be included in the summary.

6. Determine the Need for Referral to Another Health Professional

In some cases, the resident may benefit from a consultation by a qualified specialist. This could be a psychologist, dentist, audiologist, the facility dietitian or pharmacist, or other professional.

7. Document the Location of Information

Use the "location and date of CAA documentation" column on the CAA summary (Section V) to note where the CAA information and decision-making documentation can be found.

CAA Summary

The CAA summary form (on the next page) provides information on which CAAs were triggered, where the CAA review information can be found, and whether or not the team has decided to proceed with care planning. Completion is required with each comprehensive assessment MDS.

The location and date of the CAA review documentation is entered on the form in Section V0200 A. Only the primary source of documentation is listed. It is not necessary to list secondary sources used to assess. An entry may be

- CAA review 3/11/18, or
- Activity progress note 3/11/18

The care planning decision column is completed after the interdisciplinary team meets and discusses the care planning focus. The required completion date is seven days after the V0200B2 date.

Resident ______________________ Identifier ______________ Date ____________

Section V — Care Area Assessment (CAA) Summary

V0200. CAAs and Care Planning

1. Check column A if Care Area is triggered.
2. For each triggered Care Area, indicate whether a new care plan, care plan revision, or continuation of current care plan is necessary to address the problem(s) identified in your assessment of the care area. The Care Planning Decision column must be completed within 7 days of completing the RAI (MDS and CAA(s)). Check column B if the triggered care area is addressed in the care plan.
3. Indicate in the Location and Date of CAA Documentation column where information related to the CAA can be found. CAA documentation should include information on the complicating factors, risks, and any referrals for this resident for this care area.

A. CAA Results

Care Area	A. Care Area Triggered	B. Care Planning Decision	Location and Date of CAA documentation
	↓ Check all that apply ↓		
01. Delirium	☐	☐	
02. Cognitive Loss/Dementia	☐	☐	
03. Visual Function	☐	☐	
04. Communication	☐	☐	
05. ADL Functional/Rehabilitation Potential	☐	☐	
06. Urinary Incontinence and Indwelling Catheter	☐	☐	
07. Psychosocial Well-Being	☐	☐	
08. Mood State	☐	☐	
09. Behavioral Symptoms	☐	☐	
10. Activities	☐	☐	
11. Falls	☐	☐	
12. Nutritional Status	☐	☐	
13. Feeding Tube	☐	☐	
14. Dehydration/Fluid Maintenance	☐	☐	
15. Dental Care	☐	☐	
16. Pressure Ulcer	☐	☐	
17. Psychotropic Drug Use	☐	☐	
18. Physical Restraints	☐	☐	
19. Pain	☐	☐	
20. Return to Community Referral	☐	☐	

B. Signature of RN Coordinator for CAA Process and Date Signed

1. Signature

2. Date ☐☐ – ☐☐ – ☐☐☐☐ (Month, Day, Year)

C. Signature of Person Completing Care Plan Decision and Date Signed

1. Signature

2. Date ☐☐ – ☐☐ – ☐☐☐☐ (Month, Day, Year)

MDS Section V

The MDS for Reimbursement

The Balanced Budget Act of 1997 created widespread payment and regulatory reform for many health care providers. CMS's goals were to enhance access to care, improve equity and predictability of payment amounts, streamline the payment processes, and improve quality of patient care.

Prospective Payment System (PPS)

The Prospective Payment System is used by all facilities for Medicare Part A reimbursement. In some states, the Medicaid reimbursement is also based on the PPS system. This payment system is based on a patient classification system known as the Resource Utilization Group system version IV (RUG-IV). It is a case-mix system that uses Minimum Data Set (MDS) assessment data to classify residents into different payment groups or RUG categories. A set dollar amount per day — the per diem rate — is assigned to each RUG category. The reimbursement rate is based on the skilled services needed and the amount of care the resident requires. This rate is adjusted by region and urban and rural settings.

Briefly the process is as follows: an MDS assessment is completed for the appropriate billing period and the MDS is entered into the facility MDS software program. A feature of the software, referred to as the grouper software, "groups" the resident into a RUG-IV category based on the MDS coding. Grouper software is specially designed computer software that takes the information from the MDS assessment and, after analyzing the information, assigns the resident to a RUG (or payment) category. The RUG-IV code, which can be found in Section Z0100 of the MDS, is entered on the appropriate billing form, and the MDS is electronically transmitted to the Medicare fiscal intermediary.

Timing of PPS Assessments

For the Medicare resident there is a potential for completion of as many as seven assessments in the first three months of stay. Setting the assessment reference dates and completion dates is critical for reimbursement. Failure to meet the completion dates will result in receiving the default rate, the lowest reimbursement rate. It is important that the interdisciplinary team meet daily to review the time frames for the assessment reference dates and completion of each MDS.

For Part A, an MDS must be submitted for each Medicare billing period, on discontinuation of all therapies if the resident continues to meet skilled coverage requirements, and for significant change in condition. Refer to the RAI Completion Date Schedule for calculating specific completion dates. Note that completion of CAAs and the care plan is not required for a PPS assessment unless it is combined with a comprehensive assessment.

The Resource Utilization Groups Version IV (RUG-IV)

As stated above, the MDS is used as a case mix payment system for Medicare. States also have the option to use the RUG system for Medicaid reimbursement.

Reimbursement is based on the resident's nursing needs, ADL impairments, cognitive status, behavioral problems, and medical diagnoses. Residents with higher needs are assigned to a higher group in the RUG-IV hierarchy and are reimbursed at a higher level.

There are eight major classification categories: Rehabilitation plus Extensive Services, Rehabilitation, Extensive Services, Special Care High, Special Care Low, Clinically Complex, Behavioral Symptoms and Cognitive Performance Problems, and Reduced Physical Functioning.

Accurate assessment and observations by all staff are needed to assure that the level of reimbursement is appropriate for the resources used in caring for the resident. The activity professional can assist by reporting any noted changes in ADL dependency or changes in behaviors or cognition. Any new indicators of depression should be reported as well. These can be evaluated using the Resident Mood Interview (PHQ-9(c)) or the Staff Assessment of Resident Mood (PHQ-9-QV(c)), as described earlier in this chapter in Section D: Mood.

The MDS for Quality Assurance

Several reports are generated from the MDS submission. These include the Facility Measure/Indicator Report, the Quality Measures, and the Nursing Home Compare website.

Facility Measure/Indicator Report

Commonly referred to as the Quality Indicators (QIs), this is a monitoring system for evaluating care in nursing homes. The QIs are organized into domains, such as pressure ulcers, weight loss, and little time in activity. The statistics provided compare the facility with comparison groups by providing state and national averages for each domain. They are used to focus quality monitoring and quality improvement activities by federal and state regulatory agencies.

The QIs are flags to draw attention to potential problem areas that need further review and investigation. QIs can help facilities identify areas or delivery systems in the facility that may be improved through the facility's Quality Assurance program. The QIs are also used to focus onsite Quality Indicator Surveys (QIS) on potential problem areas.

The QI domains that require attention by the Activities professional are

- Falls
- Behavior/Emotional Patterns
- Cognitive Patterns
- Weight Loss
- Pain
- Physical Functioning — Bedfast
- Psychotropic Drug Use
- Quality of Life — Restraints and prevalence of little or no activity

The Quality Indicators are used in the new version of the survey process. To read about the survey process, refer to page 386

Quality Measures

These are a modified set of MDS data similar to the QIs but accessible to the consumer on the Nursing Home Compare website.

Nursing Home Compare

In an effort to provide the consumer with information to make an informed decision when choosing a nursing home, CMS has developed the Nursing Home Compare website. The site provides information regarding recent surveys, staffing, and quality measures. The site is www.medicare.gov/NHCompare/home.asp

13. Care Planning

This chapter will look at how to create a care plan from the assessment process. The goal of care planning is to aid the resident in attaining or maintaining his/her highest practicable physical, mental, and psychosocial well-being. This is the concept of the person-centered care plan. While care plans identify problems to be managed or eliminated, they also identify strengths to be built on to help the resident achieve the highest possible quality of life and to meet his/her desired goals. These areas are pinpointed in the MDS and brought forward for further assessment in the CAA process.

The care plan is the culmination of the assessment process. It is the final distillation of the resident's problems, needs, and strengths. The care plan provides a "road map" to the resident's caregivers describing conditions to be treated, expected outcome, and the care to be given. It is, most importantly, where the resident's voice is heard.

Time Frames

The comprehensive care plan is mandated to be completed seven days after completion of the MDS and CAAs (the VB2 date). This is 21 days after the day of admission. It is reviewed and updated as necessary with change in resident status and at least quarterly with the MDS review. The federal guidelines now require an interdisciplinary baseline care plan to be written within 48 hours of admission. This gets the process going and then the team continues to assess and then create the 21st-day care plan.

Components of the Care Plan

There is no mandated format or language for care planning. The only required components are

- Measurable objectives
- Time frames
- Services to be furnished

Care plans should be simple. Remember the purpose of the care plan is to deliver care to the resident. The entries should be written at a level that can be understood by all caregivers and the resident or his/her family. There is no magic number of required care plan entries. The resident's functional level and medical needs will determine the number of entries.

In order to keep a care plan simple and concise, problems are often merged or blended. Very often a problem may present many manifestations. For instance, a resident that is depressed may have a decline in activity participation, weight loss, use of an antidepressant, and more dependency with ADLs. If each of these problems were written up separately, there would be five problems on the care plan. It is likely that each of these problems would have similar interventions. None of these problems will resolve individually until the resident's depression is resolved. By merging or blending these problems into one entry, the interdisciplinary team can work toward a common goal.

When merging problems, there may be several goals. Each discipline will be adding interventions to meet these goals. The examples of care planning that follow give an idea of how a merged problem might look.

How to Write a Problem, Need, or Strength Statement

- Be specific in your description of the resident.
- Use words found in the MDS and CAA documents.
- Needs will be suggested by the CAAs, but do not rely on these alone. All conditions requiring intervention identified in the assessment process should be included in the care plan.

How to Write a Goal

- Be realistic.
- State the desired outcome using descriptive words so that it is obvious when the goal has been met.
- Make the goal measurable.
- Include a time frame to indicate when the goal should be reevaluated.

How to Write Interventions

- Be specific about how the intervention applies to the resident.
- Do not list interventions generic to all residents such as "need to escort to activities," "calendar in room," or "provide calm environment."
- Do not list one-time interventions such as "psych eval."
- Include the discipline responsible for providing the care with the intervention statement.

Gathering Data for the Care Plan

Although the RAI is the major source for care planning, the team should not neglect problems or risks identified through other sources. Data gathered from the individual disciplines' assessments, risk assessments, and information from families should always be considered when developing the care plan. For example, if a risk assessment identifies the resident as a high risk for falls, this should be considered for care planning even though the Falls CAA was not triggered.

Using the CAAs to Create a Care Plan

Completing a CAA almost writes the care plan by itself. The following CAAs will illustrate this concept. Note the underlined words — these are the beginnings of the care plan. Note that this care plan also combines the discharge plan (marked in *italics*). Social services and activities have merged entries with common goals.

Types of care plans

Care plans can be functional or person-centered. In this section we will look at examples of each type.

Functional Care Plans

The first set of care plan examples is based on a functional model. These care plans focus on the functional needs or strengths of the resident as identified by the MDS and CAA review. They are resident specific but do not reflect the resident voice. The resulting plan is shown in the box on the next page.

Triggered due to <u>not wanting to do favorite activities</u>. <u>Energy reserves are low</u> after therapy. Prefers to <u>rest in bed</u> and not pursue usual interests of knitting and gardening. Short-term stay with goal to <u>work with therapy and return home</u>. Care plan will support goals for discharge.

Need Statement	**Goal**	**Intervention**
Does not want to participate in usual activities As evidenced by: prefers to rest in bed when not involved in rehab Contributing factors: new to facility reduced energy reserves Strengths: focused on rehab program	Will not manifest complications of boredom as seen by: No apathy towards discharge or rehab plans for the next 2 weeks *Discharge to home with in-home health care in the next 2 weeks*	1. Daughter to bring husband to visit 3x wk for dinner. (SSD/CNA) 2. Short daily visits from AD and SSD to provide her with company.. 3. Calendar in room to mark off days until return home. AD to use pink highlighter with daily visits. (AD) 4. Radio by bedside. Tune to easy listening station. (AD/CNA) 5. Daily visits from SSD to *review discharge plans*, and progress in rehab. (SSD)

ː plan will combine ADL, Mood, Psychoactive Drug Use, and Activities CAAs in care
'e plan for this CAA review will look like the one in the box below.

o calling out for help, crying, and sad pained expression. Her mood is not easily altered
sponded to antidepressant therapy. She is in obvious distress and her mood is affecting
psychosocial functioning. Will create a care plan to address her need for relief from her
sympt... efer to psychologist and pharmacist for medication review.

Need Statement	Goal	Interventions
Decline in Mood, ADL, and psychosocial functioning As seen by: • calling out for help, crying, sad, pained expression • does not respond to attempts to alter mood • current antidepressant ineffective • decline in activity participation and socialization • more dependent with ADLs Contributory factors: • dementia (NCD) • memory and decision-making skills impaired Strengths: Strong family support	Will demonstrate benefit from antidepressant and relief of symptoms of distress as seen by: No side effects from change in antidepressant in 2 weeks Return to participation in AM coffee social and PM sensory awareness group in 4 weeks Improvement in dressing to limited assist in 4 weeks	1. Follow psychologist plan for mood alteration: see attached interventions. (All Staff) 2. Observe for side effects of new medication: Prozac. (LN) 3. Visit with resident daily for AM coffee. Bring out to group if resident expresses willingness. (AD) 4. Ambulate resident to sensory group daily. Allow to watch and participate if willing. (CNA/RNA) 5. Use task segmentation for dressing. Do not overwhelm with choices in daily attire. (CNA) 6. Engage family in mood alteration plan with weekly visits. (SSD)

This care plan demonstrates several points about care planning. In intervention #1 the psychologist's plans are referenced but not repeated on the care plan. If specific detailed plans for care have been outlined by a discipline, it is not necessary to repeat them. A copy can be placed behind the care plan entry, which can then be referred to by all caregivers. Also note that all of the interventions begin with an action verb and are related to the goals. This is the idea behind care planning. State specifically what needs to be done with the resident to accomplish each goal.

The next page shows a care plan for Barbara Best based on the information presented in the previous chapter.

Sample Care Plan for Barbara Best

Need Statement	Goal	Interventions
Limited Response to Stimulation Contributory factors: • Advanced Alzheimer's • Inability to understand/be understood • Decreased energy reserves • Frequent periods of sleep and rest with eyes closed Strengths: • Family involved • Makes eye contact • Behaviors resolved with current plan	Will continue to respond to staff/family visits as seen by smiling in response to visits by next review	Staff to visit often for short periods for handholding. (All) Big band/musical CDs at bedside. Play softly during the day. (AC) Gentle hand massage with lotions. (AC, RNA) Encourage verbalization in her "own language." (All)

I-Care / Person-Centered Care Plans

The second set of care plan examples are based on I-Care Plans or Person-Centered care plans. These plans are written from the resident's perspective — in their voice. They can be used with a standard care plan form as above or they can follow a different format as seen in the following example. They don't focus on functional limitations but on the areas that are important to the resident in choices regarding daily care and activities. Note that the care plan includes the resident's desired interventions and desired goals that meet regulatory requirements.

I Care Plan

NAME: HENRY JOHN DOE DATE: 08/10/2018 ADMIT DATE: 06/06/16

ADDRESS ME AS: JOHN OR MR. DOE BIRTH DATE: 06/29/1936

SOCIAL HISTORY:

I was born in Peoria Illinois. My grandfather moved there from Switzerland. He was a bicycle maker. My father was a dentist and we moved to Chicago when I was 10 years old. I attended Northwestern University, then University of Iowa for my advanced degree. I have advanced degrees in electrical and mechanical engineering. I worked for Bell Telephone Laboratories during the war. I am proud of the fact that I helped develop the equipment for radar that was used during the war.

I was married for 45 years to the light of my life, Betty. I miss her every day. I have 4 children — 3 boys and one girl. We stay in touch. My daughter will be visiting me often.

SPECIAL CONSIDERATIONS:

MEMORY ENHANCEMENT: Overall I do pretty well. I get fuzzy on dates and the day of the week but it doesn't bother me. I've always mixed names up — if I get yours wrong don't assume it's because I am getting senile.

I like to stay up with the news through the TV and radio. Please deliver my newspaper daily. I've always been a reader and like books on WWII, trains, and American history. I don't need big print yet. I'd like to go to the library.

My goal is to stay mentally active through daily reading and conversation for my stay here.

RECREATION / QUALITY OF LIFE: I've never been interested in joining in on games or sports. My usual routine is to get up late, eat lightly, watch a little TV or read and then eat lunch. After lunch I like to take a long nap and then get up again to watch the afternoon courtroom shows, especially Judge Judy. I may stay up after dinner or may go to bed early. Just depends on how I feel and what's on the tube. I don't like to be bothered with interruptions if I am watching TV or reading. I'm happy doing these things on my own. I miss my little dog Beanie.

I do like to watch football — professional and college. I like the facility dogs. Not cats.

Please invite me to events involving food. I enjoy donuts and coffee or any kind of pastry. And don't call me honey or dear or tell me how cute I am.

My goal is to take it easy and enjoy my simple pleasures for my stay here.

Revising the Care Plan

The care plan is a dynamic tool for resident care. It should be revised as often as the resident's needs change. At minimum the care plan is reviewed every 90 days with completion of the quarterly MDS. Changes in coding on the MDS may indicate a need to revise the care plan either due to an improvement or due to a decline in functional status. The process for determining if the care plan needs to be revised is as follows:

- Review all sections of the MDS for coding changes from the previous assessment
- Review the care plan entry specific to the MDS section with coding changes
- Determine if the problem statement is accurate or needs to be revised, rewritten, or discontinued
- Determine if the goal is still realistic, if it has been met, if the time frame needs to be changed, or if a new goal is needed
- Determine if the interventions are still appropriate and in effect or if a revision is needed. As a rule of thumb, when a goal is not met, it indicates that interventions were not effective. It may also mean that the goal was not realistic or achievable.

Procedures for changing the care plan vary for each facility. What need to be evident are the changes made, the date of revision, and a signature. Electronic records will provide a method to do this. On paper forms this can be accomplished by using a highlighter pen, a red line, or some other method that meets with legal documentation principles. If the care plan is reprinted, the changes made should be evident on the old copy of the care plan.

Updating the care plan for a temporary change of condition

When a resident experiences a temporary change in condition, such as the flu, urinary tract infection, or pressure ulcer requiring bed rest, the activity professional needs to assess the resident for a risk of decline due to increased isolation or decreased activity. Most care planning systems have a short-term problem care plan separate from the comprehensive care plan. If after assessing the resident for increased risks it is determined that a temporary change in interventions is needed, the activity professional should add to the problems on the short-term care plan.

Care Plan Examples

Getting a feel for writing a care plan can take some practice, so here are a few more examples of care plans. Each is written in a slightly different style to help you find a way of writing care plans that is comfortable for you.

Mrs. Y has triggered the Mood, Psychosocial, ADL, Activities, and Nutritional CAAs. The Interdisciplinary Team has decided that her most acute need is to resolve her mood problem as this is causing most of her other problems and impeding her rehabilitation goals. The team care plan merging all of the above CAAs is shown below.

Sample Integrated Care Plan

Problem, Need, Strength	Objective	Interventions	Dsc
Alteration in Mood as evidenced by: • Expresses sadness over lost status • Anger at nursing home placement • Spends little time in activities • Leaves over 25% uneaten • Lacks interest in rehab • Frustration over lack of speech Contributory factors: • Recent CVA with dysphasia • Recent decline in ADLs • Recent nursing home placement Strengths: • Close family and church group support • Good rehabilitation potential	Will eat 80% of breakfast & lunch QD by 1/20/18 Will verbalize acceptance of disability and need to participate in rehab by 1/20/18	Hipro with each meal SSD to provide substitutes for food refused Encourage husband and friends to bring in favorite foods Introduce to stroke support group Visit with facility dog Discuss Discharge Plan in positive terms Ask yes/no questions Allow time to express thoughts Psych visit 1x wk PT to describe interim goals to be met to achieve discharge Space to be arranged for daily visits from friends	D D All SS AC DC All All Psy PT AC

Sample Activity Care Plan Entries

The *Care Planning Cookbook for Activities and Recreation* by Nolta contains problem/need statements, goals, and over 300 care plan approaches and interventions. A sample care plan on anxiety is shown below. Choose the entries that are appropriate for the resident and integrate them into the care plan. Tie in with existing problems and needs if possible. The *Care Plan Guide for Person Centered Dementia Care* is also available from this company.

Category: Emotional Issues Subtopic: Anxiety

Problem Description, Concern, Need, or Strength	Goal/ Objective	Approach/ Interventions
Resident often appears to become anxious during activity programs evidenced by wringing hands, jumping at every sound, rigid posture, frequently yelling for help, ________________. Resident often states, "I'm not sure I should be here. I have lots of things to do in my room." Resident needs one-on-one attention to promote participation during activity programs secondary to displaying anxious behaviors.	Resident will not exhibit anxious behavior of ____________________, for ____ minutes, at ____________ group activities, ____ times per week. Resident will participate in ______________ activity programs by following the group's general directions, ____ times per week.	Invite, assist Resident to group activities of interest (i.e. __________________ ____________________). Explain the activity program's format to Resident prior to the start of program. Allow Resident to choose seating placement at program. Introduce to other alert peers. Identify similarities between Residents to promote conversation and friendships. Ask the Resident direct questions to promote participation. Refocus the Resident's attention to the specific activity task of ____________ if anxious behavior is exhibited. Compliment the Resident for following the activity program's directions.

Nolta, Michele M. 2010, *MDS 3.0 Care Plan Cookbook*. p. 5–5, Recreation Therapy Consultants, San Diego, CA.

The chart below shows more possible entries in a resident care plan specific to activities. These could be combined with existing problems/needs on the care plan.

Problem/Need	**Goal**	**Approach**
Poor pathfinding skills — needs to go between room and dining room	Resident will be able to go between room and dining room without assistance within 3 months.	1. Visual cue on door. 2. Walk with Resident to and from dining room. 3. All staff to praise efforts of Resident.
Sensory deprivation — needs tactile stimulation	Resident will receive a minimum of 20 minutes of tactile stimulation a day.	1. Pet visits 2x weekly. 2. Massage hands with lotion 3x weekly. 3. 1:1 with sensory stimulation kits 2x weekly
Personal appearance sloppy, beard stubble, uncombed hair, body odor — needs to improve grooming	Resident will shave at least every two days, comb hair daily, and bathe daily.	1. AC to visit with grooming items 2x weekly. 2. Grooming group 2x weekly. 3. CNAs to assist with AM care.
Hearing impairment — needs to be seated next to group leader	Resident will learn to sit next to leader where s/he can hear and respond to reminiscing questions.	1. Seat Resident next to leader in Current Events 1x weekly. 2. Reinforce advantages of sitting where s/he can hear. 3. Use visual cues.
Blindness and deafness — needs increased social contact	Resident will have at least 20 minutes of structured social contact 7x weekly.	1. AC to assist weaving hand over hand 4x weekly. 2. Resident will roll yarn ball for project. 3. Include in cooking, gardening, and outdoor events for social interactions 5x weekly.
Self-stimulation — needs to keep hands busy due to dementia	Resident will fold napkins for social events by 3 months.	1. AC to set up folding station for Resident 1x daily. 2. AC/volunteer to visit Resident with tactile stimulation 2x weekly.

Other Resident Care Plan Considerations

If your facility uses hand-written resident care plans, you can leave a few lines between your entry and the ones above and below. As the resident's needs change and interventions are revised, there is room to add new entries.

Be realistic, both in your identification of a problem and the approach. Do not enter "will visit 4x weekly" on the care plan, if you realistically cannot visit more than two times weekly.

Be specific in your interventions. For example, do not enter "Group activities 1x wk," but rather "Go to sing-along 1x week."

Be sure that the goal that is stated on the care plan is the same as the one discussed in the quarterly note. You must be sure that all parts of the care plan come from observations in the assessments and that every observation of problems or needs in the assessments — especially triggers in the MDS if the team decides to proceed — are addressed in the care plan. The team may choose not to proceed with a triggered CAA, but they must document why they made that decision.

There are some terms to avoid in identifying a problem on the care plan. The following chart offers some alternatives that are more descriptive and offer clearer connections between the problem and the treatment.

Don't say this	Say this to be more descriptive
social isolation OR loneliness	needs to be aware of people around him/her OR needs to feel useful to others
non-responsive	fear of answering inappropriately in a group setting
confusion	needs to improve problem-solving skills
short attention span	needs to follow one directive in exercise class OR needs to stay on task with project for 5 minutes
disorientation	needs to locate room
too tired	needs energy conservation techniques due to COPD
boredom	needs to develop one new leisure interest
lack of awareness	needs to stimulate short-term memory retention
anxious	cries easily due to CVA or has anxiety due to CVA
need for diversional activities	needs diversion to decrease agitation
needs sensory stimulation	needs to respond to _____ stimulation as seen by blinking eyes, holding object, etc. Be specific as to what type of stimulation — tactile, visual, auditory, etc.
refuses to attend	This is the resident's choice and is not a problem for the resident. Your problem is to devise activities that the resident will choose to participate in.
needs transportation to activities	This is your problem to solve not the resident's problem.

14. Monitoring the Treatment Plan

Assessing the participant and writing the care plan are not the end of the treatment process for the individual's care. There must be an ongoing process to monitor the status of each participant. You must make notes in the participant's chart whenever there is any change of condition that affects the individual's functioning or ability to participate in programming. Every quarter the care team must meet to perform a quarterly review of each participant's care plan, which includes determining if the most recent assessment of the participant's condition is still correct.

Monitoring Tools — Activities

There are several ways to make sure that your treatment plan is still appropriate for the participant. The methods include:

- Daily Activity Attendance (Participation) Records
- One-to-One Log Notes
- Progress Notes
- Quality Indicators

Participation Records

Records must be kept on each individual's participation in activities and treatment programs. The records must be kept seven days a week. Just documenting that an individual attended or participated in an activity is telling only part of the story. You also need to document the level of participation. The following pages show a set of forms you can use to keep a record of participation. We recommend that the activity professional use two different kinds of forms for documentation of participation:

- Activity Participation Sheet
- Special Programming/One-to-One Log

The first form, the *Activity Participation Sheet*, shows a way to keep track of each individual's participation in group activities. You don't have to use this exact form, but it includes the set of information that you do need to keep. (You, of course, need to have the activities from your facility listed.) The important components to include are participant name, type of activity, date, and length of time. You also want to use a code that shows the level of participation (active or passive). When an individual refuses an invitation to an activity or room visit, be sure to mark "R" for refuse. This will document that you attempted to include him/her and that it is his/her right to refuse.

For individuals who are restricted to their beds or who do not attend activities 2–3 times per week, you need to keep additional documentation to show their involvement in activities. One way to do this is with a bedside log shown in the second form. Whatever type of log you decide to use, it must describe the type of visit (what you did), length of the visit, date, and the individual's response.

Activity Participation Sheet

Participant Name ______________________________ **Room #**__________

Active = A **Observed = O**
Refused = R

Month __________

Activity	1	2	3	4	5	6	7	8	9	10	11	12	13	14	15	16	17	18	19	20	21	22	23	24	25	26	27	28	29	30	31

Special Programming, One-to-One Log

The activity professional must provide specialized and individualized programs for participants unable and/or uninterested in attending group activities at least 2–3 times per week.

Each participant who needs in-room activities will have a One-to-One Log Form. The form is used and kept by the month and the year.

Activity Code: These are the types of activities that you may be providing. They need to be the same as on the care plan "approaches." Numbers 17 and 18 are left blank in case you wish to add an activity not listed on the form.

Activities should be at least fifteen minutes in duration and two to three times per week in frequency. After the visit you record onto the log.

Example:

Date	**Length of Visit**	**Code**	**Participant Response**
1/16/18	20 minutes	2 and 4	Mrs. Idder held and petted the kitten and afterwards we wrote a letter to her son. She expressed thanks and enjoyment for the visit.
OR			
1/16/18	15 minutes	15 a, c	Mr. Miller opened his eyes when I turned on relaxation CD. He visually followed my movement around his bed and seemed to be intent on listening to the sound of my voice while I was talking to him.

These records can be kept either behind the individual's attendance participation records or in a separate binder. If the bedside logs are not in the attendance participation records, you should note in the participation records where the bedside logs can be found.

Special Programming: One-to-One Log

Name ____________________ **Month/Year** ______/______

Activity Code:

1. Reality Awareness
   a. Oral
   b. Written
   c. Picture book/board
2. Pet visits
3. Art projects
4. Creative expression
5. Exercise
6. Music
7. Religion
8. Games
9. Reading material
10. Grooming
11. Participant volunteer
12. Community involvement
13. Work type activities/project oriented
14. Discussion, conversation
15. Sensory stimulation
    a. Scent
    b. Tactile
    c. Sound
    d. Visual
16. Rehab goal support
17. ____________________
18. ____________________

Date	Length of Visit	Activity Code	Initials	Participant Response

Monitoring Tools — Social Services

Keeping up with a participant's needs (psychosocial and concrete) and changing conditions (health and behavior) is an ongoing challenge. It is only partly done if you know what the need/concern/problem is. To complete the cycle you must reflect your knowledge and your plan in writing in the participant's record.

Although this is not a regulation and will not even appear in any of the surveyors' guidelines, it is a good social services practice to make an entry in the participant's chart every week for at least the first two months. You can start it with each new participant and use it as a form of tracking his/her adjustment to the facility. Chart each week on some significant clue to the adjustment (or lack thereof) by indicating such things as knowledge of the facility: various rooms; recognition of faces, if not names, of staff and roommates; and familiarity with the approximate routine within the facility.

This charting will help you track the participant's moods, find behavior patterns which might escalate into problems, or begin to work toward appropriate discharge planning. Very importantly, you can determine if your current entry on the participant care plan is still a reflection of the participant's needs. Use a standard social services progress note form. A narrative style of documentation seems to work best for most social services entries.

If you find that weekly charting is not necessary because the participant's overall independence and adjustment or, at the other extreme, very poor orientation and inability to respond to standard reality orientation, you can record this observation in the chart by making a note to that effect and change the frequency of the tracking.

Another way to document social services interventions is to keep a Social Services Log for each participant. This log is a record documenting services and counseling provided to the participant by the social services professional. The form could be a narrative or it might be similar to the Bedside Log used by the activity professional. Be sure to identify date, nature of service, participant's response, and the follow-through that is required.

Quarterly Review

Care conferences for each resident are held quarterly to discuss current status and effectiveness of the care plan. The formal part of this process is the requirement to update the MDS for the resident. It is a chance for the interdisciplinary team to meet together with the resident and/or responsible party and review the resident's progress toward the care plan goals. The team needs to be sure that the information about the resident's condition is up to date and that the care plan reflects the resident's current condition.

Your responsibilities are to write a quarterly progress note, complete your part of the MDS, and then carefully read the MDS and notes for the other disciplines before you attend the care plan meeting.

Each facility has a sign in sheet for all participants (staff, resident, and family) as well as areas to review. These include, but are not limited to, a check of the face sheet for accuracy including addresses and phone numbers of family and other responsible persons and choice of mortuary. A medication review update, therapy status, if applicable, weight, intake patterns, and ancillary services received or needed are areas shared during the meeting.

As the resident advocate, the social services professional uses this opportunity to ask capable residents if they would like to execute an Advance Health Care Directive/Durable Power of Attorney for Health Care. This might require an explanation as to the value of making end of life treatment choices. The question must be asked at each q/a meeting.

Questions from residents and family can be answered at the care conference but the conferences are usually time limited. Residents and families with further concerns can make an appointment with the appropriate department head to discuss these issues in-depth.

Quarterly Progress Notes

When you write your quarterly progress notes and complete the MDS, realize that you are reflecting on three months of a participant's life. It is essential, therefore, that you take the time to do a comprehensive review of all of the most recent entries in the medical chart including the doctor's progress notes, nursing summaries, dietary and therapy entries, and your own interventions. Also check the resident care plan for any changes, the medication book for new drugs or discontinued ones, and, when indicated, behavioral monitors that reflect a resident's mood or behavior. Review your last quarterly note to ensure that you have addressed unfinished issues from the last quarter.

The note should be ended with a goal for the new quarter. This goal will be reflected on the care plan and should be person-centered.

Quarterly Progress Notes — Activity Professional

Below you will find a checklist for a comprehensive activity quarterly progress note. Follow these guidelines for a note that identifies all of the important areas of an individual. If areas do not need attention, such as special diets, skip them in the note.

The Care Plan

Now it is time to reflect on the care plan entry.

- Does any change in the MDS require a change in the care plan?
- How closely did the problem/need/concern actually reflect the individual's need(s) during the quarter?
- How close is the participant to the goal you established for him/her?
- Have the planned approaches been successful/adequate?
- Does the problem, need, or concern still reflect your assessment of the participant?
- Have things changed enough so that you

Quarterly Progress Note Content Areas

	Cognitive Status
	Communication Deficits and Needs
	Behavioral Issues and Interventions
	Mood and Behavior, Depression
	Family Involvement and Relationship with Roommate and Staff
	Previous Leisure and Lifestyle Interests
	Specific Involvement in Activity Program
	Level of Responsiveness in Group Activities
	Strengths and Abilities
	Necessary Information About Vision, Hearing, and Speech
	Psychoactive Medications
	Restraint Use
	Special Notes About Diet
	Therapy
	All Areas on Care Plan with Activity Approaches
	CAA Information
	Activity Treatment Plan and Quarterly Goal

Directions: When writing your quarterly note, review the necessary areas of information on this checklist form. Include as many of these areas as possible in order to document in a *comprehensive* manner.

need to start again or add to the care plan?

Your quarterly entry is the place to answer these questions. It is okay to change; in fact, it is essential to change any part or even all of the individual care plan entry if it is no longer a reflection of the individual. If the goal will never be accomplished, change it. Then alter the approaches to support the goal. Remember that all changes in the care plan require input from the individual and/or surrogate.

When you have done this, support your changes in the progress note. If you have been honest in your updated assessment of the individual, you will know whether the care plan needs changing. Remember — the individual care plan goal must be reflected in your progress notes. If your entry does not help to paint an accurate picture of the individual, it needs to be changed.

A few sample quarterly progress notes for activity professionals and social services are shown on the next pages.

Activity Quarterly Progress Notes

6/10/18 Activity Quarterly Progress Note

Mary is alert and aware of people and things around her. She has occasional periods of confusion, which seem to occur in the late afternoon. When in a group setting, she is hesitant to speak up due to an embarrassment about her word retrieval skills.

She spends most of her day in her room, feeding birds on the patio, and waiting for her daughter to visit.

During one-on-one visits 2x weekly, she converses and expresses interest in our conversation.

Mary has a wonderful sense of humor and a strong sense of curiosity. She is receiving speech therapy 1x weekly for language deficits due to a mild left CVA. The speech therapy goals for her will be reinforced in one-on-one conversation and word/memory games. She will also be encouraged to join in the small morning discussion group for social interaction and communication building skills.

E. Best CTRS

9/10/18 Activity Quarterly Progress Note

Mary is alert with periods of confusion reported about 1x per day, usually in the early afternoon. Some progress is being made in conjunction with the speech therapist to solve problems pronouncing words, but she still has significant difficulty being understood at times.

Most of the day, she can be seen looking out of her window, waiting for her daughter or feeding the birds out on the patio. Her daughter visits weekly and she receives mail monthly from a distant relative in Iowa.

She seems to enjoy our visits 2x weekly and has enjoyed participating in the small morning discussion group. She has contributed a lot of insight to our discussions and is much appreciated. I have had to interpret what she said to the other members about 20% of the time (down from almost 50% when she first joined the group), but this has not been a problem for the group. We have worked with the speech therapist on the continuing areas of difficulty.

One thing that I have continued to appreciate is Mary's strong sense of curiosity and a wonderful sense of humor.

GOALS:

Res. will continue to practice communication techniques (see speech therapy goal for revised plan) during the small discussion group 2x per week for the next three months. Activity professional will assist participant to practice new communication skills learned in speech therapy during the small discussion group.

Check more carefully to try to pinpoint time of confusion. Nursing is considering the possibility that it may be related to medication.

E. Best CTRS

Social Services Quarterly Progress Notes

6/08/18 Social Services Quarterly Progress Note

Lydia has been here for three months and has worked hard to make an adjustment to this environment. She came here from a loving home environment which could no longer support her, given the escalation in her personal care needs related to a compression fracture in her spine, which compounds the existing circumstance related to a CVA she suffered in 2008. She very appropriately mourned the loss of her life as she had known it and SSD spent at least an hour a week with her reminiscing, dissecting the pros and cons of her present situation, and gradually looking to a future (something she had verbalized to me after about six weeks into her admission that she had no sense of).

Lydia has rejected the idea of an antidepressant (which her physician had asked her to consider) feeling instead that she would rather "feel her emotions and deal with the issues now — not prolong the pain of separation." There have been no observed indications of depression; Lydia has maintained an excellent appetite (gaining eight pounds over the quarter), sleeps well at night, and says she has "nice dreams," all counter indications of the usual signs and symptoms of depression. Her weight gain of eight pounds keeps her well within range of her normal body weight. (For further clarification, see dietary note.)

Lydia's family, husband, and one of two daughters who lives nearby, visit several times a week and have made her room homey, reflecting Lydia's love of clowns and flowers.

Lydia remains oriented, interested in her care, and gradually has entered into an activity of her choosing.

Her placement remains appropriate at this level of care because of her dependence for care, her incontinence, and her non-ambulatory status. Lydia's advance directives are in the chart: she has expressed clear end-of-life wishes.

There are no apparent unmet concrete needs at present: she has new glasses, her dentures fit well, and she is not hard of hearing.

SSD goal of visiting at least once a week to allow her to verbalize her feelings related to adjustment, with the additional intention of establishing a trusting relationship with at least one staff member, has been met thus far. Because she is becoming more independent, emotionally and physically, within the facility, this goal will be revised to biweekly visitation for the next quarter.

M. A. Weeks, SSD

6/08/18 SS Quarterly Progress Note

John is a very stable participant of three months duration in the facility. He has a diagnosis of Alzheimer's disease (probable). His signs and symptoms are consistent with that as he is no longer able to identify himself, find his room, or ask for what he needs. He is alert, however, and seems interested in his surroundings; he is a passive observer in most activities, responds to his name by making eye contact, and appears to recognize his wife when she visits (daily at lunch) because he will smile and reach for her.

John had been receiving Ativan for agitation and anxiety BID [two times a day]. He had been placed on this medication at home because of his behavior and the physician chose not to discontinue it upon admission, choosing instead to monitor and assess his behavior on the drug in this new setting.

At first John would become very restless, moving himself in his chair, reaching out to passersby, and pulling at his clothes. This was noted especially in the evening, beginning at about 7 PM. After several weeks of a trial with the medication, the staff was not noticing a major change in his behavior pattern and it was decided to attempt behavioral interventions to address John's anxiety. The goal of reducing his episodes of nightly anxiety was addressed by removing John from the main activity room and putting him in the room where there was quiet music being played and there were never more than five other participants in attendance. Staff would speak very calmly and softly and if John began to show any signs of motor restlessness, he would be calmed with a gentle and reassuring touch to his hand. These approaches have been successful to the extent that the physician discontinued the Ativan at his last monthly visit.

All concrete needs have been addressed at the present time: John has a new upper denture; he used to use glasses only for reading but no longer reads, thus is not in any way dependent on glasses. He has a hearing aid in his right ear, which he tends to remove. It can usually be found in his pocket. His family is aware of the risk of loss and feel that, at this point in his diagnosis, he wears the aid out of habit, not for "hearing." The hearing aid is kept in the medication cart at night.

John's care needs require the supervision necessary at this level of placement. He has a Durable Power of Attorney in the medical chart.

SSD goal has been revised; John is visited at least monthly and during those visits, the goal is for him to respond in conversation by making eye contact when his name is used; he is also assessed for any personal care or clothing needs. If there are any, contact is made with his wife.

M. A. Weeks, SSD

The best advice we can give you on actually getting these done is to stay organized and try not to let progress notes pile up. Doing progress notes each week before the MDS review and participation in care conference is desired. It is your responsibility to do your reports and provide other members of the interdisciplinary team with your unique perspective as they, too, comply with quarterly entry requirements.

Progress Note Updates for a New RAI

Not only must you comment on the reason for the new Resident Assessment Instrument (RAI) when an individual's health status changes, but you must also discuss any impact that this may have had on the psychosocial well-being of the participant. For example, if the participant has had a stroke, s/he may have lost some of his/her ability to socialize. Clearly this can have an effect on his/her ongoing orientation and a new plan must be developed to address this.

Remember, because the MDS starts the clock anew, this update note will in essence be a quarterly progress note. If it has been a while since you have written a comprehensive note, now is the time to write one.

Annual Review

Once a year you will participate in an annual review of each individual. The purpose of the annual review, unlike the quarterly review, is to completely reassess the individual. An annual full MDS with CAAs is completed. New, rather than revised, care plans are generally written.

Your participation is the same as it was in the initial assessment of the individual: supplying information for your section of the MDS, assisting with CAAs, reading through information from all the other disciplines, and participating in the care plan conference.

Social services professionals are responsible for an annual update in the progress notes. This note is an overall summary that reflects change over the entire year. The annual date is determined by the date of the previous full, validated MDS.

Social Services Annual Progress Note

9/6/18 Social Services Annual Progress Note

Lydia has continued to make progress with an adjustment that started out with difficulties related to her mourning her previous life at home. She has been consistently verbal and able to express her feelings and has maintained an ongoing relationship with me, which has included at least biweekly "check-in" visits after the first quarter of weekly visits.

Her health has remained stable with no further fractures or indications of new problems related to her original CVA. Her mood is optimistic and she has reached out to other alert individuals and they have formed a dining group that meets every day at lunch. This group is also the nucleus of the Resident Council and Lydia seems delighted to use her organizational skills as the elected secretary.

Her daughters offer love and support to her; her husband has himself suffered some major health problems during the year and his pattern of visiting four times per week has been reduced to two times per week. Lydia has been able to accept this new pattern without evidence of a setback in her mood, probably, she says, because she realizes that her husband, after so many years of focusing on her, must allow others to tend him now. She misses him but is always so happy to see him when he does visit that they spend their time catching up on events in their separate lives.

There have been no new medications needed; the MD's progress notes regularly reflect Lydia's stability and good humor.

SSD goal of biweekly visits has been revised to quarterly visits, which is a reflection of a well-integrated individual.

M. A. Weeks, SSD

9/8/18 Social Services Annual Progress Note

John has had an expected decline due to his diagnosis of probable Alzheimer's disease. He is no longer alert as evidenced by his keeping his eyes closed much of the time and he does not seem to respond to his wife any longer, not even opening his eyes when she speaks to him. He spends much of the day out of his room with the possibility that he will receive some form of stimulation. John seems calm with no restlessness or aimless body movements noted. He is nonverbal and all of his needs must now be anticipated. Additionally, John has had a weight loss over the year representing about 10% of his body weight. He remains well within range of his ideal body weight but a gradual weight loss is not inconsistent with his diagnosis. The weight loss continues even though he is fed all of his meals, consumes 75–90% of each and receives protein drinks between each meal and at bedtime.

John signed a Durable Power of Attorney for Health Care when he was well and his wife is able to make decisions regarding his care. She has asked that all possible comfort measures be provided, including relief of pain if necessary; he will remain with us, even if he develops further health care problems. She does not wish him transferred out to the acute care hospital.

John's physician has noted the obvious decline during the past five monthly visits to him; there is no medication indicated.

The SSD goal has been revised to reflect these changes: during monthly visits with John, his concrete needs are assessed, he is monitored for any obvious change which should then be discussed with his wife.

M. A. Weeks, SSD

Scheduling Updates

The quarterly and annual reviews must be completed using the MDS care plan schedule. This is generated by the Resident Assessment Coordinator (RAC) and a copy is given to each department for the upcoming month. This allows the activity and social services departments to schedule ahead of time for the month. The time needed for completion of the chart review and for attending care conference can be built into the month's work management schedule.

Other Considerations for Documentation

Many of the issues in this section have been discussed in detail elsewhere in the book. This section is a reminder about and suggestions for the best way to document that all of the concerns have been covered in treatment. As always, if it isn't in writing, surveyors will assume it didn't happen.

Quality Indicators

The areas addressed in Chapter 12 are to be reviewed by the activity professional when completing the quarterly and annual reviews. Because the Quality Indicator report is generated after transmission of the MDS, the most current copy may not be available at the time the quarterly note is written. It is the activity professional's responsibility to obtain a copy of the report from the RAC and review the appropriate domains. The significance of the triggered areas needs to be addressed in a progress note and reflected in the care plan. This is the opportunity to "tie in" to the care plan. As an example: if a resident is triggered on the QI report for Domain 9.2 most of time in bed or chair, the activity professional would address the cause of the resident's behavior and make sure that it is reflected in the care plan. The reason for the behavior might be a physician's order, end of life status, or simply resident preference not to get up. In each case, the activity note would reflect opportunities offered to the resident and these would be added to the care plan as well.

Unnecessary Drugs, Tags F757, F758, F605

For the activity professional an important part of this regulation is the mandate to include, as a part of all medication management, documentation that shows non-pharmacological interventions were considered. Examples that pertain to activities programming include:

- Increasing the amount of exercise
- Following a toileting plan
- Eliminating boredom
- Individualizing sleep routines
- Accommodating behaviors through "activities reminiscent of lifelong work or activity patterns, such as providing early morning activity for a framer used to awakening early"
- Providing interventions specific to abilities and needs such as "simplifying or segmenting tasks for a resident who has trouble following complex direction"
- Addressing pain through imaging, lotion massage, or distraction
- Providing appealing environment for meals, opportunities for finger foods, and appetite enhancement

The residents who need to be addressed in the documentation can be identified through the QI report, a medication order report, and through review at the quarterly care conference. It is mandatory that the activity professional participate in the development of the behavior management plan and that the behavior care plan include the type of activity interventions listed above. This list is not all-inclusive but suggests the areas where activity programming can help to eliminate the use of psychoactive medications. Documentation that interventions besides medications were tried is a requirement.

Psychosocial Outcome Severity Guide

This guide provides criteria for determining levels of negative psychosocial outcomes that developed, continued, or worsened because of the facility's failure to provide adequate service. It is used in conjunction with the scope and severity grid and is similar to the citation process for negative physical outcome.

Because this guide instructs surveyors to determine if mood and behavior problems are due to lack of assessment and failure to develop an adequate care plan, it is very important that preexisting mood and behavior problems be well documented and that new mood and behavior problems be addressed immediately by the team.

Once a surveyor identifies what might be a negative psychosocial outcome, a connection must be established between the outcome and noncompliance by the facility. This is done through observation, record review, and staff and resident/representative interviews.

During the record review the surveyor will look for an assessment for resolvable causes of the behavior, non-pharmacological interventions, a care plan that is interdisciplinary, staff knowledge of the care plan interventions, and ongoing assessment and revision of the care plan if the mood or behavior does not resolve.

As with F757, F758, F605 above, the activity professional needs to work with the team to develop a plan to address the psychosocial conditions.

Areas of particular concern are

- Depression
- Suicidal ideation
- Not eating or drinking in order to kill oneself
- Self-injurious behavior
- Persistent anger
- Expressions of humiliation or dehumanization
- Recurrent debilitating anxiety or fear
- Expressions of unrelenting, excruciating pain that is overwhelming
- Apathy and social disengagement
- Complaints of boredom, nothing to do

F679 and F680

The guidance to surveyors is now specific to activities being integral to a resident's quality of life. As has been discussed in other sections of the book, the emphasis is on the person rather than the environment or facility routine. Documentation needs to reflect the person-centered approach.

The key points to address in documentation that demonstrate a person-centered approach are

- Dignity

- Self-esteem
- Independence
- Positive self-image
- Choice of activities
- Activities that amount to something

The kinds of activities that surveyors look for to demonstrate the quality of the program include activities that:

- Produce or teach something
- Use skills from former work
- Contribute to the nursing home
- Are gender specific
- Are physically active
- Are non-traditional
- Are part of "culture-changed" homes
- Show involvement in chores, preparing foods, interacting in ways that reflect daily life

Surveyors will also be checking the documentation to be sure the assessments include information about:

- What activities the resident prefers and what adaptations are needed
- Relevant information such as lifelong interests, spirituality, life roles, strengths, and needs
- How life roles can be continued
- New interests and hobbies to be learned
- How the resident can connect with the community

Care Plan Documentation

When you are writing your care plans there are some guidelines you need to follow. Some are new terms that surveyors are looking for. Others include ways to demonstrate that you have covered all of the requirements in the assessment and planning process.

The description of interventions has changed from "age-appropriate" to "person-appropriate" or "person-centered."

"Person-centered" interventions are based on history, preferences, strengths, and needs. When you document the interventions, you need to describe why the intervention was chosen. Interventions are selected in response to the individual. The individual is not shoehorned into existing programs such as large groups or reality orientation.

Goals have measurable objectives and are focused on desired outcomes — not on attendance in programs.

Documentation must show that all relevant departments helped to develop the care plan considering:

- Medication administration times
- Meal times
- ADL care schedules
- Therapy schedules
- Toileting schedules
- Transportation needs

Documentation must show that the interventions include adaptations necessary for each individual's needs including consideration of:

- Visual impairment
- Cognitive impairment
- Hearing impairment
- Language barriers
- Physical limitations
- Cultural barriers
- Loss of use of one side

If certain conditions exist, there needs to be documentation of how the care plan will help the person we serve or clear descriptions of why the condition is not included in the care plan. Some of the conditions that need to be covered include:

- Pain
- Sleeping disorders
- Room-bound
- Short-stay admission
- New admissions
- Younger residents

Interventions are also required for particular behaviors. The documentation must show that these behaviors, if they exist, are addressed:

- Constant walking

- Withdrawal
- Physical or verbal abuse
- Attention-seeking
- Rummaging
- Lack of safety awareness
- Delusions or hallucinations
- Aggression
- Disruption
- Anger
- Sensitivity to stimulation

The following are some sample care plan notes that show how the care plan is working, how it was individualized for the particular resident, and where changes need to be made to continue to provide appropriate care.

Barbara is responding well to 1-1 activities provided. She is meeting her goal of handholding with the activity staff on walks. Her walks last from 15 to 30 minutes and she seems to enjoy the conversation provided about the plants, birds, and anything else that is seen. A ritual stop for a high-cal cookie is included, which she seems to look forward to. Staff has identified behaviors that are precursors to her elevated agitation such as rattling doorknobs and muttering under her breath. At these times, the activity department or staff provides 1-1 to reduce stimulation and manage her behaviors. She responds very well to a photo album of her family. Finger foods are provided with decaf coffee, which she loves. Night shift is reporting that she is starting to wander more around bedtime (10 PM). Family will be requested to call her at this time and a CD player with classical music, which she likes, will be tried at bedtime to help her relax.

Jean has been in the facility for 3 weeks. She is very unhappy and expresses dislike of all of our interventions offered as being "infantile" and "demeaning." She has recently learned that she will not be able to return home. Her past history includes a career in education and a very active community life. Through this difficult adjustment period we will offer active listening. The long-term goal will be to build on her educational experience by involving her in choosing our adult ed classes and possibly developing new programs for current events, reading groups, and discussion groups. We will also explore her desire to attend her old groups such as Soroptimist.

August is a retired dairy rancher. He is a bachelor who lived with his brother on the ranch for all of his life. He has no family or close friends and is comfortable with this. He is not interested in pursuing past roles related to ranching. He states, "I've had a lifetime of that and I just want to rest now." He wants to catch up on his reading and following world events through the newspapers and radio. He needs a magnifier for the paper. An extra reading light and his chair from home have been added to his room. He does want to get "out" and be involved in the facility, but not in any organized activities. He states that he does like to tinker with things and would be glad to help with fixing up anything that "needs fixing." We will provide him with tools and projects for repair and involve him with accompanying the maintenance dept. on rounds. He said he might be interested in the small engine repair group, but only if they are not a bunch of know-it-alls. He also likes the facility dog and enjoys daily visits, but is not interested in caring for the dog. Will continue to monitor for his satisfaction with this program.

Two care plans are shown on the next page as examples of how to document person-centered care.

Concern	Objective	Intervention	Who
Persistent wandering in halls	Will not enter others' rooms	1. Barrier on doors of neighbors 2. Wander guard	All N
Behavior escalates in the afternoon		3. Daily walks at 3 PM	Act
Occasional elopement attempts	Will not exit unescorted, handholding during daily walks	4. Walks outside as weather permits	CNA
Very short attention span — candidate for 1-1 activities that reduce external stimuli	Will show + response to 1-1	5. 1-1 activities as needed to divert behaviors — reading to resident, walking, pictures of family	Act All
Low body weight with gradual wt loss due to excessive movement and calorie burning	Will not lose weight beyond 110# +/- 5%	6. Finger foods and snacks to allow for food on the go 7. Family to call at bedtime 8. CD player w/classical music at bedside	D Act Act CNA
Contributory factor: Alzheimer's	x 90 days		

Concern	Objective	Intervention	Who
Difficulty adjusting to new living situation	Will verbalize acceptance of placement	1. Meet with res daily to discuss facility issues, allow venting	SSD
Expresses dissatisfaction with current lifestyle choices	Will develop a program of her own choosing	2. Psych services 3. Accommodate family and friend visits in alcove	SSD All
Anger over lost roles and active social life and community involvement	Will regain connection with community activities	4. Transport to (meetings) (days) via Senior Bus 5. AD to meet weekly w/ res to discuss activities that support continuation of life roles, new skills until res is satisfied with individualized program	SSD AD

Health Insurance Portability and Accountability Act (HIPAA)

The Health Insurance Portability and Accountability Act of 1996 established federal privacy regulations and paved the way for development of electronic health records. It is designed to protect the resident's personal information. Activity professionals need to be sure they understand the importance of protecting that information and how serious the government is regarding enforcement.

Health care practitioners are liable to disciplinary action for violation of the federal privacy rules, up to and including immediate termination. In addition, the violator may be subject to civil or criminal fines and penalties. Civil penalties can be $100 per incident, up to $25,000 per person per year. Criminal penalties can be $50,000 to $250,000 and up to 10 years in prison.

The regulation pertains to all personal health information (PHI). This includes the reason the resident is admitted, information about medications, treatments, and past and current conditions. Any information that can be used to identify the resident, including name, age, social security number, or address is considered PHI as well.

PHI is confidential and protected under HIPAA against unauthorized release. Each facility appoints a privacy officer who is responsible for overseeing correct handling of PHI. Any observations of violations of confidentiality must be reported to this privacy officer.

Good practices such as shredding all documents containing PHI, keeping conversations private, and following the "need to know" rule (obtaining only as much information as is needed to do your job) will result in protecting the privacy and confidentiality of the residents' PHI.

15. Councils

The people we serve have the right to form and run a self-governing council. This council usually takes one of two forms: a Resident Council run for and by the residents of a facility and a Family Council run for and by the family members of residents who live in a facility. The idea is that residents (and their families) should be involved in policy decisions that affect resident life. These councils provide the residents (and their families) with opportunities to participate in decision making through voicing their views and helping resolve issues and concerns.

Resident Council

According to OBRA '87, every long-term care facility is required to have a Resident Council. Other facilities, including adult day programs, assisted living centers, and hospitals may also have some type of council. The activity or social services professional is usually the chairperson for the council and is responsible for assuring that this very important meeting occurs each month and that minutes are kept and issues resolved.

What is the Resident Council?

The Resident Council is the political voice of the individuals who use or reside in your facility. Many of the residents are *unable* to voice their opinions and/or concerns and need to rely on residents who are capable and interested in facility events to speak for them.

A president, vice president, and secretary/treasurer should be elected from the group. Because the Resident Council is so important, during the annual survey process, the survey team will ask to meet the president and/or vice president of this council. The surveyors will also lead a Resident Council meeting with only residents involved to determine whether there are issues that residents wish to confide in them without staff present.

The regular monthly meeting consists of all interested residents, representatives from the Ombudsman program, any guests that the residents invite and/or request to speak, and the chairperson (the staff person responsible for assisting the resident council). The resident council members need to approve any staff member or visitor to these meetings. They can also request to have time alone without any staff present in order to discuss issues confidentially.

Many residents will be hesitant to take on the responsibility and leadership of a council position, as it may be a new and intimidating experience. Because of this, be sure to explain how the meetings work, what the responsibilities are and encourage members to share a position if they are interested. The president is the spokesperson for the council. This resident sits at the head of the group along with the chairperson and other officers. Each council has its own personality. Create the positions to meet the needs of the current group along with the stated responsibilities of the council.

The Resident Council is required to take place *one time per month.* In large facilities, additional meetings may be called as the need occurs. The chairperson keeps the minutes of these meetings. A copy of the minutes always goes to the administrator for review so that s/he is always current on issues, concerns, and resolutions.

How Should a Meeting Be Organized?

Each meeting should begin with attendance and recognition of each member. The chairperson usually opens the meeting unless the president wishes to open. Because this is an official meeting, there should be an agenda to follow. An example of an agenda would be:

- Attendance.
- Review of last month's minutes including resolutions to each issue addressed.
- Department heads speak on any issues that may have come up. Residents need to know that when an issue is addressed, the responsible discipline follows through with the concern and speaks to the group in regards to policy, changes, and educational information.
- Review of one or more specific resident rights.
- Review of one or more quality of life issues.
- Reminder of the right to review the past year's survey results and where they are located. These should be both available and accessible for review.
- Discussion of activity planning so that the residents have a voice in future events and evaluation of the program.
- Voting issues should always be mentioned so that all members know that they can register to vote, can request assistance with absentee forms and change of address forms. A current list should always be kept of residents who are registered to vote.
- Open forum for any and all residents in the council to voice an opinion and offer additional information and recommendations for group projects.

New discussions: every six months or so, review with the resident council all of the concerns/grievances that have arisen during those six months. Are they still concerns or has the facility addressed them to the satisfaction of the residents. If not, keep trying. The surveyors will certainly want to know that there are ongoing attempts to address concerns and it is the facility's responsibility to correct any problems.

As with any group, if complaints and concerns are the only agenda, members will become disinterested in attending. Find worthwhile projects for the council to become involved in. Some examples could be welcome cards and visits to new residents, Employee of the Month award voted by council members, in-service training, invitations to outside speakers, congratulation letters to community groups and individuals recognized for special efforts, recognition projects for staff and other residents in the facility, a council newsletter, inspirational announcements each morning, and the list goes on and on.

What if Only a Few Residents Attend the Meetings?

In relationship to the census in a facility, the number of council members is always on the low end. Some very alert and independent individuals may be found in their rooms because they are not interested in attending these meetings. Others may not attend because the effort required is too great. Sometimes it is appropriate to bring the meeting to them. After the official meeting is adjourned, go individually to the rooms of residents so they can review issues and address concerns with you on a one-on-one basis. Keep a record of these council room visits attached to the council minutes.

If there are issues addressed, be sure to document these and have the responsible department head write up the resolutions. These should be signed and dated also.

How Do You Document Tough Issues in the Minutes?

As the legally responsible chairperson, your duty is to document the facts and issues verbalized by the council members. There must be an atmosphere of trust and responsibility in these meetings. If a resident requests to remain anonymous, this is his/her right and you must respect this right. If there are individuals who are "chronic complainers" even when the issue has been resolved, discuss the resolution during the meeting and add this to the minutes. This documentation will substantiate both the resolution and the fact that this resident needs to vent at each meeting regardless of past resolutions. Be sure that this resident does not have the opportunity to take over the meeting. The chairperson may have to designate a five-minute period near the end of the meeting for this member's voice to be heard.

When documenting tough issues in the minutes, be specific but not narrative. The minutes are not the place to write the story, but to record the information so that the responsible department head can address and help find resolution to the issues and concerns. Ask your administrator for assistance in writing these minutes when the issues get complex.

What Exactly Are the Chairperson's Responsibilities?

The chairperson is responsible for scheduling the monthly meeting, announcing the meeting and posting an invitation to family members, creating the agenda, facilitating the meeting, recording the minutes and typing them up, and, most importantly, taking the issues and concerns to the responsible department head for review and resolution. This is not *your* meeting. This is a legal requirement of the facility and you are the designated chairperson.

All grievances and concerns need to be resolved by identified departments. You must get these staff members to write a plan of action, date it, and sign it on the council forms. These minutes are kept on file and are always available for surveyor review, corporate review, administrative review, and ombudsman review. They are never thrown away as they are legal documents for the facility.

Policy and Procedure — Resident Council

Purpose

To provide residents with an opportunity to meet and discuss issues that affect their daily lives and quality of life as residents in long-term care facilities.

Policy

It is the policy of this facility to provide a regularly scheduled resident council meeting as required by federal and state regulations.

Procedures

1. Resident Council meetings will be held at least one time per month.
2. Additional meetings can be scheduled per special request or need.
3. The activity coordinator or social services coordinator will chair the monthly meetings.
4. All residents are invited and encouraged to attend the monthly meetings.
5. The council members can request and recommend specific visitors, guests, staff, or speakers to attend the next month's meeting if approved by the members.
6. The council members can request to meet privately without staff or visitors present during each meeting. The chair will add this to the minutes.
7. Attendance records and minutes of the resident council shall be written or compiled by the activity coordinator and secretary of the council.
8. Two resident rights are reviewed, discussed, and documented in each month's minutes. The right to vote and the right to review previous survey results should be addressed at each meeting as a reminder.
9. Resident Council members will review the activity program and give input to programs, special events, and requests at each meeting.
10. The original copy of the council minutes will be kept on file in the activity office. The original copy should include the plan of action.
11. A copy of meeting minutes will be given to the administrator for review and comment.
12. All issues addressed by the council need to be documented with a plan of action written, signed, and dated by the responsible discipline. This plan needs to be written only by

the department representative responsible for follow through.

13. The past month's issues will be reviewed with a discussion of resolution as old business at the next meeting.
14. The agenda for each meeting should include the following:
    a. Welcome
    b. Attendance
    c. Review of past month's minutes
    d. Review of past month's resolutions to issues
    e. Review of specific departments such as nursing, dietary, social services, activities, maintenance, therapy, and administration
    f. New business and issues
    g. Request for visitors for the next month's meeting

Use of the Resident Council Forms

The Resident Council form on the next page has an area for attendance, old business, review of resident rights, activity review, and new issues. The new issues area is very important. Write the issue and then have the responsible discipline write the plan of action. Attach the plan of action to the minutes. Add the title of the plan of action to the new issues section of the minutes and have the person who wrote the plan of action date and sign the appropriate box. You can also use the Department Response to Issues form shown after the one-on-one form. Your signature is on the bottom of the form along with the date. The one-on-one form needs to be completed by the chairperson also. Any issues that come from the one-on-one form should be addressed the same way as issues from the Resident Council meeting.

This form is meant to show you what areas need to be addressed. Depending on your facility, you may need to add more space for different parts of the form. Having the form as a template in your word processing program and typing the information after the heading is probably the most efficient way to use the form.

Resident Council Meeting Minutes

Attendance: ____________________ ____________________ ____________________

____________________ ____________________ ____________________

____________________ ____________________ ____________________

____________________ ____________________ ____________________

____________________ ____________________ ____________________

____________________ ____________________ ____________________

Business

1. Review of Past Month's Issues/Resolutions:

____

____

____

____

2. Review of Resident Rights: Review at least two specific rights per meeting

____

____

____

3. Review of Quality of Life Issues: Review at least two specific quality of life issues per meeting

____

____

____

____

____

4. Activities: Review of Calendar/Input by Residents:

____

____

____

____

5. New Issues

Issue	Responsible Department	Plan Completed Signature and Date

Resident Council Chair ________________________________ **Date** ____________

Resident Council Meeting
In-Room Form

Resident Name	Comments/Concerns

Resident Council Chair Date

Department Response to Issues

Department: ____

Date of Meeting Referring to: ____________________________________

Issue(s) Identified by ☐ **Resident Council** ☐ **Family Council** ☐ **Resident**

____

____

____

____

____

____

____

____

Department Response

____

____

____

____

____

____

____

____

____

____

____

____

____

____

____

____

Department Supervisor ________________________ **Date** ____________

Administrator ______________________________ **Date** ____________

Sample Resident Council Agenda

Areas to Review	Check off
Attendance	
Introduction of guests or speakers	
Review of past month's meeting	
Review of 1 or 2 resident rights	
Resident input to activity calendar	
New Issues	
Plan of action	
Responsible discipline	
Review of 1 or 2 quality-of-life questions What assistance is staff providing to help you get to activities of choice? Are you notified of all activity opportunities and offered transportation as needed or requested? Does this facility accommodate resident choices so there is not a conflict with care, treatment, and activity choices? Do you have any activity requests currently not provided? Do all staff help you with adaptations as needed?	

Resident Council Interview — Critical Element Pathway

This form on the next four pages is used by the surveyors as part of their new investigative protocols when they are interviewing the resident council. Add some of these questions to your resident council meetings so that residents feel comfortable and confident during survey process.

Resident Council Interview

Resident Council Interview - *Complete an interview with active members of the Resident Council early enough in the survey to afford the team enough time to investigate any concerns. If there is not a resident council, determine whether residents have attempted to form one and have been unsuccessful, and if so, why.*

- [ ] Introduce yourself to the president of the council and ask for assistance in arranging the meeting. If there is no president, ask for a list of active resident council participants and select a resident to assist in arranging the meeting. Try to keep the group manageable, no more than 12 residents. Explain the survey process and the purpose of the interview using the following concepts. It is not necessary to use the exact wording.

  "*[Name of facility]* is inspected periodically by a team from the *[Name of State Survey Agency]* to ensure that residents receive quality care. While we are here, we make observations, review the nursing home's records, and talk to the residents and family members or friends who can help us understand what it's like to live in this nursing home. We appreciate that you are taking the time to talk with us. We would like to know more about the Resident Council and interactions of the group and staff."

- [ ] At all times, be cognizant of resident confidentiality. Obtain permission from the Resident Council President or Officer to review the Resident Council minutes and become familiar with some of the issues that have been discussed. Review three months of minutes prior to the interview to identify any unresolved areas of concern.
- [ ] Review the grievance policy to ensure prompt resolution of all grievances and that the facility has maintained results of grievances for a minimum of 3 years.
- [ ] It is suggested that the interview begin with some discussion of issues that have been discussed during the most recent Council meeting and how the facility has responded. For example, "I read in the minutes that you had discussed noise at night during the last meeting. Has the facility responded to your concern?" or "During the last meeting, several participants brought up an issue with food being cold. Has that situation been resolved to your satisfaction?" This initial discussion of current issues before the Council may prove helpful to establish a rapport with the Resident Council President (or Officer) and help make the remainder of the interview more informative.
- [ ] Document the names of residents in the meeting.
- [ ] Follow up on any concerns that are within the scope of the long-term care requirements with reference to specific F-tags identified on this pathway. Further investigation should include interviews with appropriate staff members to determine how concerns are resolved.
- [ ] Team meetings will provide opportunities to share concerns and focus on particular problematic areas. Any potential concerns noted during the interview should be shared with all team members.

DEPARTMENT OF HEALTH AND HUMAN SERVICES
CENTERS FOR MEDICARE & MEDICAID SERVICES

Resident Council Interview

Interview		
Council		
	Resident Council Response	**Is the Facility in Compliance?**
1. Does the Resident Council meet on a regular basis?	☐ Yes ☐ **No**	☐ Yes ☐ **No F565**
2. Does the facility help with arrangements for council meetings?	☐ Yes ☐ **No**	☐ Yes ☐ **No F565**
3. Is there enough space for everyone who wants to attend?	☐ Yes ☐ **No**	☐ Yes ☐ **No F565**
4. Can you meet without staff present, if you desire?	☐ Yes ☐ **No**	☐ Yes ☐ **No F565**
Grievances		
	Resident Council Response	**Is the Facility in Compliance?**
5. Does the facility consider the views of the resident or family groups and act promptly upon grievances and recommendations?	☐ Yes ☐ **No**	☐ Yes ☐ **No F565**
6. Does the Grievance Official respond to the resident or family group's concerns?	☐ Yes ☐ **No** (If Yes, Skip Question #7)	☐ Yes ☐ **No F565**
7. If the facility does not respond to concerns, does the Grievance Official provide a rationale for the response?	☐ Yes ☐ **No**	☐ Yes ☐ **No F565**
8. Do you know how to file a grievance?	☐ Yes ☐ **No**	☐ Yes ☐ **No F585**
9. Do you feel a resident or family group can complain about care without worrying that someone will 'get back' at them?	☐ Yes ☐ **No**	☐ Yes ☐ **No F585**

DEPARTMENT OF HEALTH AND HUMAN SERVICES
CENTERS FOR MEDICARE & MEDICAID SERVICES

Resident Council Interview

Resident Specific Areas		
	Resident Council Response	**Is the Facility in Compliance?**
10. Have staff made you feel afraid, humiliated, or degraded? (If concerns are identified, refer to the Abuse Pathway)	☐ Yes ☐ **No**	☐ Yes ☐ **No F600**
11. Do you get the help and care you need without waiting a long time? Does staff respond to your call light timely? (If concerns are identified, refer to the Sufficient Staffing Pathway)	☐ Yes ☐ **No**	☐ Yes ☐ **No F725**
12. Do you receive snacks at bedtime or when you request them?	☐ Yes ☐ **No**	☐ Yes ☐ **No F809**
13. Ask about concerns identified during survey:		

Rules		
	Resident Council Response	**Is the Facility in Compliance?**
14. Have you (residents) been informed of the rules at the facility (such as are there restrictions on visiting hours)?	☐ Yes ☐ **No**	☐ Yes ☐ **No F563**
15. If the Resident Council makes suggestions about some of the rules, does the facility act on those suggestions?	☐ Yes ☐ **No**	☐ Yes ☐ **No F565**

DEPARTMENT OF HEALTH AND HUMAN SERVICES
CENTERS FOR MEDICARE & MEDICAID SERVICES

Resident Council Interview

Rights		
	Resident Council Response	**Is the Facility in Compliance?**
16. Does staff talk about and review the rights of residents in the facility?	☐ Yes ☐ **No**	☐ Yes ☐ **No F572**
17. Are residents able to exercise their rights?	☐ Yes ☐ **No**	☐ Yes ☐ **No F550**
18. Do you feel that the rights of residents at this facility are respected and encouraged?	☐ Yes ☐ **No**	☐ Yes ☐ **No F561**
19. Is mail delivered unopened and on Saturdays?	☐ Yes ☐ **No**	☐ Yes ☐ **No F576**
20. Without having to ask, are the results of the State inspection available to read?	☐ Yes ☐ **No**	☐ Yes ☐ **No F577**
21. Do residents know where the ombudsman's contact information is posted?	☐ Yes ☐ **No**	☐ Yes ☐ **No F574**
22. Does the facility allow you to see your medical records if you ask?	☐ Yes ☐ **No**	☐ Yes ☐ **No F573**
23. Have residents been informed of their right (and given information on how) to formally complain to the State about the care they are receiving?	☐ Yes ☐ **No**	☐ Yes ☐ **No F574**
Other		
Investigation of responses from this question should be conducted through initiation of a care area, if available. If an applicable care area is not available, a direct F-tag initiation is appropriate.		
24. Do you have any questions, or is there anything else you would like to tell me about the Resident Council?	☐ **Yes** ☐ No	☐ Yes ☐ **No (Display all F-tags)**

Family Council

Organizationally, the Family Council is wide open and its success is dependent upon the available family population and their energy level and interest. Theoretically, it is a self-governing body, which serves in an advisory capacity to the administration. Underlying its motivations is the support that can only be given and received by people sharing situations in common. Because each council sets its own standards and determines its own needs, each is unique.

Family Council provides a wonderful opportunity for personal support within the group and also forms a ready and willing audience for giving information about the facility, the staff, and the long-term care system in general. The ideas generated by those most directly affected by facility policies can make a difference in the overall atmosphere. When the group is part of the decision-making process (from remodeling to laundry problems), everyone — the people we serve, families, and staff — benefits.

The presence of staff should be occasional and limited to one to two people who have been invited or have a direct purpose for being in attendance (e.g., explanation of a program or policy). The social services professional is the appropriate resource person and his/her presence will be monitored by those in charge of the Family Council.

It can be very difficult to convene an entirely autonomous Family Council. For some, any leadership commitment is an additional drain on an already taxed spirit and some feel the transitory nature of their involvement in the facility. The size of the group doesn't matter. Whether it is five or fifteen members, regard the council as the body that speaks for all of the families. As the members begin to become involved in the facility through the family council, they will be the best advertisement for new members.

Family Councils are not mandatory, but facilities must allow such organizations to exist. The support required by the facility is space for meetings, privacy, and, by invitation only, staff. The other obligation is to follow up on grievances and recommendations, which are directly related to the person we serve and his/her quality of life.

The meeting can be announced by direct mail, e-mail, newsletter, and/or posters within the facility. Vary the time, the day, and the topics in order to appeal to the schedules and interests of a number of family members. Coming together for a meal will frequently create the informal, relaxed atmosphere desired in the early stages of a Family Council. Speak with your dietary manager, plan a meal or a snack, choose a program (the Ombudsman, Medicare, your rehabilitation program, etc.), announce the meeting, and see what happens.

Once convened, families will soon realize what a relief it is to share with others. Long-lasting friendships are often made through these meetings because most find that their concerns, complaints, recommendations, and emotional highs and lows are remarkably similar. Proceed from this point of sharing; encourage varying agendas, projects (e.g., a facility garden), a newsletter, or legislative activity. Be creative.

Even if no one agrees to take on the leadership roles, you do not need to abandon the Family Council concept. You must simply assume more responsibility yourself, at least temporarily, especially if it appears that there are very interested families and very real concerns. Be mindful always of not imposing on the families' right to privacy.

The Family Council may be one of your most frustrating ventures — not because it isn't worthwhile, but because of the turnover of families and the frequent lack of interest in being in charge. We find that families really enjoy coming together and they like receiving new information. When the time is right and someone feels that s/he would like to do more, step aside. Until then, continue to provide a welcoming environment yourself.

Someone once told us to expect it to take 18 months for a Family Council to get organized. We think that's an underestimate, but keep at it and it will get done.

The form on the next page can be used to record the minutes of a Family Council meeting. You can use the same Department Response to Issues form, shown in the Resident Council section, to record responses to issues raised by the Family Council.

Family Council Meeting

Meeting Date: ______________________________

Attendance: ________________ ________________ ________________

________________ ________________ ________________

________________ ________________ ________________

________________ ________________ ________________

________________ ________________ ________________

________________ ________________ ________________

Agenda: ____

____

____

____

Minutes: ____

____

____

____

Action Items:

Concern: ____

Department: ____

Response (including Plan of Correction): ______________________

____

Concern: ____

Department: ____

Response (including Plan of Correction): ______________________

____

Recommendations:

____

____

____

16. Volunteers

"Volunteers" is the first word that you will hear from the administrator after you accept the position of an activity professional. Not only do you need volunteers as part of your departmental team, the people you serve need a variety of personalities and a collection of talents to enhance the quality of their interactions. It is important, however, to inject a word of caution. Do not begin recruiting volunteers until there is a structure to your program. In terms of priorities, the department needs to be well organized and structured and you need to know both the resident needs and the volunteer needs. If you encourage volunteers without a vision for how the experience will benefit them and the people you serve, it will be disappointing to all involved. And most importantly, the volunteer will not stay long.

Both federal and state regulations identify the need for volunteers and address this as a function of the activity department. Volunteers can help with groups or provide one-on-one support. LITA, which is a good example of a one-on-one volunteer program, is discussed at the end of this chapter.

Activity Department Volunteers

There are many excellent resources on designing and developing a volunteer program. Contact the local volunteer center in your community and request brochures and job descriptions. Arrange to go to training sessions that they offer. Go to facilities and organizations that have strong and successful programs in place. Although the settings and needs are different, the basic development of a volunteer program is similar.

Steps in Developing a Volunteer Program

- Identify what needs the department has for volunteers.
- Write volunteer policies and procedures.
- Design a job description with specific responsibilities, qualifications, and time needed.
- Have a choice of possible work and responsibilities for volunteers to choose from.
- Identify volunteer skills, talents, and strengths for the growth of both volunteer and program.
- Create forms for applications, orientation to facility, work, attendance records (sign in and keep track of hours), and evaluation.
- Recruit and select volunteers. This process should be as structured as it was for you to be interviewed and selected.
- Train and orient all volunteers well. The more information that a volunteer has, the better able s/he is to meet the demands of the work, the people you serve, and the setting.
- After orientation, have the volunteer sign the orientation form to document that they were oriented and understand the requirements and limitations of the position. Keep this on file.
- Supervise. By working with a volunteer on site you continue his/her training and assure follow through with the responsibilities of the work.
- Evaluate. It's easiest to evaluate volunteers according to the duties and outline of the specific work. Everyone needs feedback on how s/he is doing and this is one of your responsibilities as the volunteer coordinator.

Evaluation should be done on a regularly scheduled basis.

- Recognize. Individuals who volunteer are doing so for personal reasons. There is a personal goal that they have identified as being important in their lives. For most it is the opportunity to help others in need or to build work skills that can be transferred to employment. There are other volunteers who are completing hours either for school or to work off minor violations through a community service program. These volunteers also need feedback and recognition for their work. There are many ways to recognize volunteers. What are more important than "prizes," are recognition and individual honors. Volunteers need to know that they are making a difference to the organization and lives of the people you serve. Having the people you serve involved in this recognition is very meaningful.

If you have ever volunteered, you know how important it is to manage this time into your already busy schedule. Be clear on how much time is needed per day or week or month. If a volunteer feels that there is not enough organization or direction, s/he will seek out another agency that is better prepared.

Another important area to consider is how you identify needs to determine what volunteer jobs should be created. Think beyond the needs of group activity and individual visits. These both are very important and demand assistance from volunteers. However, there are many other ways that individuals and groups can be involved. Some ideas are

- Writing and typing the newsletter
- Decorating the facility
- Shopping
- Letter writing
- Sewing and mending
- Caring for facility pets
- Sharing talents in performances
- Creating visual aids and cards for residents who are sensory impaired
- Making the new month's calendar of activities
- Monitoring residents who are confused and disoriented in structured parallel sensory activities
- Filing and organizing the office
- Reaching out to the community with presentations and flyers
- Developing an intergenerational exchange program with a local school or agency
- Having a business or agency adopt your facility one time monthly

The list is endless so the best way to begin is with a wish list. Volunteers help create a quality activity program! It takes work to recruit and supervise a good set of volunteers, but all staff, residents, and families feel the benefits.

> Sometimes our light goes out, but is blown again into flame by an encounter with another human being. Each of us owes the deepest thanks to those who have rekindled this inner light.
>
> *Albert Schweitzer*

Social Services Volunteers

The social services volunteer differs significantly in function from the volunteer in the activity program mainly because emphasis is on one-on-one contact as opposed to group involvement. This means that a volunteer who wishes to interact directly with an individual must maintain contact with the social services professional to stay abreast of changes in the emotional or physical status of the individual s/he visits.

In our experience, however, it can be difficult to recruit and train the true social services volunteer — the person who is not threatened or intimidated by the ongoing contact with one person at a potentially intimate emotional level. There is a high turnover rate with one-on-one volunteers as they begin to feel that they are not qualified or are not prepared to interact with an individual so intensely. Often a volunteer will come to the facility with some time to share but with no idea of how emotional this experience can be. Also, some volunteers begin to relate too personally in this setting because they themselves are elderly or have an aging relative. These factors also contribute to the high turnover rate among volunteers.

When we are fortunate enough to find individuals who are willing and able to take on the role of social services volunteers, they act as a direct adjunct to the social services program and extend the contact that the social services professional is able to have with the person.

The social services volunteer may be a Friendly Visitor (some begin in this casual role and stay for years), a support to someone in an adjustment crisis, a source of support for someone in a terminal state, or a variation on these themes. The key to success in terms of individual needs is a solid mix of warmth, compassion, consistency, and a true interest.

The social services professional has the responsibility of providing ongoing support for the volunteer, beginning with a well-rounded orientation to the facility and a definition of role expectations. An introduction to Resident Rights, especially confidentiality, is essential. After that, a weekly check-in is vital. The volunteer can offer "untrained" insights and ask questions which will assist in a better overall psychosocial plan for the individual. The social services professional can share information from a professional perspective and elicit feelings and concerns from the volunteer.

Your support may be what makes the difference in keeping a volunteer in your facility — for the benefit of all concerned.

One-on-One Friendship Programs

One of the most important gifts that you can give to an individual is the gift of ageless friendship. A volunteer not only adds to the services provided by the activity department, s/he also adds to the quality of life of the individual. The losses associated with being in a care setting are profound, and depression is prevalent in every setting. One way to lessen the loneliness is to bring in volunteers of all ages to visit on a one-on-one basis and match them with a person who has no family or visitors close by.

Such a volunteer program has existed in California under the name of LITA (*Love is the Answer*) for the past thirty-five years. The mission statement of this non-profit organization is to lessen loneliness in long-term care settings by providing one-on-one friends for isolated residents. The concept is a simple one, to be a friend. The commitment for the volunteer is a weekly visit of at least 15–30 minutes with the matched resident friend. Matches are made with only one resident at a time as developing relationships takes time and attention.

We encourage you to look within your geographic area and identify agencies and programs that offer volunteer services to the elderly. This may be a volunteer organization, church affiliated program, or a service provided through your community's agency on aging. Find ways in which to link onto an already existing program if possible. Also, contact other skilled nursing facilities and assisted living settings to see if they would be interested in organizing a program similar to LITA. It makes such a difference.

Volunteer Resources

Album for Activity Compliance, Michele Nolta, Recreation Therapy Consultants, 6115 Syracuse Lane, San Diego, CA 92122. (858) 546-9003. (This publication has excellent forms for volunteer programs.)

17. Quality Assurance and Performance Improvement, Infection Control, Risk Management, and Emergency Preparedness

This chapter covers important aspects of working in any health care setting: quality assurance and performance improvement (QAPI), infection control, risk management, and emergency preparedness. *QAPI* looks at the ability to provide the highest quality services and treatment. *Infection control* is concerned with the ability to eliminate the spread of infection from one individual to another. *Risk management* discusses the ongoing process of making the environment safer. *Emergency preparedness* assures that each community is ready to respond to a variety of emergency situations with protocols and procedures in place and regular in-service training

Providing the individual with quality services — meeting his/her needs — does not happen by accident. It takes knowledge, thoughtfulness, and some old fashioned self-evaluation to do good work. And, it does not matter how good your services are or how successful your treatment is if you cannot guarantee the person you serve a basic level of safety while s/he is in your facility. Each individual has the absolute right to be free from bodily harm or psychological damage while receiving care. It is up to each staff person to act in a manner that ensures that each of the people we serve is safe. An effective quality assurance and performance improvement program, knowledge of the basic principles of infection control, a solid understanding of risk management, and being prepared for emergencies are required to ensure a good program.

Quality Assurance and Performance Improvement

Quality assurance and performance improvement is a process of continually self-evaluating the services you provide and then improving the services based on problems you have identified and corrected. In order to continually evaluate your department, you must have a QAPI Program in place.

Quality assurance is not a new term but is much more frequently used in nursing homes now that OBRA '87 regulations (Tags F865, F866, F867, and F868) have mandated that each nursing facility have a QAPI program. Almost every type of facility will have some kind of quality assurance program.

Section 6109 (c) of the Affordable Care Act requires all skilled nursing care centers to develop a Quality Assurance and Performance Improvement Program. QAPI is defined by CMS as "an initiative that goes beyond the current Quality Assessment and Assurance (QAA) provision, and aims to significantly expand the intensity and scope of current activities in order to not only correct quality deficiencies (quality assurance), but also to put practices in place to monitor all nursing home care and services to continuously improve performance" You can access more information on QAPI at www.ahcancal.org/quality_improvement/QAPI/Pages/default.aspx.

A QAPI program must include policies and procedures for quality assurance and a committee that meets at least quarterly to review current studies and issues.

A long-term care facility must maintain an ongoing assessment of the quality of services provided and have a QAPI committee to monitor the overall effectiveness of the facility's program. The QAPI committee consists of:

- The director of nursing services,
- A physician designated by the facility, and
- At least three other facility staff members.

The quality assurance committee must meet at least quarterly to identify areas that could and should be improved and to develop and implement appropriate plans to correct identified quality deficiencies.

Assuring Success

Quality assurance and performance improvement (QAPI) is the process of internally monitoring your own work. It is an ongoing program that looks at the quality of the services provided, as well as the cost effectiveness of those services. Performance improvement was added to quality assurance because it is required by CMS under the Affordable Care Act.

It is not enough to find out at survey time that there are problems. We should always know, during the entire year, what our weak areas are. And we should always be working on improving our services by taking a systematic approach to problem solving. Just as we have written out care plans identifying ways to meet resident needs (with measurable objectives), we need a written quality assurance program that identifies ways to improve our services.

The best way to begin the process is by educating all staff on the importance of monitoring their performance. Stress that they are not only a part of the process but also accountable for the end results.

Starting a Program or Study?

Your facility already has a QAPI program, policy and procedure manual, and QAPI committee. If you are not a member of the committee, ask to sit in on these meetings to better understand the process. Each professional should be a strong element of this committee because of his/her involvement in the area of *Quality of Life*, *Resident Behavior and Practices,* and *Quality of Care.*

The QAPI process is, by definition, an interdisciplinary process. When the committee has identified an area needing attention, all departments will work to solve the problem. But in addition to working on identified problems, each department should be on the lookout for potential problems and issues specific to its service.

Types of Studies

There are many areas to study. Some of these might include:

- Does the current program meet the needs of the current population?
- Are some individuals having difficulty getting to activity groups of interest? If the individual is not getting to the activity, this is an issue to address in QAPI.
- Is there a clear definition of the role of activity professionals in the behavior management programs to decrease the use of psychoactive medications?
- Is there a clear definition of the role of activity professionals in the physical restraint reduction programs during groups or one-on-one activities?
- Are the people we serve satisfied with their rooms, food, opportunities, interactions with staff, or any other quality of life issues?
- Is the space where activities are held large enough? Is the lighting at the proper level for individuals who have visual impairments?
- Are all levels of cognitive and functional needs being met in group or individual settings?
- According to the percentage of men or younger residents in the facility, are there appropriate and available leisure activities for their interests?

There are specific steps involved in the design of a quality assurance study. The chart on the following page shows the five steps you need to take for a successful QAPI program. For more information about quality assurance programs see Cunninghis and Best-Martini's book, *Quality Assurance for Activity Programs, Second Edition* (1996) from Idyll Arbor, Inc.

The following forms can be used as quality assurance review forms for survey preparedness. The first two forms provide a review of what you should be doing that will help you prepare for survey. The third and fourth forms can be used to review your activities. It can also be used as a time management tool and for orienting new employees to their duties.

Steps of QAPI Programs[55]

Step 1	*Identifying Issues and Selecting Study Topics*	Obviously it is essential to begin with a determination of what service needs to be improved to provide quality service. This first step has you look closely at the problem to specifically identify what is not right. Unfortunately, many quality assurance programs concern themselves with issues that are not important or with procedural items that can be easily remedied, rather than those that justify being part of long-range planning.
Step 2a	*Establishing Indicators*	Identifying elements that can be monitored to measure changes made. The elements or characteristics of the service you select to measure should be a general statement about what the service would look like if there were not a problem.
Step 2b	*Developing Criteria*	Developing criteria for each indicator. Writing a plan that spells out exactly what should be found and ideally in what quantity and in what time frame.
Step 3a	*Determining Methodology*	Establishing the exact method to be used to collect information: from which sources, by whom, how often, how long, and how the results are going to be used.
Step 3b	*Collecting Data*	Implementing the chosen methods of data collection.
Step 4a	*Understanding the Problem*	Reviewing and assessing collected data to see what, where, and how serious the problems are. Deciding which problem areas should be the focus of further study.
Step 4b	*Setting Standards*	Standards are set to describe the desired outcomes in a measurable way.
Step 4c	*Finding Solutions*	Searching for possible ways to reach the standards set.
Step 4d	*Writing an Action Plan*	The methodology for implementing a change is determined along with decisions about who is to have the responsibility and what the time frames will be.
Step 4e	*Implementing*	Putting into action the strategies that have been developed.
Step 5a	*Assessing the Outcomes*	Did the plan work? Do the problems still remain? Has there been some improvement? This procedure often entails a repeat of steps 3 and 4: going back and re-collecting the data and then analyzing the results to see if the standards have been reached.
Step 5b	*Identifying New Issues or Continuing to Work on the Old*	If the problems are not solved, new strategies must be planned. If, however, the process has been successful, a new plan should be developed for the next area of focus. As stated earlier, quality assurance is an ongoing process and does not stop once a particular problem is corrected. It is also necessary to periodically go back and monitor earlier plans and see if the goals are continuing to be met. Two or three past issues may be chosen at random for an ongoing audit in addition to the main topic of study. These could be changed periodically on a rotating basis to assure that new problems have not arisen in any of these areas.

[55] Cunninghis, R. N. and E. Best-Martini, 1996, *Quality assurance for activity programs, second edition*, pp. 18–19, Idyll Arbor, Inc., Ravensdale, WA.

QAPI Checklist for Activities

Reviewed by: ____________________________ Date: ________________

Review this list to determine the level of compliance for your department.

Staff **Yes/No**

1. Proof of training/qualifications ______
2. Consultation reports and qualifications ______
3. Job descriptions ______
4. Weekend coverage ______
5. Evening coverage ______
6. Professional involvement ______
7. In-service training ______

Documentation

1. Initial activity assessment form ______
2. MDS form, activity portion (LTC) ______
3. Input to CAA summary sheet (LTC) ______
4. Care plan entry ______
5. Daily attendance (7 days per week) ______
   Did you include level of participation and refusals? ______
6. Bedside log ______
   Did you include type, frequency, and response to visit? ______
7. Individual included in assessment and care plan process ______
8. Quarterly activity progress note ______
   Did it end with a goal? ______
   Is this the same as on the care plan? ______
9. Change of condition note ______
10. Physician's orders for activities, outings, and work related activities ______

Physical Environment

1. Large calendar posted and legible to visually impaired ______
2. Individual calendars in each room ______

Program Evaluation

1. Activity Analysis Form completed for all activities offered ______
2. Activity Program Review completed ______
3. Programs offered that meet the diversity of resident needs and abilities ______

Resident Rights

1. Resident Council minutes ______
   Proof of resolution to issues ______
   Posted invitation to monthly meetings. ______
2. Review of resident rights ______
3. Review of last survey results ______
4. Accessibility of survey results to interested residents ______
5. Opportunity to register to vote ______

Notes

QAPI Checklist for Social Services

Reviewed by: ____________________________ Date: __________________

Review this list to determine the level of compliance for your department.

Staff **Yes/No**

1. Proof of qualifications .... ______
2. Job description .... ______
3. Consultant reports and qualifications .... ______
4. Professional improvement .... ______
5. In-service training .... ______

Documentation

1. Social history .... ______
2. Initial psychosocial assessment .... ______
3. Initial discharge plan .... ______
4. MDS form, psychosocial aspects (LTC) .... ______
5. CAA summary sheet input (LTC) .... ______
6. Care plan entry .... ______
7. Quarterly social services progress note .... ______
8. Annual social services progress note .... ______
9. Annual discharge plan update .... ______
10. MDS update (change of condition) (LTC) .... ______
11. Care conference attendance sign in .... ______
12. Durable power of attorney for health care, living will directive to physicians, and/or conservator papers .... ______
13. Advance directives signed (such as no CPR) .... ______
14. Surrogate decision maker listed .... ______
15. Room change notification; introductions made .... ______

Optional Recommendations

1. Community resource file .... ______
2. Family council minutes .... ______
3. Theft and loss log .... ______
4. Social services groups .... ______
5. Social services newsletter .... ______
6. Social services log .... ______
7. Social services volunteers .... ______
8. Grievance log .... ______
9. Log for marked dentures, glasses, and hearing aids .... ______
10. Client follow-up after discharge .... ______

Notes

Activity Department Checklist

Activity Professional ________________________________ **Starting Date** ____________

Daily — Areas To Be Completed	Mon	Tue	Wed	Thu	Fri	Sat	Sun
Attendance							
MDS —CAA Summary							
Initial Interviews and Assessments Completed							
Schedule Changes and Revisions							
Quarterly Progress Notes							
Volunteer Sign-in and Supervision							
Room Visits/Bedside Log							
Office/Department Readied for Next Day							
Other							

Weekly	
Shopping and Inventory	
Community Contacts	
Care Conference	
Completion of Special Planning	
Interdepartmental Meetings	
Calendars/Decorations/Newsletter	
Department Head Meetings	

Monthly	
In-service Training	
Resident Council Minutes	

Notes:

Social Services Department Checklist

Social Services Professional ____________________________ **Starting Date** _____________

Daily — Areas to be completed	Mon	Tue	Wed	Thu	Fri	Sat	Sun
Department Head Meetings							
Complete Assessments on New Admission							
Complete Multidisciplinary Discharge Summary							
Paperwork Related to Room Changes							
Introduce Residents to New Roommates							
Fix Up Room Changes with Visit about Move							
Chart Room Changes and Adjustments							
Document Significant Behavior Changes							
Document Significant Changes in Condition							
Record Lost Dentures, Glasses, and Hearing Aids							
Clothing and Personal Care Needs							
Transportation Needs							
Family and Resident Counseling							
Deaths							
Discharge Planning							

Weekly	√
Quarterly, Annual Progress Note Updates (Including MDS)	
Attend Resident Care Conferences	
Attend Rehabilitation Meetings	
Organize Rehabilitation Meetings with Resident and Family	
New Resident Adjustment Issues	
In-service Training	
Staff Meetings	

Monthly	√
Send Out Notices for Next Month's Resident Care Conferences	

Notes:

Infection Control, Tags F880-F883

The spread of infection requires three elements: 1. a source of infectious material, 2. a resident who is susceptible to the infectious material, and 3. a means of transmitting that infectious material to the susceptible resident. Just by the nature of health care facilities it is not possible to exclude infectious material (people come in sick), nor is it possible to exclude individuals who might be susceptible to infection. The only way to truly control the spread of infection in facilities is to control the transmission.

There are four main routes of spreading infections:

1. Contact transmission
   - Direct contact (staff to resident or resident to resident)
   - Indirect contact (germs transmitted by touching an object, e.g. a CD player passed from one resident to another)
   - Droplet contact (transmission of germs from a person sneezing, coughing, or talking within a distance of three feet)
2. Vehicle route transmission through contaminated items (food, water, drugs, blood)
3. Airborne transmission (infectious materials which adhere to moisture or dust in the air and are suspended for long periods of time)
4. Vector-borne transmission (infection spread through an insect or animal as in mosquito-transmitted malaria)

Hand washing is the best way to control the spread of infections. Staff will need to wash their hands after coming into physical contact with any resident, using the restroom, or coming into contact with activity supplies that may have contaminated surfaces. It would not be unusual for activity professionals to wash their hands over 30 times a day — activity assistants even more.

Using good hand washing technique is important. First, get the hands wet. Place soap in the hands and lather up the soap. Once the soap is lathered, scrub all parts of the hands while slowly counting to ten. The hands should be rinsed under running water while continually rubbing the hands, again counting to ten slowly. Dry the hand using disposable towels or air-dry them. Turn off the water using the paper towels, not the newly cleaned hands, to turn the handles.

Many of the supplies used by activity professionals are considered to be "reusable equipment" versus "disposable equipment." Nursing and other health care professionals have turned to using disposable equipment to help significantly reduce the spread of microorganisms, but this would prove too costly for activity departments. It is therefore important that the activity professional learn the basics of good disinfecting techniques.

When cleaning items that can tolerate getting wet, use the following technique:

- The staff or volunteer doing the cleaning should wear waterproof gloves while cleaning all items.
- When using equipment that has moving parts or comes apart to be cleaned and has body secretions on it, take apart the item immediately after it is used. This allows cleaning to take place later without the pieces becoming stuck together after the secretions dry.
- When rinsing the item to be washed, always use cold water first. Body secretions are more likely to coagulate (to thicken and become glue-like) when placed in hot water versus cold water.
- Soap and sudsy water work well for loosening up dirt. Let items soak if possible.
- When doing the actual cleaning, use water as hot as your hands will tolerate. Hot water and soap help break the dirt into tiny particles, making them easier to rinse off.
- Use a cloth or sponge if you need to clean using friction (scrubbing). This friction,

combined with hot water and soap, breaks down the dirt and microorganisms into even smaller pieces, allowing for easy rinsing.

- Use a stiff bristled brush to remove dirt and microorganisms from grooves in the equipment, being careful not to allow any of the dirt to fly up into your face. Wear a face shield or a mask and goggles for extra precautions.
- Use abrasive cleaners to remove stains that soaking doesn't remove. Use alcohol or ether to remove oily stains that don't come out with just soap and water. Remember to rinse items cleaned this way thoroughly.
- Rinse all items under hot, running water to detach any remaining dirt and microorganisms.
- Thoroughly dry all supplies prior to putting them away.
- Clean all of your cleaning supplies and then wash your hands, even though you wore gloves.

For items that cannot be washed using water and soap, follow your agency's disinfecting or sterilization techniques. When using disposable equipment, dispose of the equipment immediately after use to reduce the chance of further contamination of other equipment.

Risk Management

Risk management is the act of identifying situations in the workplace that may harm the person we serve, the staff, or the facility. Most facilities will have many policies and procedures related to making the workplace safe. This section will talk about how the staff controls for risk.

Controlling risk is like placing a safety net under the person we serve. It requires around-the-clock management by each staff person — on duty as well as off duty. Krames Communications, in the booklet "Risk Management: Your Role in Providing Quality Care" (1989) lists eight areas of around-the-clock management. Specific questions for the professionals have been added to Krames Communications' categories.

Around-the-Clock Risk Management

On the Job

Safe Environment

- Are the activity supplies appropriate for the individual's abilities?
- Are all the fire exits unblocked?
- Is the water temperature below 110°F?

Ongoing Monitoring

- Do individual assessments represent the individual's actual abilities and needs?
- Are staff diligent in changing the individual's care plan as the individual's abilities change?
- Are staff continuing to be careful about individual safety and infection control?

Clear Communication

- Do staff communicate important information to each other concerning an individual's status and workplace concerns?
- Do staff communicate with the people we serve and their families in a timely and appropriate manner?

Handling Incidents

- Do all staff know the facility's policies and procedures well enough to implement them all of the time?
- Have staff had the proper training to be able to carry out the administration's intent for handling the different types of incidents?

Off the Job

Continuing Education

- Have you kept your knowledge and skills up-to-date by continually seeking out new information?

- Are you seeking continuing education in the areas where you have the weakest knowledge and skill, not just the areas that are convenient or interesting to you?

Journals

- Do you regularly (e.g., at least monthly) spend an hour or more reading up on new information and developments in your professional journals?
- Do you support the body of knowledge by writing up important information or developments and submitting them for publication?

Professional Groups

- Are you an active member in at least one national and state/local organization?
- Do you find time to discuss issues with other professionals outside of your facility, especially if you are a one-person department?

Healthy Lifestyle

- Are you responsible enough to make sure that you get enough sleep prior to going to work to reduce the chance of mistakes being made?
- Do you eat food that is good for your physical health and exercise on a regular basis to be able to perform your job well?
- Do you balance your work life with your play life to be able to be refreshed?

Standards of Practice

How do you ensure that each individual is safe while s/he is in your environment and receiving your services? One of the most successful ways of ensuring that the individual is receiving quality care and services is to make sure that your department is adhering to professional standards of practice. Standards of practice usually outline minimum standards for management of the service, minimum standards for delivery of the service, and minimum qualifications for staff. However, even when you seem to be following standards of practice completely, you may still run into problems. Risk management and quality assurance are similar — only on different ends of the continuum. Quality assurance is the process of improving good services to make them better. Risk management is the process of reducing or eliminating harmful or dangerous situations. There are six steps:

1. To recognize that there is a problem.
2. To be able to identify what in the system is causing the problem.
3. To be able to identify who is impacted by the problem.
4. To be able to identify if the problem is changeable (or if other systems need to be changed to accommodate for what cannot be changed — a long-term care facility cannot decide to exclude all individuals who are HIV positive, so they need to change their systems of infection control to accommodate those individuals).
5. To develop a method of correcting the problem.
6. To develop a means to measure if the problem was corrected.

joan burlingame studied the worst breakdowns in resident safety in her 1992 study of Immediate Jeopardy citations. She was able to identify ten basic principles of reducing risks to resident safety. By being aware of these risks, the activity professional can help manage harmful or dangerous situations within his/her own facility. These basic principles are

- Water temperature at the taps should never be over 110° Fahrenheit.
- Fire doors and fire routes must always be free of clutter. Fire safety standards must always be followed.
- Floors should be free of objects that may cause the individual to slip or to trip.
- Walkways (including hallways) must be free of protruding objects — many individuals have poor vision and may walk into a protruding object and injure themselves. (Protruding objects may stick out only 4 inches

from the wall between the heights of 27" to 80" from the floor. Exceptions are made for drinking fountains or telephones that are mounted on posts. They may stick out 12 inches.)

- The building must be maintained in a manner that ensures it is always structurally safe.
- Staff must always talk to and treat each individual respectfully.
- Only life threatening events should get in the way of any staff helping an individual resident move/turn who is at risk for pressure sores and is in need of movement/turning.
- Staff should always practice good infection control principles.
- Staff should always ensure the physical safety of each individual — including protecting him/her from self-inflected injuries.
- Food and fluid should always be treated as if they were a prescription item — never given to an individual unless in a manner which follows the medical orders.

The most important thing for staff to remember is — if something doesn't seem right, it probably isn't. Even if your supervisor assures you that the way a resident is being treated is all right because the treatment team agreed to the treatment, if you feel that it may be abusive or neglectful treatment, *act!* Approach your facility administrator. If that doesn't work, each state has a law that says a staff person must report a potential case of abuse or neglect, usually in 24 hours or less. It is not up to that staff person to obtain proof that the treatment is abusive or neglectful. If the staff person suspects abuse or neglect, s/he is to leave it up to the state investigators. When you call, you do not need to give your name. Remember, you may be the best advocate that the resident has!

Immediate Jeopardy

Surveys are conducted, in part, to assess whether your facility follows appropriate risk management practices. When a survey is conducted, the surveyors determine whether or not a facility meets the Conditions of Participation (the federal regulations) for receiving Medicare and Medicaid funding by assessing whether the facility meets all of the requirements in the federal regulations. Usually, a deficiency means that the provider must submit a plan of correction to be acted upon within 30 days.

Sometimes the surveyors discover situations that are so severe that stronger sanctions are required. In these cases, the guidelines for determining "immediate jeopardy" (also known as "fast track") are applied. The provider must correct a condition of "immediate jeopardy" immediately or "immediate termination action" will be taken; i.e., the residents will be removed and the facility closed.

To assist surveyors in determining when circumstances pose an "immediate jeopardy" to an individual's health and safety, a set of criteria has been developed. This guide is intended to provide greater consistency among surveyors when reviewing specific situations and assessing provider failures.

The standards for the funding for health care services (and therefore, the standards of health care practice) in the United States depend heavily on the actions of the Congress of the United States. For administration purposes, health care is divided into two separate entities, the Centers for Medicare and Medicaid Services and the Public Health Service. Almost every activity professional who works in a clinical setting is under the auspices of the Centers for Medicare and Medicaid Services or CMS.

Specific minimum standards are set for each type of facility, e.g., hospitals, home health care, long-term care (nursing homes), etc. All changes and new health care laws are released on October 1 of each year in the government publication called the Code of Federal Regulations or CFR. While most regulations are facility-type specific, there are two federal health care regulations that apply to all health care under the jurisdiction of CMS. The first regulation is the Civil Rights Act (Title Six). The second regulation, the most stringent, is called *Immediate Jeopardy*, also known as Appendix Q.

With just a few exceptions, every facility that is surveyed either by the Joint Commission or by CARF: the Rehabilitation Accreditation Commission falls under the jurisdiction of CMS. The loss of CMS certification is actually more severe than the loss of accreditation either by the Joint Commission or by CARF. A facility may maintain its business license without Joint Commission or CARF Accreditation. Without CMS certification, it is not likely that a facility can maintain its business license. In such a case, it often requires legislation on the state level to maintain the facility.

Definitions from Appendix Q and Appendix J

Immediate and Serious Threat. An immediate and serious threat is defined as a situation having a high probability that serious harm or injury to residents could occur at any time or already has occurred and may well occur again if residents are not protected effectively from the harm or the threat is not removed.

Patients. Includes all persons receiving treatment, care, or services from the provider.

Physical Abuse. Refers to any physical motion or action (e.g., hitting, slapping, punching, kicking, pinching, etc.) by which bodily harm or trauma occurs. It includes use of corporal punishment as well as the use of any restrictive, intrusive procedure to control inappropriate behavior for the purpose of punishment.

Provider/Facility. Means all Medicare providers and suppliers and Medicaid only facilities (intermediate care facilities for the mentally retarded — ICF-MR).

Psychological Abuse. Includes, but is not limited to, humiliation, harassment, and threats of punishment or deprivation, sexual coercion, intimidation, whereby individuals suffer psychological harm or trauma.

Verbal Abuse, Refers to any use of oral, written, or gestured language by which abuse occurs. This includes pejorative and derogatory terms to describe persons with disabilities.

Guiding Principles. (taken directly from Appendix Q)

1. An immediate and serious threat need not result in actual harm to the resident. The threat of probable harm is perceived as being as serious or significant.
2. The threat could be perceived as something that will result in potentially severe temporary or permanent injury, disability, or death and must be perceived as something, which is likely to occur in the very near future.
3. Mental abuse can be as damaging as physical abuse and may constitute an immediate and serious threat.
4. Only one resident needs to be jeopardized; the entire or large percentage of resident population does not have to be threatened or injured.
5. The absence of adequate staff training does not, in and of itself, pose the threat. However, if the staff lacks the skill or knowledge necessary to properly care for the residents, this may present the same serious problems as when there are insufficient numbers of staff and will make it more difficult for the provider to correct or eliminate the problems.
6. The situation is severe enough that it outweighs potential concerns of resident transfer to another facility.
7. The situation may or may not be a threat considering such factors as season of the year and geographic location.
8. The deficiency cannot be corrected quickly to prevent a resident from being severely harmed.
9. Immediate and serious threat termination is the only response to the problem.

Immediate Jeopardy may be "called" without having to close a facility. By citing Immediate Jeopardy the survey team is stating that there exists an unacceptable threat to a resident, which must be corrected within hours or days, or else termination action will begin. Termination action usually does not officially occur (with public notification) until the fifth day after Immediate Jeopardy has been called.

Emergency Preparedness

Each care community is responsible by federal, state, and county regulations to be ready for any emergency and to assure the safety of all residents, staff, and family members. The emergency could be a power outage, hurricane, earthquake, fire, active shooter situation, etc. Whatever the emergency, there needs to be a clear and concise list of protocols to follow. These protocols need to be familiar to all staff and be in-serviced on a regular basis. Below is a form created by CMS to outline some of the emergency protocols.

U.S. DEPARTMENT OF HEALTH AND HUMAN SERVICES CENTERS FOR MEDICARE & MEDICAID SERVICES

Survey & Certification
Emergency Preparedness for Every Emergency

EMERGENCY PLANNING CHECKLIST
RECOMMENDED TOOL FOR PERSONS IN LONG-TERM CARE FACILITIES & THEIR FAMILY MEMBERS, FRIENDS, PERSONAL CAREGIVERS, GUARDIANS & LONG-TERM CARE OMBUDSMEN

Part I:		**For Long-Term Care Residents, Their Family Members, Friends, Personal Caregivers, & Guardians**
Target Date	Date Completed	
		• **Emergency Plan:** Prior to any emergency, ask about and become familiar with the facility's emergency plan, including: ✓ Location of emergency exits ✓ How alarm system works and modifications for individuals who are hearing and/or visually impaired ✓ Plans for evacuation, including: ▪ How residents/visitors requiring assistance will be evacuated, if necessary ▪ How the facility will ensure each resident can be identified during evacuation (e.g., attach identification information to each resident prior to evacuation) ▪ Facility's evacuation strategy ▪ Where they will go ▪ How their medical charts will be transferred ▪ How families will be notified of evacuation ✓ Will families be able to bring their loved one home rather than evacuating, which is often less traumatic than a move to a new facility? ✓ How family members can keep the facility apprised of their location and contact information (e.g., address, phone number, e-mail address), so the facility will be able to contact them, and family members will be able to check with the facility to meet their loved one following an emergency ✓ How residents and the medicines and supplies they require will be prepared for the emergency, have their possessions protected and be kept informed during and following the emergency ✓ How residents (if able) and family members can be helpful (for example, should family members come to the facility to assist?) ✓ How residents, who are able, may be involved during the emergency, including their roles and responsibilities. **Note**: It is important for staff to know each resident personally, and whether involving him/her in the emergency plan will increase a sense of security or cause anxiety.. For example, residents may have prior work or personal experience that could be of value (health care, emergency services, military, amateur ham radio operators, etc.) Provide the opportunity for residents to discuss any fears and what actions may help to relieve their anxiety (e.g., a flashlight on the bed, water beside the bed, etc.).

Note: Some of the recommended tasks may exceed the long-term care facility's Federal regulatory requirements.

U.S. DEPARTMENT OF HEALTH AND HUMAN SERVICES — CENTERS FOR MEDICARE & MEDICAID SERVICES

Survey & Certification
Emergency Preparedness for Every Emergency

		• **Helping Residents in a Relocation:** Suggested principles of care for relocated residents include: ✓ Encourage the resident to talk about expectations, anger, and/or disappointment ✓ Work to develop a level of trust ✓ Present an optimistic, favorable attitude about the relocation ✓ Anticipate that anxiety will occur ✓ Do not argue with the resident ✓ Do not give orders ✓ Do not take the resident's behavior personally ✓ Use praise liberally ✓ Be courteous and kind ✓ Include the resident in assessing problems ✓ Encourage family participation ✓ Ensure staff in the receiving facility introduce themselves to residents
Part II:		**For Long-Term Care Ombudsmen**
Targeted Date	Date Completed	
		• **State Ombudsman Responsibilities:** ✓ Become generally familiar with state emergency plans pertinent to long-term care facilities, including the state or federal agency that may be established to serve as a clearinghouse for facility evacuations: know the name, telephone number and e-mail of the person to whom long-term care facility evacuations and evacuees' names should be reported. If no clearinghouse has been established, advocate for one. ✓ At least annually, ensure that all regional ombudsman coordinators and local ombudsmen and/or representatives read, are familiar with and have the opportunity to discuss resources, such as the two recommended CMS emergency preparedness checklists pertaining to long-term care facilities: the *CMS Emergency Preparedness Checklist – Recommended Tool for Effective Health Care Facility Planning* and this *CMS Emergency Planning Checklist – Recommended Tool for Persons Living In Long-Term Care Facilities, Their Family Members, Friends, Personal Caregivers, Guardians, & Long-Term Care Ombudsmen.* ✓ Maintain at home and office hard copies of current regional ombudsman contact information, including cell phones. ✓ Prior to an anticipated disaster, if the state ombudsman program has regional coordinators and/or other program representatives in the areas likely to be affected, call them to make sure they have assigned representatives to carry out the responsibilities listed in the section below pertaining to local ombudsman programs. ✓ Immediately following a disaster, contact regional ombudsman coordinators/representatives in the affected areas to provide support and

Note: Some of the recommended tasks may exceed the long-term care facility's Federal regulatory requirements.

18. Management

This chapter discusses some of the important management issues not covered in the rest of the book. The issues include resident rights, restraints, behavior management, time management, budgets, writing policies and procedures, OBRA '87 regulations, surveys, and medications for the elderly.

Resident's Rights

Residents in both assisted living centers and nursing facilities have specific rights outlined in federal and state laws. This section discusses some of the most important rights.

The primary right of a resident is to make decisions and exercise their rights. If the resident is no longer competent to make decisions, another individual is named to represent the resident's wishes.

The resident rights section of the federal regulations has the most changes of any other section. This is a list of the entire 483.10 Resident Rights F-Tags for your review. Each new resident is also required to receive his/her own copy of these regulations.

Resident's Rights, CMS, and Culture Change

These guideline revisions helped to intertwine the culture change movement and federal regulations. By doing so, CMS was able to reflect their interest in seeing and being a part of this very important movement. In addition, since the revisions more clearly define expectations, surveyors and community staff members can all be working on the same concepts and protocols to better empower those individuals living in long-term care settings.

Be sure to read each revision and keep a copy for your department as these revisions play a significant role in the resident council.

483.10 Resident Rights

F550 Resident Rights/Exercise of Rights
F551 Rights Exercised by Representative
F552 Right to be Informed/Make Treatment Decisions
F553 Right to Participate in Planning Care
F554 Resident Self-Admin Meds-Clinically Appropriate
F555 Right to Choose/Be informed of Attending Physician
F557 Respect, Dignity/Right to have Personal Property
F558 Reasonable Accommodation of Needs/Preferences
F559 Choose/Be Notified of Room/Roommate Change
F560 Right to Refuse Certain Transfers
F561 Self Determination
F562 Immediate Access to Resident
F563 Right to Receive/Deny Visitors
F564 Inform of Visitation Rights/Equal Visitation Privileges
F565 Resident/Family Group and Response
F566 Right to Perform Facility Services or Refuse
F567 Protection/Management of Personal Funds
F568 Accounting and Records of Personal Funds
F569 Notice and Conveyance of Personal Funds
F570 Surety Bond-Security of Personal Funds
F571 Limitations on Charges to Personal Funds
F572 Notice of Rights and Rules
F573 Right to Access/Purchase Copies of Records
F574 Required Notices and Contact Information

F575 Required Postings
F576 Rights of Forms of Communication with Privacy
F577 Right to Survey Results/Advocate Agency Info
F578 Request/Refuse/Discontinue Treatment: Formulate Advance Directives
F579 Posting/Notice of Medicare/Medicaid on Admission
F580 Notice of Changes (Injury/Decline/Room etc.
F582 Medicaid/Medicare Coverage/Liability Notice
F583 Personal Privacy/Confidentiality of Records
F584 Safe/Clean/Comfortable/Homelike Environment
F585 Grievances
F586 Resident Contact with External Entities

In addition to the Resident Rights, there is a separate section, 483.12 Freedom from Abuse, Neglect, and Exploitation.

Determining Capacity

Capacity is defined as "the ability to make choices that reflect an understanding and appreciation of the nature and consequences of one's actions." If the resident is unable to make decisions for himself/herself, these rights are granted to his/her legal representative. Many states have provisions for representation of the resident who has no legal representative or who may not have any interested family member and is not capable of making decisions. The capacity of the resident may be established in several ways. A court may determine that the resident is unable to make his/her own health care decisions and formally declare him/her incompetent. In this case a conservator of person will be appointed. If an individual is not available to act as conservator, a public guardian may be appointed. It is important when reviewing conservatorship papers to determine whether the conservatorship is for person or property or both. Only a conservator of person can make health care decisions for the resident.

In the absence of a court order, the physician may make the determination of capacity. On admission it should be assumed that the resident has capacity unless there is documentation to prove otherwise. If the staff is not aware of any court ruling concerning the resident's ability to make decisions and if the staff questions the resident's capacity, the nursing staff or the social services professional should contact the physician for a determination. The physician should get feedback from family and close friends when evaluating the resident's capacity. The determination of decision-making capacity should then be documented in the health record.

If the resident has executed a durable power of attorney, the durable power of attorney for health care (DPAHC) agent has authority only when the resident loses decision-making capacity. Depending on the laws of the state, the physician may appoint a surrogate in the absence of conservatorship or a DPAHC.

Often when making changes in the treatment plan or obtaining informed consent, the staff will defer to an involved family member and neglect to discuss the changes with the resident with decision-making capacity. It is very important for the professional to be sure that the resident is allowed to exercise his or her right to free choice.

Informed Consent

The overriding principle governing informed consent is that residents have the right to control what happens to their bodies. Informed consent is a legal term that means that the resident or surrogate has the right to understand both the positive reasons for making a decision and also the possible negative consequences of any decision made. This includes informed consent for psychoactive medications and physical restraints.

To meet the legal test of informed consent, the resident must have been presented five types of information. The first type of information is a clear description of the problem presented in a language and manner that the resident can understand. The second is a description of the suggested solution presented in a language and manner that the resident can understand. The third is an explanation of the possible negative consequences (or possible side effects) of going along with the proposed solution. The fourth piece of information is the possible negative consequences of not going along with the proposed solution. The fifth type of information is other, possible treatment options. When the resident is given these five different types of information, s/he should be able to make a decision about the proposed solution.

The professional is required to document in the health record that informed consent has been obtained. Except in a few situations outside the scope of practice of activity professionals and recreational therapists, when informed consent is required, the staff cannot initiate treatment until the consent is documented in the record. As in all circumstances of resident's rights, the staff must be sure that the resident is being afforded the right to exercise free choice.

Advance Directives

The Patient Self-Determination Act (PSDA) of 1991 requires that all skilled nursing facilities accepting Medicare or Medicaid funding inform residents of their rights to accept or refuse treatment and to formulate advance directives.

Definition

An advance directive is a written instruction relating to the provision of health care when an individual is incapacitated. It can be a living will, a durable power of attorney for health care, or other instrument recognized under state law. Simply put, an advance directive makes your wishes for health care known when you are not able to express them.

A Durable Power of Attorney for Health Care does not require that an agent/surrogate be named in order for it to be a valid document. However, if someone is named, it is important to name an alternate in case the primary agent cannot fulfill the obligation. With a living will choices about treatment are stated in advance of an incapacitating illness. The two functions can also be combined in a single document.

Documentation

There are two requirements that must be addressed on admission:

- The staff must determine if the resident has executed an advance directive. The answer must be documented in the health record. If s/he has, a copy must be obtained and filed in the record.
- The resident must be informed of the right to formulate an advance directive. If the resident is incapacitated on admission, the provider may give advance directive information to the legal representative or the family. A PSDA pamphlet explaining advance directives is available from most medical societies or local hospitals.

During the stay at the facility, a capable resident without any advance directive should be asked at each care conference if s/he would like to execute one. There is never an obligation nor is it a condition of continuing to stay in the facility, but the staff needs to educate the resident about the importance of making end-of-life care decisions while s/he is still able. Document that the resident received the information.

Honoring an Advance Directive

Providers are not required to provide care that conflicts with an advance directive. Life-sustaining treatments such as feeding tubes and antibiotics may be withheld if stipulated in the advance directive.

The provider can conscientiously object to implementing the advance directive if state law allows. In this event, the resident may be transferred to another facility or to another physician's care. The notice of transfer regulations would apply.

When there is a disagreement between the surrogate decision maker and other interested parties, every effort should be made to reach consensus. The parties may need to consult an institutional or regional bioethics committee.

Conservatorship vs. Durable Power of Attorney

The agent appointed by a resident in the DPAHC takes precedence over all others, including the court-appointed conservator, family, and close friends. The only person who can overrule the DPAHC is the resident who possesses current decision-making capacity. The DPAHC agent only has authority in the event that the resident loses decision-making capacity.

Right to Participate in Care Planning

An important right the resident has is the right to participate in the plan of care *including the right to refuse a treatment or a service* (Tags F552, F553, and F656). In other words, the resident must give consent before any treatment or service is initiated. In some cases, informed consent is required (e.g. for a restraint program). The regulations specify that even if the resident's ability to make decisions is impaired or the resident is formally declared incompetent by a court, the resident should still be informed of changes in his/her plan of care and consulted about preferences. OBRA '87 requires that a resident be fully informed in advance about care and treatment and of any changes in that care or treatment that may affect his/her well-being (483.10 (d) (2)). The resident must receive information necessary to make health care decisions, including those involving activity services. When planning an activity program for a resident, be sure to include the resident or the surrogate decision maker in the planning.

Residents (or their legal representative) have the right to refuse any and all treatments or services. When a resident refuses medication, treatments, food, fluids, socialization, or activities, the professional must assess the cause of the refusal and discuss with the resident or surrogate decision maker the risks and consequences of refusal. The counseling of the resident must be clearly documented. The refusal must be shown to be consistent and persistent. Alternative treatments must be offered and all attempted interventions should be documented in the progress notes and on the care plan. Every effort should be made to safeguard the resident's health and safety while also respecting his/her right to refuse treatment.

Right to Be Restraint-Free

The resident has the right to be free from any physical or chemical restraint not used to treat medical symptoms (Tags F604 and F605). In fact, the resident is guaranteed the right to make an informed choice about the use of restraints. Except for a few situations (e.g., medical crisis), informed consent must be obtained before restraints can be used. Posy vests and lap belts are easily recognized restraints, but bed rails, geri-chairs, and seizure medications may also be used to modify a resident's behavior. Any piece of equipment, furniture, or medication that is used to control any aspect of the resident's behavior is considered to be a restraint and requires specific consent.

Before using restraints, the facility must show that reasonable attempts were made to determine the cause of the problem and that non-restraint interventions were exhausted. It must be determined if the resident's behavior is due to a lack of a meaningful activity program or the need to manipulate his/her environment. Is the resident's behavior due to environmental factors — e.g., too hot, too cold, too noisy, too crowded — or is it related to a recent loss, such as the loss of a family member or a roommate? Perhaps individual needs are not met or customary routines are not being followed. Activity and recreational therapy professionals, because of their expertise in these areas, should participate in these assessments and interventions. See the section on restraints in this chapter for more information on when and how restraints may be used.

Visitation Rights

The resident must be given immediate access to his/her immediate family or relatives, his/her physician, the state ombudsman, or other individuals of his/her choosing. *Restricted visiting hours are not legal!*

Transfer and Discharge Rights

Resident rights safeguard the resident from discharge at the facility's discretion. This is an area that is scrutinized very closely by survey agencies.

The local Ombudsman is often asked if there are any problems surrounding transfers or with residents being allowed to return to the facility. Family members of former residents may be interviewed as well to determine if the discharges met legal guidelines and facility policy.

During closed record review, surveyors are instructed to look for appropriate notices for residents transferred to the hospital or absent on a therapeutic leave. The notices must meet the requirements specified in federal regulation 483.12.

The facility policies for discharge must be discussed with the resident and family on admission. Any transfer of the resident to another room or to another setting must be discussed before it happens as described below.

Room Transfers

The resident's preferences must be taken into account when a change in room or roommate is proposed. Federal regulations require that the resident be notified in advance of any changes. Frequent room transfers can be very disorienting to residents. Surveyors review these closely to determine if the changes are being made for the facility's benefit or to accommodate resident needs.

Documentation of room change should show that the notice was given in advance of the transfer, that the resident or legal representative agreed to the transfer, and that family was notified. The reason for the transfer should be clearly documented. The resident should be assessed for adjustment to the new room a few days after the transfer and the findings must be documented in the records.

Notification of family is very important. It can be very awkward when a family member comes in to visit and the resident's bed is empty and his/her belongings are no longer in the room.

When a change in roommate occurs, the documentation needs to show that the roommates were introduced to each other prior to the move. If this is not reasonable, at least inform and describe one roommate to another.

Following the move, there needs to be charting on the resident who was moved and the resident who received the new roommate. Most facility Policies and Procedures require charting follow-up satisfaction at least twice in the first week.

If the SS is not in the facility when the move occurred, s/he is still responsible for the follow-up documentation per facility policy.

Bed-Hold Notice

A bed-hold is the period the resident has to return and resume residence in the nursing facility after leaving for the hospital or other therapy. State law defines the number of days the bed will be held. If the resident does not exceed the duration of the bed-hold, s/he must be allowed to return to the same bed as soon as s/he is discharged from the hospital or returns from therapy.

Residents who exceed the duration of the bed-hold must be readmitted to the facility when the next empty bed is available. They must require skilled nursing care and be Medicaid eligible.

Federal regulations require that the nursing facility notify the resident and a family member or legal representative of the facility's bed-hold policies. This notice must be provided twice — on admission and when a facility transfers a resident to a hospital or allows the resident to go on a therapeutic leave.

The notices must be in writing and a copy kept either in the financial file or in the health record. The second notice must document whether or not the resident or legal representative wishes to pay for the bed if the absence exceeds the bed-hold duration. For non-Medicaid residents, the resident or legal representative is asked if s/he wishes to pay for all days of the bed-hold.

The facility's bed-hold policy needs to be explained to all residents and their families. The explanation should include how the resident is afforded the right to return if the bed-hold duration is exceeded.

Notice of Transfer and Right to Appeal

Federal regulations specify when the resident may be discharged. These regulations exist to prevent the facility from discharging a resident for reasons such as difficulty of care, expensive treatments, abrasive personality, or refusing treatment. The resident or legal representative may appeal any discharge.

Criteria for Discharge

A transfer or discharge is allowed when:

- *The resident's needs cannot be adequately met in the facility.* The resident needs emergency treatment and is transferred to the hospital.
- The resident's health has improved so that the resident no longer needs the services provided by the facility. The resident no longer needs skilled nursing and can return to a lesser level of care.
- *The safety of individuals in the facility is endangered.* The resident is assaulting other residents. Documentation shows that all attempts to manage the behavior have failed.
- *The health of individuals in the facility is endangered.* The resident has an infectious disease that cannot be managed in the facility.
- *The resident has failed to pay for a stay at the facility.* Documentation supports that payment has not been made after reasonable and appropriate notice.
- The facility ceases to operate.

When the facility initiates a discharge or transfer of a resident they must:

- Record the reason for the discharge or transfer in the resident's clinical record and include a copy of the notice sent to the resident, family, or legal representative.
- Provide 30 days advance notice or, as soon as practicable, if it is an emergency transfer or the resident has not resided in the facility for 30 days.
- Include in the notice: the effective date of transfer or discharge; the location of discharge; the right of appeal; the name, address, and phone number of the Ombudsman and appropriate protective and advocacy agencies.
- Notify a family member or legal representative of the proposed transfer or discharge.

Facility initiated discharges are usually for reasons 1, 3, 4, 5 and 6 listed above. Note that a transfer within the facility from the part that handles Medicare residents to another part of the nursing home is considered a discharge and requires the above notification.

Resident/Family Initiated Discharges

When the resident or family initiates a transfer or discharge and the facility anticipates the discharge they must:

- Provide adequate counseling and referrals.
- Provide a recapitulation of the stay that summarizes the resident's status and provides for continuity of care (commercial forms are available to meet this requirement).
- Provide a post-discharge plan of care.

Resident/family initiated discharges are usually for reason 2 listed above. Their preferences for discharge are usually clear on admission. Initial and subsequent discharge planning notes should clearly indicate that it is the resident's or family's desire to return to a lesser level of care.

Although not required, in some cases where the success of discharge may be questionable, the facility may want to provide the Notice of Discharge to the resident or family.

The recapitulation of stay and discharge summary is required for all discharges to home, board and care, or to another nursing home.

If the resident/family-initiated discharge is considered inadvisable, documentation should reflect the alternatives offered and notification of appropriate advocacy and protective services. The physician may choose to document that the resident left against medical advice (AMA).

Protection of Resident Funds

The long-term care facility may not require that the resident deposit his/her personal funds with the facility.

If the resident does choose to deposit his/her funds with the facility, there are strict guidelines for the handling of the resident's funds. If the resident's funds are in excess of $50, they must be deposited in a separate account and the resident must receive all interest earned on the deposited money. If a resident's deposited funds stay under $50 at all times, they may be deposited in a non-interest bearing account or in a petty cash fund as long as full accounting is kept.

The facility has five legal responsibilities for the funds deposited:

1. To assure a full and complete, separate accounting of each resident's personal funds
2. To maintain a written record of all financial transactions involving each resident's personal funds deposited with the facility
3. To provide the resident or his/her legal representative with reasonable access to the record of deposits, withdrawals, and interest
4. To convey promptly the resident's personal funds and final accounting record to the administrator of the resident's estate upon the resident's death or transfer
5. To purchase a surety bond to provide assurance that the resident's funds are protected from staff theft

Theft and Loss: An Issue of Identity

Theft and loss occur in facilities. The way to handle situations of theft and loss are part of both federal and state law. It serves a facility well to explain its philosophy about theft and loss very early in the admission process to prepare individuals and families for the reality of the situation. It also behooves all of us in the facility to take very seriously any claims concerning missing items and to use the quality assurance process to reduce the number of incidents of theft and loss by eliminating situations that allow theft and loss to occur.

The prevailing philosophy is that everything, from a misplaced robe to a lost radio, is assumed stolen until it is found again. It is our experience, however, that episodes of theft are less frequent than episodes of loss. The number of items that are lost far outweighs the number of items that are stolen. Additionally, it is assumed that anything that is not found has been taken by a staff member when in fact individuals are known to wander into rooms and "rearrange" other peoples' radios, clocks, glasses, dentures, watches, etc. This is especially true in facilities that have individuals who are able to walk freely but, due to dementia, lack judgment. In any case, before accusations of any kind are made, a thorough search of the facility is in order.

Another common occurrence is misplaced laundry. Our advice: In the short run, be patient. In the long run, fix the system. Laundry has a way of finding its way back to one's closet although the route can be circuitous, taking several days, even weeks. When that happens, the facility needs to put procedures in place to prevent the delays. It can be very difficult to keep track of laundry, but the facility is expected to do it, even the socks and underwear.

Never negate the impact on a family of seeing their mother's clothes on someone else — or vice versa. This is a terrible shock and a very emotional experience when this happens (and all too frequently, it does). Try to prepare both the person you serve and family about this in advance; it may ease the trauma.

If everything fails after an item has been reported missing, time spent in room searches, and laundry area forages, families and the people you serve may be entitled to some compensation. The circumstances governing this must be very clearly defined in the facility theft and loss policy using federal and state mandates as guidelines.

Never forget that inherent in all of this is the fact that everything, including items of clothing, has an intrinsic value. We must treat all possessions as prized items because the fewer "treasures" left to us, the greater the trauma associated with any loss.

Voting

Every individual has the right as both a citizen of the United States and as a resident covered by the Resident Bill of Rights to continue his/her responsibilities through voting in local and national elections. The information regarding whether an individual is interested and registered is gathered upon admission either by the admissions clerk or through the activity assessment process. The activity assessment form in Chapter 11 has a space on the upper right side for this information.

The activity professional needs to know the following information regarding voting:

- Is the individual interested in being registered to vote?
- Is s/he currently registered to vote and, if so, at what address?
- Would s/he like to vote by absentee ballot?
- Is s/he capable of making this decision or does s/he have a power of attorney?
- Does s/he need any special devices or assistance in order to use voting equipment?
- How many individuals in the facility are registered?
- Where do you keep this information and how do you update it?
- Do you know whom to contact in the community to assist the individuals with current issues and initiatives? (League of Women Voters, Registrar of Voters)
- Would you like the facility to be a polling place for the community? If so, contact the Registrar of Voters and request information on this and the guidelines necessary.

The box above shows a sample policy and procedure for voting. As you can see, there are many important issues to address regarding voting. The form on the next page will assist you in keeping this information up to date. Add every resident's name onto the form and identify his/her current voting status.

Voting Policy and Procedure

Policy:

It is the policy of this facility that each resident, according to federal and state regulations, has the right and the opportunity to vote as a citizen of the United States.

Procedures:

1. Upon admission, the resident will be asked about voting status. Are they registered to vote and would they like to be registered to vote?
2. The activity coordinator will document this information on the activity assessment form.
3. This name will be added to the current list of voters.
4. The activity coordinator or social services coordinator will send in a change of address notification for all interested residents.
5. The activity coordinator or social services coordinator and other staff members will assist residents with completing their absentee ballots.
6. The staff will assist in encouraging and informing residents of issues and the importance of their vote.

Voting Status Form

Record each resident's name on the form. Answer the questions and date the information when completed. List also if they need assistance with voting forms.

Resident Name	Interested	Registered	Absentee Form	Help Required
	Yes/No	Yes/No	Yes/No	Yes/No

Restraints

Federal law requires that the least invasive approach be tried first before more invasive approaches to modifying an individual's behavior are tried. This is especially true when one considers restraints. Restraints can be either physical (like geri-chairs or lap belts) or chemical (like Ativan or other psychoactive medications).

While it is usually the physician, in consultation with the nursing staff, who decides if an individual is to be restrained in any manner, *it is not the staff's right to make that decision independent of the person and his/her guardians*. Any time a restraint is needed, there should be clear documentation as to the path taken to achieve consent from the person or his/her legal guardian. This documentation should also show a progression of the least restrictive restraints being tried first, before more restrictive ones.

The physician and the nursing staff may be the primary individuals initiating the use of restraint, but all professional staff are expected to be advocates for the individual and notify the treatment care team when a violation of the person's rights may have occurred. This violation is very serious. Each department head is responsible to ensure that all of his/her staff are aware of the importance of each person's rights and to notify the administrator immediately if there is a potential violation. In some states this may be considered a case of resident abuse and, by law, needs to be called in to the appropriate state agency within 24 hours.

Restraint Reduction

The interdisciplinary team (IDT) needs to look for ways to reduce restraints and find alternatives to guarantee the highest possible quality of life. Modification of behavior works best when the entire team and environment are working together in a unified and integrated approach. As a member of the interdisciplinary team, the activity professional plays an integral role in providing the best possible quality of life to the people we serve. Because an individual will be in the activity program for some portion of the day, the IDT works together to determine the specific role that the activity professional will be playing as part of this program.

A facility should have a set of procedures in place to initiate a restraint program for individuals who would benefit from a restraint program and another set of procedures that allow the frequent review of possible reductions in the use of restraints for every individual who is currently involved in a restraint program. This may include having a specific group of staff (including the activity professional and recreational therapist) to help identify strategies for restraint reduction. This restraint reduction committee should be well versed in ways to reduce the use of restraints based on each person's abilities and strengths.

After the IDT or restraint reduction committee has tentatively identified a resident as needing a reduction of restraint, six steps are taken. The steps are

1. Assessment to determine if the individual would benefit from a restraint reduction program
2. Approval from the individual's physician for a restraint reduction program
3. Identification of the possible levels of reduction
4. Identification of responsibilities
5. Approval from the individual (or surrogate)
6. In-service for the staff on the specific aspects of the program

The first step is to assess if the person is a good candidate for a reduction in his/her restraint program or if alternatives to the current program are indicated. "Good candidates" are usually people who are doing exceptionally well or exceptionally poorly on their current program. If a person is doing exceptionally well on his/her restraint program, it may mean that s/he could tolerate and even thrive with a less restrictive program. If an individual is not doing well on his/her current program (e.g., the desired results are not being achieved), then a change in the restraint program is definitely called for. A checklist for behaviors that make an individual a "good candidate" can be used or other types of assessment forms can be created by staff. The "scoring" or data placed on the assessment tool should include input from all disciplines.

The second step involves the individual's physician. The physician needs to give approval and orders for any reduction. The orders need to be signed and in the medical chart.

The third step is to identify possible levels of physical restraint reduction or alternative strategies. There will be different levels of reduction within any restraint reduction program. These include the removal of the restraint (least restrictive), alternatives to provide maximum freedom within safety margins (moderately restrictive), or the identification that a restraint is required (most restrictive). If the team (and the individual/surrogate) recognizes that some kind of restraint is required, effort can be made to minimize the time and type of restraint being used.

The fourth step is to identify who is responsible for implementing the various parts of the individual's restraint/restraint reduction program. Clearly define which staff member is responsible for each duty. Communication is crucial for the security of the person and success of the program. When the individual participates in an activity, it is important to identify who is responsible to release the restraints and who will re-secure them at the end of the group.

Informed consent is step five. In the ideal situation, the person and/or his/her surrogate will have helped define the restraint reduction process. Sometimes this is not possible, but at this point, once the restraint reduction program has been formally defined, s/he must give informed consent.

The sixth and last step of a restraint reduction program is to let all the staff know what they will be expected to do. Each restraint reduction or alternative program will likely follow similar guidelines but vary according to the individual's needs, teamwork goals, and individual goals. All staff need to be educated about the goals of the program, the program structure, and expectations of staff involved.

In addition to the specifics of each person's restraint reduction program, the training of all staff needs to include gait belt use; restraint options, use, and techniques; positioning; and transfer techniques (when included in the policy).

You will need to determine which activities are appropriate for this reduction. You will supervise and observe responses while the person is restraint-free in a structured activity. Small groups are better than large groups for evaluating the effect of any restraint reduction on an individual's performance and affect.

The names of each participant, information regarding his/her restraint reduction needs or goals, and seating position should be available for any staff member who is assisting in the room in which the activity is held. This could be a diagram posted behind the door or on a clipboard for reference. All of the professionals working with the individual will want to be evaluating, assessing, and documenting behavior, mood, safety issues, and functional levels.

In terms of chemical restraint reduction or alternatives, a Behavior Management Program is often the most successful approach.

Behavior Management[56]

With the implementation of OBRA '87 and MDS version 3.0, staff are called upon to deal with unwanted behaviors through behavioral interventions first, before using any psychoactive medications. If behavioral interventions fail, then the use of medication to modify behavior may be tried. Gone are the days when we saw an unwanted behavior and called the attending

[56] This section is by Kay Garrick, LCSW. Used with permission.

physician for a psychoactive medication to control the behavior. This change is a good thing. It asks us to pay attention to the specific behavior and to be creative and professional in dealing with it. On the MDS we are asked if a behavioral plan has been implemented. This section will provide some ways to deal with managing behavior instead of using psychoactive medications, prior to using psychoactive medications, or in conjunction with them.

A behavior is an observable action. Many behaviors are a result of experience, values, or beliefs. Others are caused by organic changes within the individual's own body (e.g., psychosis). There are three primary ways we can effect behavioral change: help the individual change his/her own behavior, change the environment that the individual is in, or use psychoactive medications (medications that change a person's behavior by changing his/her body chemistry).

Often when we look at behaviors, it is the environment that has created the behavior. For example, an individual who has moved into a facility learns that s/he gets his/her needs met quicker when s/he yells out. After a time s/he begins to yell out just to get attention. By modifying the environment (having staff respond quicker to his/her call bell) and by re-training the individual, we can decrease the yelling.

The first place to begin modifying unwanted individual behaviors is to make sure that the environment within the facility promotes positive, cooperative behaviors. It is also important to train all staff in appropriate behavioral interventions. These interventions are not necessarily part of a formal behavioral management program, but are consistent behaviors used by all staff to encourage appropriate individual behaviors. When the facility is able to offer a positive environment with appropriate staff behaviors, the need for formal behavioral modification programs will drop significantly. This is a win-win situation. The individuals have a better, more social place to live and the staff spend less time with the paperwork required of a formal behavioral management plan.

Environmental Management

Environmental management means changing the environment to affect the behavior. This may be as small a change as playing classical music versus rock and roll in the activity room to painting the double door that leads off the unit to look like a bookshelf. (Painting a mural of a bookshelf across the door that leads off the unit confuses individuals with dementia who wander, making it less likely that they will leave the unit.) By using environmental management we may be able to deal with unwanted behaviors without using psychoactive medications. It could mean changing rooms, roommates, the showering schedule, or meal times. Be creative and listen to what the individual is telling us through his/her words and actions.

This is an example that happened during one of my consultations. A long time resident of a nursing home became a little more agitated than normal. She had a long history of psychiatric problems. The behaviors associated with her psychiatric diagnosis were generally not disruptive but included episodes of hallucinations. While I was there, the nurse received a phone call from the individual's physician with an order for Haldol 1 mg BID for three days for agitation with delusions. This order was unexpected, as the individual's behavior did not seem significantly different from her normal baseline — a baseline that seemed well within the facility's ability to accommodate without the use of psychoactive medications. As the nurse did some detective work, she found that the individual had called her daughter and told her the nursing home was making her stay in a room with a dead person. Because of the individual's psychiatric history, the daughter assumed the individual was becoming psychotic and called the physician. The nurse came to me with the dilemma of whether to implement the physician's orders or to call the physician back to discuss the situation. The nurse was concerned because she felt the individual was not hallucinating, as the individual's roommate was in the process of dying. I suggested we check with the individual to see if she wanted to move to another room. The individual gladly accepted the move. We called the daughter, explained the situation, and then called the physician who canceled the medication order. The individual was moved to another room. By being sensitive to the individual's concerns and what was happening in her environment, we were able to solve the problem without using medications.

Behavioral Intervention

Behavioral intervention is just another term for providing the person with gentle, normal consequences for inappropriate behavior. Staff frequently create unrealistic "community" standards for social skills within the facility. Instead of ignoring grabbing behavior, the staff should be taught how to respectfully ask the person not to grab them and, just as important, figure out why the individual felt the need to grab.

Behavioral interventions can be used when the behavior is seen in limited situations — when the behavior is not pervasive. An example would be an individual who yells when s/he is in an activity and not at other times. Talk to the individual about the behavior when the behavior is not happening. If an individual calls out in group, talk to him/her before the group. Tell him/her what behavior you have noticed and then ask what s/he thinks is causing the behavior. (This is for individuals who have the mental ability to understand.) Let him/her know that it is affecting other people and how it is affecting them. Ask the person if s/he has any suggestions to solve the problem. Perhaps his/her hearing is bad and if s/he sits in the front of the group, s/he would not yell out. If s/he has no suitable ways to solve the problem, let the person know what you will do. If s/he disrupts the group again, you will need to remove him/her from the group.

Remember to maintain the person's dignity as much as possible. If the situation arises where you must remove an individual from an activity, do not discipline him/her in front of the group. Simply go to the person and take him/her out of the activity. Outside of the group remind him/her that the behavior was disruptive to others. Use a consistent simple phrase that describes the behavior and use it every time the behavior happens. Do not touch, smile sweetly, or show anger. In our guilt at taking this kind of action, our behaviors can reinforce the wrong behavior. Keep your facial expression blank. Later, visit privately with the person to see how s/he responded to the intervention.

Make a plan to meet the needs of the individual. If you have a person who consistently yells out in group and not when s/he is in his/her room, why do you continue to bring him/her to group? Perhaps one-on-one visits would be more effective. Often individuals with dementia get over-stimulated in large groups. Try smaller, quieter activities. Physical activities may be successful also.

In one facility a newly admitted resident with a diagnosis of dementia called out constantly, "Nurse, nurse, nurse." It was her first admission to a nursing facility and the Director of Nurses was ready to discharge her on her date of admission because of her calling out. The resident loved to receive hugs. I pulled the clock at the nurses' station off the wall and went to the resident and put the clock in her lap. I used simple phrases but told her she needed to be quiet for five minutes and that if she was quiet she would get a big hug. I showed her the clock and where the hands of the clock would be when she would get a hug. Her face lit up. I left her in her wheelchair across from the nursing station and sat nearby but out of her range of vision. When she called out, I got her attention and made a quiet signal and verbally cued her to three more minutes until her hug. I kept my face blank and did not touch her. At the end of five minutes she had called out three times and I went to hug her and praised her for the good job she did being quiet. Then I increased the time to ten minutes with the "hug" reward at the end and continued increasing the time in increments of five minutes up to an hour. When the resident was up to an hour, she called out only once.

The Director of Nurses was sold on behavior management along with the rest of the staff. The Maintenance Director found a large kitchen timer that rang after the appropriate amount of time. The certified nurses' aides took the resident to her room, set the timer and when the bell rang they would go to her and give her a big hug and reward her behavior. Initially it took me all morning to work this through with the resident and staff. We were able to eliminate the yelling out behavior so that the resident felt safe and her quality of life was improved. The staff bonded with the resident and gave her attention and praise for appropriate behavior. She was able to be maintained at the facility instead of being placed elsewhere.

Behavior Management Programs

When a negative behavior is serious and frequent enough to require a systematic change, the team will need to develop a behavior management plan. Behavior management plans should be implemented when the behavior is affecting most aspects of care and the quality of life for others is impacted. It is a more complex system that involves all disciplines and the person and/or family in an organized, planned approach to eliminate the behavior.

The reason that this situation is complex is that it has reached the point where the unwanted behavior is ingrained. Instead of having just isolated occurrences, this behavior has been established as a coping pattern. To break this pattern, all staff must work together in a systematic way. Each staff person needs to know how to discourage the behavior as well as promote healthy ways of coping.

We can change a behavior *if* there is something an individual *likes*. I prefer to use positive reinforcements rather than negative. Positive reinforcements are more successful. It is often easier for staff to use positive rewards.

Many folks believe that if a person has a diagnosis of dementia, behavioral management is not effective. That is not my experience. Individuals with dementia *can* benefit from behavioral plans. Does the person really like hugs, candy, to sit outside, time with family/staff? We then use what the individual likes as a reward for the appropriate behavior and behavior can be changed.

Behavioral programs take time initially but, when they are effective, they take less time than responding to the inappropriate behavior. This may be difficult for staff to understand. Just have the staff add up the amount of time they spend answering a person who uses the call light frequently. Changing the behavior will eventually save time.

To change a behavior, we must act like a detective and find out the reason for the behavior. The best way to find out the causes is usually at a special care planning conference where all disciplines are represented and can give input related to the behavior. It is very helpful to have the certified nurses' aides who work with the person present at this meeting. Has something changed in the person's life that triggered the behavior — a new room, a new roommate, a new nurses' aide, family out of town? What is the individual's diagnosis? What are the medications the person is taking? What happens before the behavior occurs? These are called the "antecedents." Is it change of shift? Does the nurses' aide try to provide care? Does the family leave? What exactly is the behavior? We need to be very specific. Is the individual verbally abusive or did s/he raise his/her voice and yell at the staff? We cannot change the behavior if we do not know exactly what it is.

What does the person get by behaving this way — space, distance, control, power, maintaining dignity? This is often called the "consequence." Has anyone told the person that the behavior is causing a problem for others? Who on the interdisciplinary team has the best relationship with the person? Would it be better to have a male staff talk to the resident? This often works best with males who are physically, verbally, or sexually acting out. Could the family help us deal with the behavior? Do they have information about the behavior prior to admission? Can they come in and help at difficult times? Is there anything we can change in the environment to help change the behavior?

Consistency is crucial for a behavioral plan to work. That means all staff must behave the same way — all shifts need to be told of the plan and follow through with it. If we use a verbal phrase, all staff should repeat the same phrase to the resident. Keep your behavioral plan as simple as possible. Only work on one behavior at a time and choose the behavior that causes the most problems for the other people we serve and staff.

Behavioral plans are more difficult for individuals with a diagnosis of "borderline personality disorder." These are often the people who like to stir up tension among staff or family members. They usually do not have anything that is as rewarding to them as the tension they cause, so finding something else they like that will cause them to change can be very difficult.

When behavioral management plans are started, the person's behavior will often get worse for approximately two weeks. The individual is trying to hold on to what s/he knows, including old coping mechanisms and behaviors that are causing problems. Expect the first two weeks to be difficult, encourage staff to remain consistent, and only change the program during the first two weeks if it is completely clear that the program is going to fail or make matters worse.

Difficult Behavior

Every facility tends to have at least one person who exhibits difficult behavior. This part talks about three difficult behaviors that I am often asked to work with: inappropriate sexual behavior, suicidal thoughts, and violent behaviors. These behaviors are not often discussed in behavior guides. Use a team approach, define the problem, and decide your approach using some of the ideas discussed above.

Sexual Behavior

One of the most difficult behaviors to deal with is sexually inappropriate behavior. With younger individuals being admitted more frequently to facilities, sexually inappropriate behavior is becoming more of an issue for staff to deal with. Remember that this behavior can be exhibited by young and old, as well as male and female.

Sexual behavior is normal. Often what come up around the behavior are our own judgments, values, and religious beliefs. We all have sexual needs and expressing them is part of life for both old and young. It is important for us to define "inappropriate" sexual behavior. Staff walking into an individual's room where the curtain is closed to find the person masturbating is not considered inappropriate behavior on the resident's part. It could be viewed as inappropriate staff behavior. Did you allow the individual the privacy s/he wanted? Did you knock? Did the individual give the staff person permission to enter the room? Married couples have the right to share a room and are entitled to privacy.

It is crucial to know the diagnosis, as the approaches will vary depending on whether the person has mental capacity. Whether the person has capacity to make health care decisions is determined by the attending physician and can be found in the Advance Directives or in the Physician's Orders.

If an individual becomes sexually aggressive or active with another resident, determine if both individuals have capacity. If they do, they can make their own choices and consent as long as privacy is maintained. If the residents have capacity, we are not allowed to discuss this with their families unless the residents give us permission. To discuss this with the family without the resident's permission is a violation of resident rights. If the resident does not have capacity, the responsible party or agent must be informed and decide if the behavior is acceptable. Cases of sexually aggressive behavior must be reported to the appropriate reporting agency (Ombudsman, Adult Protective Services, police). Report all episodes of sexually inappropriate behavior to your supervisor.

When a resident without capacity is demonstrating sexually inappropriate behavior, you can use the following guidelines. Remember to maintain the resident's dignity. If s/he is exposed, make sure s/he is covered or dressed appropriately. If the resident is in a public place and cannot be distracted, take him/her to his/her room and pull the curtain. Make the nursing staff aware so that they respect the resident's privacy. For a resident who exposes himself or urinates in public places, consider ordering the resident a back closure jumpsuit. They are difficult for the residents to remove. A back closure jumpsuit is considered to be a restraint. Before dressing the resident in one, the facility must follow the standard procedure for placing a resident in a restraint, including informed consent.

Do not talk down to or shame the resident by saying anything that makes you want to shake your finger at the resident. The resident may not understand what you are saying but s/he may understand that you are trying to make him/her feel ashamed of the behavior. You need to look at your values about sexual behavior. Remember that you are the professional and do not personalize the behavior.

Are you doing anything to contribute to the behavior? Watch the "sweetie, honey, baby" phrases. Are you touching the resident or kissing him/her? If a resident displays inappropriate sexual behavior, do not call him/her "sweetie," or kiss him/her. Sometimes residents with this behavior ask for kisses. State professionally, "Mr. Smith I'm the Activity Director and I will not kiss you, but I will shake you hand." Remind the resident of your professional role. "Mr. Jones you must have confused me with someone else. I am the Activity Coordinator and I want to invite you to the piano recital today." Keep your face blank. Do not show shock, displeasure, laughter, smiles, or anger. Remember any facial expression could encourage the behavior. If you cannot control your facial expression, turn your face away from the resident.

Do not run to your peers and giggle about the behavior. Someone will always overhear conversations. Again, this means you need to look at your own values around sexuality. Do report the behavior to the charge nurse. Is this new behavior? Is it covered in the care plan? If so, what are our interventions to deal with the behavior?

When a resident with capacity is demonstrating sexually inappropriate behavior, you can use the following guidelines. Refer the resident to the Social Services Director who will talk to the resident about the behavior. Why is it being displayed? Does the resident need more control, power, or privacy? What is the resident's solution to the problem? One younger resident consistently exposed himself to older female visitors. When asked why he did this, he said that he had been in prison and that he had more freedom there than in the nursing home. He did this in hopes of being arrested and put back in prison. We were able to give the resident more control over his life and he stopped the behavior. Referral to a therapist, psychologist, social worker, or psychiatrist for counseling related to the problem may be helpful. Involve the Ombudsman. Sometimes someone from outside the facility can have more impact on the resident's behavior. And remember, when the resident has been determined to be capable, s/he will need to be involved in the decision-making process.

Suicidal Behavior

Suicidal behavior is another difficult behavior to deal with. If a resident is displaying suicidal behavior, it must be determined if the facility can provide for the resident's safety. If not, the resident may need to be transferred to an acute psychiatric hospital for appropriate treatment. Suicidal statements are often a cry for help and *must* be taken seriously. Report any suicidal comments to the charge nurse *and* the Social Services Director.

If a resident threatens suicide, states a desire to commit suicide, or is known to have been suicidal in the recent past, an assessment to determine whether the resident is currently suicidal will be made by the Social Services Department, possibly in conjunction with any of the following: the Nursing Department, the attending physician, a consulting psychiatrist, consulting psychologist, the social work consultant, the county's mental health specialist, or the family. Observe the resident for warning signs of suicide: prolonged depression, marked changes of behavior or personality, a sudden lifting of the mood (e.g., the resident who is depressed suddenly seems happy), making final arrangements as though for a final departure, and/or suicide threats or similar statements.

Question the resident as to motivation, method, and means. If there is a desire to commit suicide, a plan devised, and a viable way to kill oneself, the risk is greater. If a risk exists, the facility interdisciplinary team will formulate an intervention to ensure the safety of the resident. However, if the resident seems to have a clear plan as to how s/he will end his/her life, the staff should question whether they could keep the resident in the facility. Determine whether there is a need for a temporary transfer. A transfer to a psychiatric unit used to handling this crisis situation is usually a reasonable choice. Check with your county's mental health specialist.

If you decide that the resident can stay in the facility, enlist all staff in monitoring actions of resident, but have one specific staff person on each shift who is responsible for checking the resident on a regular basis. Put regular check-ins in place, usually every 15 minutes. This may require moving the resident closer to the nursing station for observation. To ensure that the frequent checks are done, a sign-off sheet should be available at the nursing station for the staff to document the resident's activity and affect every 15 minutes and then to sign off, indicating who observed the resident during those last 15 minutes and what the resident was doing.

As much as possible, reduce environmental hazards. Remove sharp objects from resident's room and reach (e.g., matches, razors, scissors). Remove the call light cord and replace it with a tap bell. Remove any belts, cords, etc. from resident's access. Replace silverware with plastic. The nursing staff should be sure that the resident swallows his/her pills and does not hoard or cheek them.

Most residents who feel like taking their own life have mixed feelings about taking action. They frequently feel like life is out of control and want to be able to "grab" onto some strength and stability provided by someone else. Knowing that someone will be there to help gives him/her a sense of security. Consider using a written contract with the resident (verbal would be fine but written is more powerful). This way the resident knows that someone will be there if s/he feels the need for support. Write a contract that states "I, ___________ (resident's name), agree that if I feel like harming myself in any way, I will not take any action to do myself harm. I agree to contact the Social Services Director _____________ (name) or the charge nurse ___________ (name)." Have a place for the resident to sign and for a staff signature. Give a copy to the resident and put a copy in the chart. Be sure to include this service/intervention in the care plan. Remember to designate staff to cover on the weekends, holidays, and during staff illness and be sure the resident knows who the staff are.

Encourage the resident to talk about feelings. Often staff avoid stating the obvious, "Do you feel like killing yourself?" It will not encourage the resident to take this action but may be seen as a relief by the resident that someone will talk about it — that someone understands. Make sure you visit the resident regularly. Often staff avoid seeing the resident because they do not know what to do. All you need to do is let the resident know that you care about him/her and sit with him/her for a few minutes. Offer touch when appropriate.

Violent Behavior

Violent behavior exhibited by one or more residents can be difficult to deal with, can endanger the other residents and staff, and can cause a facility to lose its license. Violent behaviors cannot be tolerated and need to be addressed immediately.

This behavior can be a result of inability to control one's impulses or feeling powerless over one's environment. Anger can be directed at others or the environment. The resident may be combative with staff, peers, and family or throw things such as food or furniture. This anger can be a result of feeling a lack of control, neurological damage, or inadequate coping skills. It may also be a result of impulse control problems, which arise after a head injury or stroke. Staff's first responsibility is to assure that residents involved in a violent situation are safe. Do others need to be protected, moved, or other staff called to assist?

Staff need to be safe, and you need to insure the safety of other residents. If someone is being violent, stay an arm's length away. Give the person space to calm down. Take him or her to a quiet place. If there is no mental decline, let the resident know that the violent behavior will not be tolerated and that staff need to keep others safe. The resident needs to know that staff will protect and set boundaries since the resident feels out of control. The behavior could lead to eviction if the resident cannot control the violent outbursts (although this may not be the most prudent thing to say during the middle of a resident's violent outburst).

Staff should avoid areas or topics that cause conflict. Avoid power struggles. Instead of saying, "It's time for your shower." try asking, "When would you like to shower?" This gives the person more control over his/her life.

When interacting with a resident who seems on the edge of losing control, keep a neutral manner. Do not show fear, anger, or laughter. Keep your face blank and present a calm professional demeanor. Do not try to shame the resident.

Controlling one's anger requires good coping skills and socially appropriate ways to express one's feelings. The resident may be justified in his/her feeling of anger although his/her way to express it is not appropriate. How would you feel if the same thing happened to you? It is good to identify the feeling and offer acceptance. "I can understand why you felt angry after what happened." Referral to a counselor, psychologist, therapist, psychiatrist, or social worker may help the resident explore his/her anger and ways to express it appropriately.

Violence may be a way for the resident to release energy. Offer the resident alternatives and appropriate ways to release his/her anger, thereby increasing his/her coping skills. Consider trying workouts with weights; give the resident a pillow to pound on or regular exercise such as walks around the facility.

When the violence is severe and cannot be stopped, staff may have to call 911 to have the police assist the resident. Remember, assault, no matter where it happens, is against the law. If the law is being broken, the facility may need to have professionals who are used to dealing with violent behavior take over the situation.

The following page has a sample form for a behavior management meeting. The form after that can be used by the activity professional to monitor resident behavior.

Behavior Management Meeting

Name: ________________________ **Date:** ____________

What is the individual's problem? (Do not describe the staff's problem with the individual, e.g., person is frustrated and fearful so s/he becomes combative): ________________________

____

____

How is this behavior a problem within the facility? ________________________

____

Identify the individual's strengths (e.g., is physically strong, good motor skills, maintains social etiquette, etc.): ________________________

____

Environmental stimulus to consider (Identify environmental factors — light, noise, temperature, space, other people who are present when behavior occurs): ________________________

____

____

Medications

Antipsychotic Medication: ________________________

Target Behavior: ________________________

Episodes: **Increased** **Decreased**

Antianxiety Medication: ________________________

Target Behavior: ________________________

Episodes: **Increased** **Decreased**

Antidepressant Medication: ________________________

Target Behavior: ________________________

Episodes: **Increased** **Decreased**

Successful non-drug approaches: ________________________

____

Unsuccessful non-drug approaches: ________________________

____

Last Psychiatry Evaluation: ________________________

Plan: ________________________

____

____

Behavioral Monitoring Sheet

Name: ____

Date	Behavior	Activity Intervention(s)	Response	Comments

Time Management

Time management is the process by which we manage our time so we feel accomplishment, completion, and a personal sense of well-being. Managing our lives — being on time — is something we're always going to do … tomorrow. As a result, we tend to engage in a lot of "knee-jerk" activity. We react instead of act.

Staying on a schedule seems an especially daunting objective in a profession that deals with people and their problems. In effect, a day is never linear as we are continuously diverted to mend and fix. At the end of the day, even though we have been busy, sometimes it seems that we haven't really done any work! It is only an illusion that we can never really get it all done. In fact, we have a responsibility, an obligation to do just that: to address everything our job description says we must do.

Time management is not a skill that most people are born with. It is an acquired skill that needs attention and practice. Managing time also means that the manager needs systems designed which work for him/her. All people organize their thoughts and schedules in a unique style. For this reason, each person needs to organize in the way that best suits his/her style, type of work, and personality.

Maintain a Schedule

We have attempted to give you a bird's eye view of the work in the sections entitled "Life of a …" For an activity professional, the schedule has some clear responsibilities at set times so this discussion will help you with the less structured times.

What you need to do is derived directly from your job description. Within those obligations, you need to develop a plan for when you work and decide on your own cues for completion. For example, you might try to do your computer work each morning before 9 AM; or do your quarterly notes between 4–5 PM after you have had time in the day to see each of the individuals you need to report on, jotting notes as you proceed throughout the day.

Set goals for the week. You can do this on Monday morning for the ensuing week or Friday afternoon in anticipation of the week ahead. Revise these goals each morning before you begin. Of course, no one working with people will ever get from A to B every time, but with an idea of your task load, you can do it much of the time.

Keys to Success

- Prioritize each day's responsibilities.
- Complete the least appealing work first.
- Complete one task at a time. Too much time and energy are spent trying to complete two to three things within the same amount of time. Some people are able to do this, but most find that it does not work for them.
- Discourage interruptions by scheduling calls and appointments at a good time for you. Advise staff of this schedule also. When you are leading a group, you should not be answering calls. This leaves the unspoken message to the group participants that your calls are more important than they are.
- Schedule enough time each day to complete all required documentation.
- Schedule enough time each day to visit on a one-on-one basis and record this in the bedside log.
- Keep your desk organized so that you can sort through stacks of papers according to priorities.
- Write a list of all the work responsibilities that you have. By referring to this list, you can better identify a plan and way of organizing all of the different types of duties.

Make Choices

There will always be more demands than you can possibly respond to. Be realistic as to personal goals and abilities. If the frustration becomes too great because of lack of organization, stress mounts, anxiety occurs, and there is a general feeling of loss of control. Break the cycle before this happens. There are four D's in time management: *Drop it, Delay, Delegate, Do it.*

If you are a department head, you will have greater demands and expectations. Not only are you required to provide the services expected of *you,* but you are also responsible for all the other mandated responsibilities of the department, other staff members, and volunteers.

When you go about trying to meet all of these demands, the most important thing you can do is to set priorities (act — don't react). Decide what needs to be done first, second, and so on. Then write down your decisions so you will remember what you have to do and how soon you plan to do it.

Try to find a balance between never varying your plan and having the plan disrupted by everyone who asks you to do something. A good rule of thumb is if you already have something on your list of things to do, you should do it when you planned to even if someone just asked you how soon it would be done. The only time to change your priorities is when something new comes up. Then you need to decide where it goes in your list of priorities.

When human need arises (and that's why we do what we do), get involved up to your elbows. If you have to decide between addressing a need and writing a quarterly report, the choice is obviously to attend to the need. In fact, addressing a need as it arises is really the action position. Ignoring or avoiding creates the need for reaction. However, do not allow diversion to derail you. Act, but return to your schedule of work as soon as possible. Work on your documentation skills so that you say what you need to say in a clear concise manner. Don't waste time writing too much.

Chip away at your schedule and list of goals in order to keep going forward. As you finish one project for the day or week, immediately focus on your next task. There will always be something waiting for your attention. It's the nature of work like ours where we are not only dealing with people but also with paper — lots of it.

TGIF

Before you leave work for your well-deserved weekend, check the list of goals you started with on Monday (this includes the must do's from your job description, e.g., assessments and quarterlies). Is everything complete? If not, why not? Can it wait until Monday? What will be the consequence if a task remains incomplete?

If you can safely answer that everything is done that needs doing with no ill effect from a job that might be left, then you can leave! However, you might feel better prepared to face Monday morning if you write a sketch for the coming week. That way, you will not have to dread that day or face decisions first thing in the morning after a relaxing weekend.

Time Management Calendar

One way to determine how well you are managing your time is to complete a Time Management Calendar for one month and then analyze the results. This has been a helpful tool for many professionals. Read the codes below. These represent your responsibilities. Be sure to add duties specific to your facility.

- **FM** (Facility Management) Any responsibility directly associated with office and departmental functions. In other words, everything related to keeping the department in order. This may also include resident shopping.
- **DRC** (Direct Resident Care) Direct leadership and time spent with the people we serve. This would be either in a group setting or on a one-on-one basis. If you are arranging an activity for adult education teachers or a volunteer, this is listed under coordination and not direct care.
- **D** (Documentation)
- **T** (Transportation) Time bringing individual to and from groups.

- **PR** (Public Relations) Time spent explaining your work to the public, press, or other agencies.
- **TMC** (Time Management Calendar) The time spent in completing this form each day for a month needs to be added on. It will be approximately 15 minutes daily.
- **CC** (Care Conferences) The time spent preparing for and attending care conferences.
- **C** (Coordination) This includes calendars, newsletters, interdepartmental functions, fundraising, etc.
- **PD** (Personal Development) This is the time spent reviewing program ideas, going to workshops, reading and reviewing guidelines. You should have some of this each week.
- **M** (Meetings) These could be staff meetings, MDS meetings, QA meetings. You should note what kind of meeting it was.
- **S** (Supervision) Time when you are supervising volunteers and staff in the department.
- **CV** (Consultant Visits) Add the time spent with the consultant for the department.
- **FC** (Family Concerns) The time spent working with the family and friends of the people we serve.
- **G** (Grievances) The time spent learning about and resolving grievances.
- **CL** (Clothing) Making sure participants have appropriate clothing.
- **LA** (Lost Articles) Checking on lost clothing and other articles.
- **DC** (Discharge Planning)
- **L** (Lunch)
- **O** (Other) Explain how the time was spent.

How to Complete the Calendar

At the end of each day for one month, record where your time went on any standard wall or notebook calendar. Each entry must be in an increment of no less than 15 minutes. If you find that you are doing two things at one time, you must divide the time and show each one separately. Use the codes shown above. These represent the various functions of the work. If you work more than eight hours, this must be reflected on the calendar also. In order for this to be accurate, the calendar needs to be completed each day at the end of the day.

Example of how an average day will appear on the calendar when completed:

DRC	2 hours
D	1 1/2 hours
T	45 minutes
S	1 hour
L	1 hour
C	1 hour
RCC	1 hour
PD	15 minutes
Total time	8 1/2 hours.

By reviewing an average day over a period of one month, you will be able to see what takes the longest amount of time to complete, how much direct time is spent with the people you serve in programming, what needs more time, and what may be an area of weakness.

Budgets

Every department has a budget to which it must adhere. This budget is created by the administrator and/or corporate office and is an integral part of the total facility budget. If you do not have previous experience with budgets and accounting, ask for some advice or reading materials to better educate yourself about protocols and requirements.

When you look at budgets, it is important to understand the difference between a supply item and a capital item. The capital items are large items that the department needs to provide a basic service. (In accounting terms, these items are depreciated rather than expensed.) Some of these items may include slide projectors, DVD players and monitors, headsets with CD players and/or radios, large bingo games, reality orientation boards, eraser boards, monthly calendars, typewriters, and computers. The money for capital items may not come from the budget you use to get supplies, but you need to check this out with your administrator to be sure how your facility budgets its capital funds.

In some facilities, the activity budget contains *all* costs that are incurred through this department. Some examples could be coffee supplies, paper supplies, consultant costs, entertainment, and many more. Other facilities budget some of these things separately. It is important to understand how your individual facility budget works so that you can not only plan ahead but also negotiate when you know the budget will not meet current resident needs.

As with any business, accountability is extremely important. Accountability in this instance refers to the ability of the department head to identify where every penny has gone, with receipts to back up the expenses. Without the paper backup, there is no record to substantiate purchases and payments.

At least once a year, your facility will plan the budget for the next year. You need to be part of this process. The best way to figure out what you need is to go through your records for the last year (another reason to keep these records) and add up your expenses for each category of expenditure. Make rough schedules for the next year, noting especially differences between the past year and the coming year. (Some important differences are changes in the number of participants, changes in the diagnoses, changes in requirements for consulting, or needs for capital items.) Be prepared to defend your proposed budget by showing exactly where the money will go and exactly what kind of programs you will be running. Tie the programs to assessments and to regulations to demonstrate that they need to be run.

Each state varies in its rules about budgets. Some may make no reference to the activity budget. You need to understand facility and state regulations about activity budgets.

Many of the items and supplies you buy should be ordered with a purchase order. Get in the habit of using purchase orders when sending in orders and requesting supplies. If your facility does not already have a purchasing system, you can purchase your own at any office supply store. If there is a delay or question about an order, you can refer back to this transaction by the purchase order number, the date, and the items listed.

Each department needs to keep an inventory of all supplies and equipment. The activity department should have an up-to-date inventory identifying all current supply items in the facility. For any of you who have taken a position in an unorganized facility, you know what it is like to try to figure out what you have, where it is, what you need to order, and whether you will have enough money to last the year.

Being organized in this way is like leaving a legacy in the facility for those department heads to come. Always keep things in the manner that you would like to find them.

Policies and Procedures

Policies and procedures are the framework of any organization and any department. Each department head needs to review the current policy and procedure manual used by the facility and specific departments. Review the policies specific to your department and determine if they are up to date with federal, state, corporate, and facility requirements. If not, the department head is responsible for making sure that these policies are written. After policies and procedures are written, they need to be reviewed and approved by the policy review committee in the facility. After approval, committee members sign and date the front page of the manual.

There should be a policy for each aspect of service provided through the department. When you write policies and procedures, keep in mind the following definitions:

Policy. A policy identifies and defines an administrative decision about *what* needs to be done.

Procedure. A procedure describes *how* the policy will be implemented.

Both the policy and procedure need to be written *clearly* enough to define the need while at the same time they need to be *general* enough to encompass a variety of situations. Be sure that the descriptions are realistic, as the facility can be cited during a federal or state survey for not following through with their own policies.

Many policies are designed from federal and state regulations. An example would be an individual's right to vote in elections. This is a federal law protecting the rights of the resident as a citizen and as a resident. By writing a policy and procedure, the facility is not only complying with the law, but also clearly defining how this regulation will be adhered to and implemented in the facility. An example policy and procedure statement for outings is shown on the right.

Outings

Policy

It is the policy of this facility to plan and offer resident outings away from the facility. This meets OBRA '87 Regulations.

Procedures

- Each resident participating in an outing needs a doctor's order to leave the facility.
- A list of participants needs to be reviewed and approved by the Director of Nursing or Charge Nurse to determine if they are physically, cognitively, and emotionally able to leave the facility.
- The activity professional will contact the families to update them as to the date and time that their family member will be away from the facility.
- The activity professional will arrange for appropriate numbers of staff and volunteers. The ideal ratio is one staff member to one resident.
- All medications will be administered before the departure or after the resident returns. *No medications will be transported unless an RN or LPN goes on the outing to administer them to the residents.*
- Residents who have approval for self-administration will be addressed on a case-by-case basis.
- All residents need to be signed back into the nursing station upon return to the facility. The activity professional will also share any information felt to be pertinent in regards to behavior, interaction, and/or condition changes, which may have occurred during the outing.

There are other special policies that will need attention. An example would be a policy and procedure for a facility pet. Although this is not a required area, the philosophy of many facilities is to encourage a homelike environment that includes a facility pet. A sample policy and procedure might look like this:

Facility Pets

Policy

It is the policy of this facility to provide and care for a facility pet.

Procedures

- All veterinary records and vaccination records will be kept on file in the facility.
- A designated staff member will be responsible for the feeding, grooming, and general care of the pet.
- The pet will not be in the halls, resident rooms, or dining areas during meal times for infection control purposes.
- The activity and social services departments will arrange a schedule for in-room pet visits.

Notice how the procedures are broadly written, for example, the designated staff member who will be responsible for the grooming and care of the pet. Obviously this individual will have a schedule designed for when, where, and how often this will occur. This may be a page attached to the original policy and procedure as additional information.

There is no mystery to writing policies and procedures. Look at your department and see if there is an area that needs a policy. Write the policy to meet either the regulations or current need. Write the procedures to describe how the policy will be implemented. After completion, have the policy and procedure reviewed and approved by the administrator and committee. *The Professional Activity Manager and Consultant*[57] contains a full chapter on how to write policies and procedures. It describes each step in the process in an easy-to-follow way.

OBRA '87 Regulations

The latest guidelines for the OBRA '87 law contain 21 sections with requirements for nursing homes. These sections are organized by "tags" and each tag has a number. The following is a list of the sections and their associated tags. A few of the tags are considered part of more than one section, as shown below.

1. Resident's Rights, 483.10, F550-F586, also F604, F605, and F917
2. Freedom from Abuse, Neglect, and Exploitation, 483.12, F600-F610
3. Admission, Transfer, and Discharge, 483.15, F620-F626
4. Resident Assessments, 483.20, F635-F646, also F842
5. Comprehensive Resident Centered Care Plans, 483.21, F655-F661
6. Quality of Life, 483.24, F675-F680
7. Quality of Care, 483.25, F684-F700
8. Physician Services, 483.30, F710-F715
9. Nursing Services, 483.35, F725-F732
10. Behavioral Health Services, 483.40, F740-F745
11. Pharmacy Services, 483.45, F755-F761
12. Laboratory, Radiology, and Other Diagnostic Services, 483.50, F770-F779
13. Dental Services, 483.55, F790-F791
14. Food and Nutrition Services, 483.60, F800-F814
15. Specialized Rehabilitative Services, 483.65, F825-F826
16. Administration, 483.70, F835-F851
17. Quality Assurance and Performance Improvement, 483.75, F865-F868
18. Infection Control, 483.80, F880-F883
19. Compliance and Ethics, 483.85, F895
20. Physical Environment, 483.90, F906-F926

[57] D'Antonio-Nocera, A., N. DeBolt, and N. Touhey, Eds., 1996, *The professional activity manager and consultant*, Idyll Arbor, Inc., Ravensdale, WA.

21. Training Requirements, 483.95, F940-F949

Because the survey process depends largely on the federal regulations, it is important that the professional understands how to use and interpret the regulations. Each section in the *State Operations Manual* Appendix PP — Guidance to Surveyors for Long Term Care Facilities describes the regulation and also contains a set of interpretive guidelines. The guidelines give the surveyor additional information about the meaning of the regulation and provide accepted survey procedures and probes. If you read the regulations and the critical element pathways you will have a good idea of how the surveyor will look at this section of the regulations. It will help you prepare for a survey. The Critical Element Pathways forms were created to assist the surveyor in asking specific questions in order to determine compliance. There are 40 Critical Element Pathways. They will also guide staff in better understanding the surveyor and survey team approach. You can download these at www.cms.gov/Medicare/Provider-Enrollment-and-Certification/SurveyCertificationGenInfo/Downloads/CriticalElementPathway.

It is important to note that the interpretive guidelines are guides only and not requirements. The regulations themselves are used as the basis for survey activities. When a problem is found during a survey, the problem is written up under the regulation that corresponds to the problem.

Tags Related to Activities and Social Services

While there are only two tags dealing directly with activities (Tags F679 and F680), there are many other tags that deal indirectly with activities, social services, and recreational therapy. Here are some of the areas you are expected to understand.

Activity professionals need to be aware of care plans; documentation; visual deficits; hearing loss; other sensory losses; physical limitations; language barriers; diverse ethnic, cultural, and religious backgrounds and needs; pain; palliative care; hospice care; dementia-specific needs and interventions; behavioral interventions; resident right to work; environmental factors impacting individual and group activities; and food and nutrition. The list will continue to grow as the individual and group facility assessments become more accurate.

Social service professionals need to be aware of care plans; documentation; visual deficits; hearing loss; other sensory losses; physical limitations; language barriers; diverse ethnic, cultural, and religious backgrounds and needs; pain; palliative care; hospice care; dementia-specific needs and interventions; behavioral interventions; resident right to work; environmental factors impacting individual and group activities; and food and nutrition. In addition, social services deals with advanced directives, room changes and transfers, grievances, theft and loss, family council, follow-up on psychological and psychiatric services, discharge planning, and alleged abuse investigations and documentation. The list will continue to grow as the individual and group facility assessments become more accurate.

The primary tags that could be used to measure how well the activity staff and social services professionals are meeting the needs of residents are listed below, along with a summary of the regulations and surveyor guidelines. For survey guidelines for all of the F-Tags, see https://www.cms.gov/Medicare/Provider-Enrollment-and-Certification/GuidanceforLawsAndRegulations/Downloads/Appendix-PP-State-Operations-Manual.pdf.

Asterisks in front of the tag numbers indicate that citation of the tag may lead to the facility beimg cited for Substandard Quality of Care. Surveyors use the Scope and Severity Grid to determine the scope and severity of a deficiency. Information in italics is taken from CMS Appendix PP effective November 28, 2017.

483.10 Resident Rights

The first section of the regulations pertains to Resident Rights. Each resident has the absolute right to be treated with dignity and to exercise his/her rights of citizenship. Just because the resident is no longer in "his/her own home" does not mean that s/he loses the rights associated with being an adult citizen. As described ay the beginning of this chapter, the Guidelines were changed in 2009 and again in 2017 to add more rights, which are described in the tags discussed below. These rights include the resident's right to services and activities of their choice both inside and outside of the facility.

These rights have become much more focused on the resident having a voice in all areas of care and quality of life. Many of the rights are cross-referenced with other rights and regulations so it is important to review them in their entirety in addition to this section.

***Tag F550 Resident Rights/Exercise of Rights**

All residents have rights guaranteed to them under federal and state laws and regulations. This regulation is intended to lay the foundation for the resident rights requirements in long-term care facilities. Each resident has the right to be treated with dignity and respect. All activities and interactions with residents by any staff, temporary agency staff, or volunteers must focus on assisting the resident in maintaining and enhancing his or her self-esteem and self-worth and incorporating the resident's goals, preferences, and choices. When providing care and services, staff must respect each resident's individuality, as well as honor and value their input.

Each resident must be treated with respect and dignity. The environment must maintain or enhance quality of life, as much as possible while recognizing each resident's individuality. Each resident must have equal access to persons and services inside and outside the facility. The facility will ensure that the resident can exercise his/her rights as a citizen or resident of the United States without interference, coercion, discrimination, or reprisal from the facility.

The resident also has the right to be free from negative actions or undue pressure from the facility and facility staff when exercising his/her rights in a reasonable manner. This right includes freedom from the reduction of the group activity time of a resident trying to organize a resident group or singling out residents for prejudicial treatment such as isolating residents in activities.

Tag F551 Rights Exercised by Representative

In the case of a resident who has not been adjudged incompetent by the state court, the resident has the right to designate a representative, in accordance with state law and any legal surrogate so designated may exercise the resident's rights to the extent provided by state law. The same sex spouse of a resident must be afforded treatment equal to that afforded to an opposite-sex spouse if the marriage was valid in the jurisdiction in which it was celebrated.

The resident may designate some rights and not others. If the facility feels that the representative is not acting in the resident's best interest, the facility is required to follow state law for reporting its concerns.

In the case of a resident adjudged incompetent under the laws of a State by a court of competent jurisdiction, the rights of the resident devolve to and are exercised by the resident representative appointed under State law to act on the resident's behalf.

The federal and state governments have set up specific guidelines to follow if the treatment team feels that a resident is no longer cognitively able to make thoughtful, informed choices about his/her care. This part of the OBRA '87 law provides a check and balance for residents who are at risk of well meaning staff "making choices for them." The system is meant to be set up so that a guardian can place the resident's needs first when making choices about care (not just what is convenient for the facility). This tag requires the surveyors to make sure that all consents (including photo release and outing release) are signed by the legally appointed guardian.

In all cases the resident must be included as much as possible in the care planning process.

Tag F552 Right to be Informed/Make Treatment Decisions

The resident has the right to be informed of, and participate in, his or her treatment including: the right to be fully informed in language that he or she can understand of his or her total health status, the right to be informed, in advance, of the care to be furnished, and to be informed of the risks and benefits of the treatment.

The staff and consultants at the facility must make sure that the resident is fully informed about his/her health and status in a manner that s/he can easily understand. Total health status includes functional status, activities potential, cognitive status, psychosocial status, and sensory and physical impairments.

The information must be presented in advance of the treatment and must let the resident know if the treatment will affect the resident's well-being. Unless the resident has been previously determined (legally) to be incompetent or otherwise found to be incapacitated, the resident has the right to chose his/her preferred care and treatment.

Tag F553 Right to Participate in Planning Care

This tag ensures that the facility staff facilitates the inclusion of the resident or resident representative in all aspects of person-centered care planning and that this planning includes the provision of services to enable the resident to live with dignity and supports the resident's goals, choices, and preferences including, but not limited to, goals related to their daily routines and goals to potentially return to a community setting.

The resident should be involved in the assessment and care planning process, including the discussion of diagnoses, treatment, options, risks, and prognoses. Unless the resident has been previously determined (legally) to be incompetent or otherwise found to be incapacitated, the resident has the right to participate in planning care and treatment or changes in care and treatment. The resident has the right to identify individuals or roles to be included in the planning process, request meetings, and request revisions to the person-centered plan of care. The resident also has the right to participate in establishing the expected goals and outcomes and all other aspects of care. The resident must be informed, in advance, of changes to the plan of care and must agree with them. Finally, this tag gives the resident the right to receive the services included in the plan of care.

Tag 554 Self-Administer Medications if Clinically Appropriate

A resident may be allowed to self-administer medications, if the interdisciplinary team has determined it is appropriate. Activities staff need to be aware of what is allowed.

Tag 557 Respect and Dignity/Right to Have Personal Property.

All residents' possessions, regardless of their apparent value to others, must be treated with respect.

All areas of the facility must provide a homelike environment. The resident has the right to keep some of his/her personal possessions in his/her room (including furniture) as long as its presence does not jeopardize the health and safety of the other residents.

***Tag F558 Reasonable Accommodations of Needs/Preferences.**

The accommodation of resident needs and preferences is essential to creating an individualized, home-like environment.

Residents have the right to receive services in the facility with reasonable accommodation of resident needs and preferences except when to do so would endanger the health or safety of the resident or other residents. The facility must be organized to assist the resident in maintaining and/or achieving independent functioning, dignity, and well-being to the extent possible.

***Tag F559 Choose/Be Notified of Room/Roommate Change**

Residents who are married to each other have the right to share a room in the facility as long as both partners want to share a room.

Residents have the right to share a room with his/her roommate of choice when practicable, when both residents live in the same facility and both residents consent to the arrangement.

Residents have the right to receive written notice, including the reason for the change, before the resident's room or roommate in the facility is changed.

***Tag F561 Self Determination**

The intent of this requirement is to ensure that each resident has the opportunity to exercise his or her autonomy regarding those things that are important in his or her life. This includes the residents' interests and preferences. The resident has the right to and the facility must promote and facilitate resident self-determination through support of resident choice.

The resident has the right to choose activities, health care, health care providers, and schedules (including sleeping and waking times), consistent with his/her interests, assessments, and plans of care. S/he may interact with members of the community both inside and outside of the facility; and make choices about aspects of his/her life in the facility that are significant to the resident. A resident has the right to participate in social, religious, and community activities that do not interfere with the rights of other residents in the facility. The facility, to the extent possible, should accommodate an individual's needs and choices for how s/he spends time, both inside and outside of the facility.

Tag F562 Immediate Access to Resident

Certain state and federal officials, including those providing protection and advocacy, must be allowed immediate access to any resident at any time. Immediate access is also allowed for the resident's personal physician and representative.

Tag F563 Right to Receive/Deny Visitors

The resident has a right to receive visitors of his or her choosing at the time of his or her choosing, subject to the resident's right to deny visitation when applicable, and in a manner that does not impose on the rights of another resident.

The facility may not have visiting hours that apply to any individual whom the resident wishes to visit. Visitors must be admitted 24 hours a day if the resident wishes it to be that way. If there are restrictions on visiting, they must be supported by written policies and procedures that describe why the restrictions or limitations are necessary from a clinical or safety perspective. Restricting visitors without clinical or safety reasons may result in a citation.

Tag F564 Inform of Visitation Rights/Equal Visitation Privileges

All residents have the right to visitors in accordance to their preferences. The facility policy for restricting or limiting visitors must be communicated to the resident. If limitations are placed on a resident's visitation rights, the clinical or safety reasons for the limitations and the specific individuals the restriction applies to must be communicated to the resident or resident representative in a manner he or she understands. [The facility may not] restrict, limit, or otherwise deny visitation privileges on the basis of race, color, national origin, religion, sex, gender identity, sexual orientation, or disability.

The resident must be informed of the rules regarding visitors. Failing to inform a resident, the family, and/or resident representative of their visitation rights, including any restrictions or limitations of these rights, may result in a citation.

***Tag F565 Resident/Family Group and Response**

This requirement does not require that residents organize a resident or family group. However, whenever residents or their families wish to organize, they must be able to do so without interference. Additionally, they must be provided space, privacy for meetings, and staff support. The designated staff person responsible for assistance and liaison between the group and the facility's administration and any other staff members may attend the meeting only if invited by the resident or family group. The resident or family group may meet without staff present. The groups should determine how frequently they meet.

Facility staff are required to consider resident and family group views and act upon grievances and recommendations. Facility staff must consider these recommendations and attempt to accommodate them, to the extent practicable. This may include developing or changing policies affecting resident care and life. Facility staff should discuss its decisions with the resident and/or family group and document in writing its response and rationale.

This tag outlines the residents' right to hold meetings in the facility, with adequate space for the meeting provided by the facility. The residents and their families have the right to meet in private and to present a written request to the facility to address grievances and/or recommendations. The facility is then required to address the grievances and/or recommendations in a timely manner.

Tag F566 Right to Perform Facility Services or Refuse

The resident has a right to choose or refuse to perform services for the facility and the facility must not require a resident to perform services for the facility.

The resident may not be required to work for the facility. If the resident elects to work for the facility (e.g., folding clothes, running activity groups), it must be part of the plan of care. The facility must have in writing whether the resident is working for a wage or as a volunteer, as well as documentation that the resident is knowledgeable about his/her pay status. If the resident is getting paid for the work being done, s/he must be paid the prevailing wage for the job being done.

Tag F567 Protection/Management of Personal Funds.

Residents who have authorized the facility in writing to manage any personal funds have ready and reasonable access to those funds.

The resident has the right to continue managing his/her finances after s/he is admitted to the long-term care facility. The facility may not require that the resident deposit his/her money with the facility or at a bank of the facility's choosing. Rules for where the funds may be deposited are described.

Tag F568 Accounting and Records of Personal Funds.

This tag specifies the manner in which the facility may handle the resident's money if the resident chooses to allow the facility to do so.

Tag F571 Limitations on Charges to Personal Funds

This tag limits the items and services a resident may be charged for. For activities programs, the resident may not be charged for programs required by OBRA '87. Residents may be asked to pay for some special events, but it is important to understand the restrictions.

Tag F572 Notice of Rights and Rules.

This requirement is intended to assure that each resident knows his or her rights and responsibilities and that facility staff communicates this information prior to or upon admis-

sion, as appropriate during the resident's stay, and when the facility's rules change.

The resident has the right to be informed of his or her rights and all rules and regulations governing conduct and responsibilities during his or her stay in the facility. The facility must provide a notice of rights and services to the resident prior to or upon admission and during the resident's stay. The facility must inform the resident both orally and in writing in a language that the resident understands. The facility must also provide the resident with the state-developed notice of Medicaid rights and obligations, if any. Receipt of such information, and any amendments to it, must be acknowledged in writing.

It is hard for a resident to exercise his/her rights if s/he does not know what they are. For this reason, the Federal Government requires that the resident receive a copy of his/her rights written in a language and manner that s/he can read (avoid small print) and understand (native language, if necessary). The resident must also be verbally told of his/her rights. Receipt of the rights must be acknowledged in writing.

This notice of his/her rights (both verbally and in writing) must happen: 1. right before and/or at the time of admission, 2. immediately upon any changes in those rights, 3. upon request, and 4. periodically throughout admission. The surveyors are instructed to interview some of the staff to determine if the staff know the rights and rules well enough to help implement them.

Tag F573 Right to Access/Purchase Copies of Records.

The facility must provide the resident with access to personal and medical records pertaining to him or herself, upon an oral or written request. The facility must allow the resident to obtain a copy of the records or any portions thereof (including in an electronic form or format when such records are maintained electronically) upon request and 2 working days advance notice to the facility.

The resident and/or his/her legal representative have the right to review all of the resident's records within 24 hours of the request. This request may be either verbal or in writing. The facility cannot insist that only written requests be accepted. This requirement is for the resident's medical chart as well as trust fund ledgers, contracts with the facility, facility incident reports, and any other record that may have been made on behalf of or about the resident. The facility may charge the resident for any copies of the records that s/he may request, however, the amount of that charge may not exceed what is normally charged at places like the public library, the post office, or low-cost copy shops.

Tag F574 Required Notices and Contact Information

The resident has the right to receive notices orally (meaning spoken) and in writing (including Braille) in a format and a language he or she understands.

The notices include information about personal funds, regulatory agencies, advocacy offices, adult protective services, Medicare and Medicaid eligibility, Medicaid fraud prevention, and where to file a complaint about violations of nursing facility regulations.

Tag F575 Required Postings

The facility must post, in a form and manner accessible and understandable to residents [and] resident representative: a list of names, addresses, and telephone numbers of all pertinent state agencies and advocacy groups... and a statement that the resident may file a complaint with any of the groups.

Tag F576 Right to Forms of Communication with Privacy

The resident has the right to have reasonable access to a telephone to receive and place calls in a private manner. This phone must meet ADA (Americans with Disabilities Act) standards for height and volume control (TTY or a TDD).

Phones in offices are not considered private use of phones. Instead the facility must provide jacks in the rooms or cordless phones. The facility must protect and facilitate a resident's right to communicate with individuals and entities within and external to the facility.

The resident has the right to receive mail and packages without them first being opened by facility staff. The laws that apply to the individual's right to privacy of mail received apply to residents of the facility just as it would if they were in their own homes. Because many of the residents are not able to go shopping for stationery, writing implements, and postage stamps, the facility is expected to provide them for the residents but may attach a reasonable charge to these supplies. These tags also specify that residents must receive their mail in less than 24 hours of it being delivered to the facility and that the residents' outgoing mail must be to the post office in less than 24 hours after being given to a staff person.

The resident has the right to have reasonable access to and privacy in their use of electronic communications such as email and video communications and for internet research.

Tag F577 Right to Survey Results/Advocacy Agency Information

The resident has the right to examine the results of the most recent survey...and any plan of corrections.... The facility must post in a place readily accessible to residents and family members and legal representatives of residents, the results of the most recent survey of the facility.

The resident and the public in general have the right to see a copy of the facility's most current survey along with the plan of correction written up by the facility. This copy must be easily available and either the actual survey document or a notice of its availability must be posted in a prominent place for all to see. The resident has the right to contact agencies acting as client advocates.

Tag F578 Request/Refuse/Discontinue Treatment; Formulate Advanced Directives

The resident has the absolute right to refuse to participate in any treatment (unless it is court ordered). The resident also has the right to sign an Advance Directive and have the facility honor that Directive. The resident does not have the right to receive medical treatment or medical services deemed medically unnecessary or inappropriate.

This tag leads to a philosophical discussion about whether the treatment team — especially the activity professional — can write up any treatment objective based on participation. If the activity professional has the care plan objective that the resident will participate in three activities a week, then the treatment being provided is *participation*. The resident always has the absolute right to refuse all treatment and the right to refuse to participate in facility sponsored activities.

When most residents decline the invitation to go to any specific activity, they are not usually refusing treatment in their mind; they just are not interested in going to the activity. If the care plan objective is to participate in activities, the resident says "no thank you" and yet the staff person still tries to persuade the resident to go — that staff person is violating the resident's right to refuse treatment and is trying to coerce the resident to abandon (even if for a short while) his/her rights.

The prudent professional will always separate the treatment plan (therapeutic intervention) from the normal leisure pastime of going to activities. Leave participation in the domain of a normalizing activity. When you feel that the resident needs a treatment, the care plan should be based on treating the identified need (e.g., increase frequency of initiation of social communications, increase use of fine motor skills, decrease percentage of time spent alone) and not on going to activities.

Tag F579 Posting/Notice of Medicare/Medicaid on Admission

The facility must display in the facility written information, and provide to residents and applicants for admission, oral and written information about how to apply for and use Medicare and Medicaid benefits, and how to receive refunds for previous payments covered by such benefits.

Tag F580 Notify of Changes (Injury, Decline, Room, etc.)

A facility must immediately inform the resident; consult with the resident's physician; and notify, consistent with his or her authority, the resident representative when there is an accident involving the resident which results in injury and has the potential for requiring physician intervention; a significant change in the resident's physical, mental, or psychosocial status; a need to alter treatment significantly; or a decision to transfer, or discharge the resident from the facility ... and when there is a change in room or roommate assignment or a change in resident rights.

Communication from the facility with the resident, the resident's legal guardian, or interested family member and the resident's physician is important. In situations in which the resident: 1. has been involved in an accident, 2. has experienced a significant change in health status, 3. has a need to have a change in treatment, 4. is to be discharged, 5. is scheduled to have a change of roommate, and/or 6. has a change in his/her rights, the listed parties are to be notified *immediately*. A subsection of this tag requires that the facility must periodically check to make sure that all of the phone numbers and addresses that they have for legal guardians, interested family members, and the resident's physician are current.

Tag F582 Medicaid/Medicare Coverage/Liability Notice

The facility must inform each Medicaid-eligible resident, in writing, at the time of admission to the nursing facility and when the resident becomes eligible for Medicaid of the items and services that are included in nursing facility services under the state plan and for which the resident may be charged; those other items that the facility offers and for which the resident may be charged, and the amount of charges for those services and inform each Medicaid-eligible resident when changes are made to the items and services specified in ... this section

The facility must inform each resident before, or at the time of admission, and periodically during the resident's stay, of services available in the facility and of charges for those services, including any charges for services not covered under Medicare/ Medicaid or by the facility's per diem rate.

Tag F583 Personal Privacy/Confidentiality of Records

The resident has a right to personal privacy and confidentiality of his or her personal and medical records including accommodations, medical treatment, written and telephone communications, personal care, visits and meetings of family and resident groups.... The resident has the right to refuse the release of personal and medical records except as provided at 483.70 (i) (2). The facility must allow representatives of the Office of the State Long Term Care Ombudsman to examine a resident's medical, social, and administrative records in accordance with state law.

The resident has the right to maintain his/her personal privacy and to have all of his/her records maintained in a confidential manner. With some exceptions, the resident has the right to refuse to release personal and medical records. The facility must allow the state-appointed Ombudsman access to the resident's records if the resident or his/her legal guardian gives permission.

The right to privacy in personal communications is also part of this tag.

***Tag F584 Safe/Clean/Comfortable Homelike Environment**

The resident has to a right to a safe, clean, comfortable, and homelike environment, including but not limited to receiving treatment and supports for daily living safely.

All areas of the facility must provide a homelike environment. The resident has the right to keep some of his/her personal possessions in his/her room (including furniture) as long as its presence does not jeopardize the health and safety of the other residents.

This tag also provides guidelines for the quality and comfort level of the living space for the residents. For a more in-depth review of these tags the reader should review the OBRA '87 Environmental Review Form in this book.

Tag F585 Grievances

[This tag supports] each resident's right to voice grievances (such as those about treatment, care, management of funds, lost clothing, or violation of rights) and to ensure that a policy is in place to process grievances. Facility staff are responsible for making prompt efforts to resolve a grievance and to keep the resident appropriately apprised of progress toward resolution.

The resident has the right to complain (voice grievances) about treatment received or not received or about other things that dissatisfy him/her about the facility. The facility must take these grievances seriously by 1. listening to the grievances, 2. investigating the complaint, 3. promptly trying to address the cause of the grievance (resolve the grievance if possible), and 4. monitoring to ensure that the cause does not lead to the same situation again. This includes addressing the resident's complaints about the behaviors of other residents and of staff.

The facility must make information on how to file a grievance or complaint available to the resident. The facility must establish a grievance policy to ensure the prompt resolution of all grievances regarding the residents' rights and make copies of the grievance policy available to the resident. The regulations detail what must be in the policy.

Tag F586 Resident Contacts with External Entities

A facility must not prohibit or in any way discourage a resident from communicating with federal, state, or local officials. Facility staff must ensure that residents are able to communicate freely with representatives of protection, advocacy, and survey agencies for any reason.

483.12 Freedom from Abuse, Neglect, and Exploitation

This next section of regulations guarantees resident freedom from abuse, neglect, and exploitation. Many of these violations are also crimes. The survey guidelines provide extensive guidance and protocols for investigating violations in these areas. All of the F-Tags in this section have potential for substandard quality of care with one or more deficiencies.

***Tag F600 Free from Abuse and Neglect**

Each resident has the right to be free from abuse, neglect, and corporal punishment of any type by anyone. The regulation specifies the right to be free from verbal, sexual, physical, or mental abuse, corporal punishment, involuntary seclusion, and any physical or chemical restraint not required to treat the resident's medical symptoms.

The surveyor guideline provides details of policies and procedures that must be in place and followed to handle each kind of abuse and neglect.

***Tag F602 Free from Misappropriation/Exploitation**

Each resident has the right to be free from misappropriation of property and exploitation. "Exploitation" means "taking advantage of a resident for personal gain, through the use of manipulation, intimidation, threats, or coercion." "Misappropriation of resident property" means "the deliberate misplacement, exploitation, or wrongful, temporary, or permanent use of a resident's belongings or money without the resident's consent."

***Tag F603 Free from Involuntary Seclusion**

Each resident has the right to be free from involuntary seclusion. "Involuntary seclusion" is defined as separation of a resident from other residents or from her/his room or confinement to her/his room (with or without roommates) against the resident's will, or the will of the resident representative.

During a situation in which a resident's behavior has escalated and immediate interventions are required for the safety of the resident, staff, and/or other residents, the facility must provide necessary supervision of the resident to ensure that the resident and other residents are protected. The facility must immediately consult with the resident's designated representative and the resident's physician about the behavioral symptoms.

***Tag F604 Right to be Free from Physical Restraints**

See Tag F605.

***Tag F605 Right to be Free from Chemical Restraints**

The resident has the right to be free from any physical or chemical restraints imposed for purposes of discipline or convenience, not required to treat the resident's medical symptoms. "Physical restraints" are any manual method or physical or mechanical device, material, or equipment attached to or adjacent to the resident's body that the individual cannot remove easily which restricts freedom of movement or normal access to one's body. Leg restraints, arm restraints, hand mitts, soft ties or vest, wheelchair safety bars, geri-chairs, and bed rails are physical restraints. "Chemical restraints" are psycho-pharmacological drugs used for discipline or convenience and not required to treat medical symptoms. "Discipline" is any action taken by the facility for the purpose of punishing or penalizing the resident. "Convenience" is any action taken by the facility to control resident behavior or maintain residents with a lesser amount of effort by the facility and not in the residents' best interest.

Before using restraints, a facility must demonstrate the presence of a specific medical symptom that would require the use of restraints and how the restraint would treat the cause of the symptom and assist the resident in reaching his/her highest level of physical and psychosocial well-being. Often appropriate exercise and therapeutic interventions such as orthotic devices, pillows, pads, or lap trays will be sufficient.

These less restrictive, supportive devices must be considered prior to using physical restraints. If after a trial of less restrictive measures, the facility decides that a physical restraint would enable and promote greater functional independence, then the use of the restraining device must first be explained to the resident, family member, or legal representative. If the resident, family member, or legal representative agrees to this treatment alternative, then the restraining device may be used for specific periods for which the restraint has been determined to be an enabler.

When a medication is indicated to treat a medical symptom, the facility must:

- Use the least restrictive alternative for the least amount of time;
- Provide ongoing re-evaluation of the need for the medication; and
- Not use the medication for discipline or convenience.

Any resident who requires a restraint must have a specific intervention in the care plan to ensure maintenance of his/her physical, mental, psychosocial, and functional status. To determine maintenance, the treatment team should administer the appropriate assessments to establish a baseline.

***Tag F606 Not Employ/Engage Staff with Adverse Actions**

The facility must not hire an employee or engage an individual who was found guilty of abuse, neglect, exploitation, misappropriation of property, or mistreatment by a court of law; or who has a finding in the State nurse aide registry concerning abuse, neglect, exploitation, mistreatment of residents, or misappropriation of resident property, or has had a disciplinary action in effect taken against his/her professional license. The facility must report knowledge of actions by a court of law against an employee that indicates the employee is unfit for duty.

***Tag F607 Develop/Implement Abuse/Neglect, etc. Policies**

This regulation provides protections for the health, welfare, and rights of each resident residing in the facility. In order to provide these protections, the facility must develop written policies and procedures to prohibit and prevent abuse, neglect, exploitation of residents, and misappropriation of resident property.

***Tag F608 Reporting of Reasonable Suspicion of a Crime**

The intent is for the facility to develop and implement policies and procedures that:

- *Ensure reporting of crimes against a resident or individual receiving care from the facility occurring in nursing homes within prescribed timeframes to the appropriate entities;*
- *Ensure that all covered individuals, such as the owner, operator, employee, manager, agent or contractor report reasonable suspicion of crimes, as required by Section 1150B of the Act;*
- *Provide annual notification for covered individuals of these reporting requirements;*
- *Post a conspicuous notice of employee rights, including the right to file a complaint; and*
- *Assure that any covered individual who makes a report, or is in the process of making a report, is not retaliated against.*

***Tag F609 Reporting of Alleged Violations**

The facility must report alleged violations related to mistreatment, exploitation, neglect, or abuse, including injuries of unknown source and misappropriation of resident property and report the results of all investigations to the proper authorities within prescribed timeframes.

All staff are required to report violations.

***Tag F610 Investigate/Prevent/Correct Alleged Violation**

The facility must take the following actions in response to an alleged violation of abuse, neglect, exploitation, or mistreatment:

- *Thoroughly investigate the alleged violation;*
- *Prevent further abuse, neglect, exploitation and mistreatment from occurring while the investigation is in progress; and*
- *Take appropriate corrective action, as a result of investigation findings.*

483.15 Admission, Transfer, and Discharge

Some of the tags in this section have implications for social service professionals regarding discharge planning. To help protect the rights of each resident, the Federal government has outlined the acceptable reasons for transfer or discharge and the procedures and steps required to take before, during, and after a resident is either discharged or transferred.

Tag F622 Transfer and Discharge Requirements

This tag specifies the limited conditions under which a skilled nursing facility or nursing facility may initiate transfer or discharge of a resident, the documentation that must be included in the medical record, and who is responsible for making the documentation. Additionally, these requirements specify the information that must be conveyed to the receiving provider for residents being transferred or discharged to another healthcare setting.

Tag F624 Preparation for Safe/Orderly Transfer/Discharge

The facility must provide sufficient preparation and orientation for discharge or transfers. This means it informs the resident where s/he is going and takes steps under its control to minimize anxiety.

Tag F625 Notice of Bed Hold Policy Before/Upon Transfer

The facility must ensure that residents are made aware of a facility's bed-hold and reserve bed payment policy before and upon transfer to a hospital or when taking a therapeutic leave of absence from the facility.

483.20 Resident Assessments

This section has implications for all staff involved with documentation including activity professionals and social service professionals.

Tag F636 Comprehensive Assessments and Timing

The facility must conduct initially and periodically a comprehensive, accurate, standardized reproducible assessment of each resident's functional capacity. [The intent is to] ensure that the Resident Assessment Instrument (RAI) is used, in accordance with specified format and timeframes, in conducting comprehensive assessments as part of an ongoing process through which the facility identifies each resident's preferences and goals of care, functional and health status, strengths and needs, as well as offering guidance for further assessment once problems have been identified.

The facility is required to conduct a comprehensive assessment on each resident when s/he is admitted and then at intervals during his/her stay. This assessment must done using a standardized assessment (the MDS), the findings must be accurate, the staff performing the assessment must be qualified to do the assessment, and a variety of staff must be able to get substantially similar results (reliability). This tag also explains that the testing tools that the staff use (e.g., the nursing assessment, the activity assessment) must, when put together, measure everything that is required to be written into the MDS. Each facility must use the RAI (which includes both the MDS and the CAAs). The areas measured include:

- Medically defined conditions and prior medical history
- Medical status measurement
- Physical and mental functional status
- Sensory and physical impairments
- Nutritional status and requirements
- Special treatments and procedures
- Mental and psychosocial status
- Discharge potential
- Dental condition
- Activities potential (The resident's ability and desire to take part in activities that maintain or improve physical, mental, and psychosocial well-being. Activity pursuits refer to any activity outside of ADLs that a person pursues in order to obtain a sense of well-being. Also included are activities that provide benefits in the areas of self-esteem, pleasure, comfort, health education, creativity, success, and financial or emotional independence. The assessment should consider the resident's normal, everyday routines and lifetime preferences.)
- Rehabilitation potential
- Cognitive status, including the resident's ability to problem solve, decide, remember, and be aware of and respond to safety hazards
- Medication therapy

Requirements for assessments are discussed in more detail in Chapter 11 of this book.

Tag F637 Comprehensive Assessment after Significant Change

A resident must be reassessed within 14 days after the facility determines, or should have determined, that there has been a significant change in the resident's physical or mental condition.

This is discussed in Chapter 11.

Tag F638 Quarterly Assessment at Least Every 3 Months

A facility must assess a resident using the quarterly review instrument specified by the State and approved by CMS not less frequently than once every 3 months.

This is discussed in Chapter 11.

Tag F639 Maintain 15 Months of Resident Assessments

Facilities are required to maintain 15 months of assessment data in each resident's active clinical record.

Documentation supporting MDS findings must also be maintained for 15 months.

Tag F641 Accuracy of Assessments

The assessment must accurately reflect the resident's status.

"Accuracy of Assessment" means that the appropriate, qualified health professionals correctly document the resident's medical, functional, and psychosocial problems and identify resident strengths to maintain or improve medical status, functional abilities, and psychosocial status using the appropriate Resident Assessment Instrument (RAI) (i.e. comprehensive, quarterly, significant change in status).

Facilities are responsible for ensuring that all participants in the assessment process have the requisite knowledge to complete an accurate assessment.

Assessments must be done accurately, by an appropriate staff member.

Tag F642 Coordination/Certification of Assessment

Each resident's assessment will be coordinated by and certified as complete by a registered nurse, and all individuals who complete a portion of the assessment will sign and certify to the accuracy of the portion of the assessment he or she completed.

Assessments must be signed by each person who completes a portion of the assessment.

483.21 Comprehensive Resident-Centered Care Plans

This section is an important section of regulations. It has implications for all staff involved with documentation including activity professionals and social service professionals.

Tag F655 Baseline Care Plan

Completion and implementation of the baseline care plan within 48 hours of a resident's admission is intended to promote continuity of care and communication among nursing home staff, increase resident safety, and safeguard against adverse events that are most likely to occur right after admission; and to ensure the resident and representative, if applicable, are informed of the initial plan for delivery of care and services by receiving a written summary of the baseline care plan.

This is a new requirement in the latest set of guidelines. Baseline care plans are discussed in the Documentation and Care Plans chapters of this book.

Tag F656 Develop/Implement Comprehensive Care Plan

Each resident is required to have a comprehensive care plan based on his/her needs that were identified in the assessment process.

Tag F657 Care Plan Timing and Revision

This care plan must be developed no later than seven days after the completion of the MDS. This care plan must be developed by the resident (and/or his/her legal guardian or family) working along with the treatment team and must be reviewed periodically to ensure that it is still appropriate.

Tag F658 Services Provided Meet Professional Standards

See Tag F659.

Tag F659 Qualified Persons

These two tags state that each professional in the facility must provide his/her services in a way that will meet or exceed the standards of practice published by his/her professional group, as well as any other governmental or accrediting standards that apply. For facilities who are surveyed by either the Joint Commission or CARF: the Rehabilitation Accreditation Commission, the professional must comply with the standards of those groups to comply with this tag. The services must be culturally competent and trauma-informed. Tag 659 will be implemented in 2018.

Tag F660 Discharge Planning Process

See Tag F661.

Tag F661 Discharge Summary

These two tags outline the requirements for discharge summaries. See the discussion on discharge summaries in Chapter 11.

483.24 Quality of Life

This section on quality of life specifies the facility's responsibility to create and sustain an environment that humanizes and individualizes each resident's quality of life by:

- Ensuring all staff, across all shifts and departments, understand the principles of quality of life, and honor and support these principles for each resident.
- Ensuring that the care and services provided are person-centered, and honor and support each resident's preferences, choices, values, and beliefs.

Violations of any of the tags in this section may be considered substandard quality of care.

***Tag F675 Quality of Life**

Quality of Life is a fundamental principle that applies to all care and services provided to facility residents. Each resident must receive and the facility must provide the necessary care and services to attain or maintain the highest practicable physical, mental, and psychosocial well-being, consistent with the resident's comprehensive assessment and plan of care.

This tag states that the resident must receive the types and quality of care indicated as needed by the assessment and outlined in the care plan.

***Tag F676 Activities of Daily Living (ADLs)/Maintain Abilities**

Based on the comprehensive assessment of a resident and consistent with the resident's needs and choices, the facility must provide the necessary care and services to ensure that a resident's abilities in activities of daily living do not diminish unless circumstances of the individual's clinical condition demonstrate that such diminution was unavoidable. These ADL's include Hygiene, Mobility, Elimination, Dining, and Communication.

***Tag F677 ADL Care Provided for Dependent Residents**

A resident who is unable to carry out activities of daily living receives the necessary services to maintain good nutrition, grooming, and personal and oral hygiene.

***Tag F678 Cardio-Pulmonary Resuscitation (CPR)**

Personnel provide basic life support, including CPR, to a resident requiring such emergency care prior to the arrival of emergency medical personnel and subject to related physician orders and the resident's advance directives.

***Tag F679. Activities Meet Interest/Needs of Each Resident**

The facility must provide, based on the comprehensive assessment and care plan and the preferences of each resident, an ongoing program to support residents in their choice of activities, both facility-sponsored group and individual activities and independent activities, designed to meet the interests of and support the physical, mental, and psychosocial well-being of each resident, encouraging both independence and interaction in the community.

Research findings and the observations of positive resident outcomes confirm that activities are an integral component of residents' lives. Residents have indicated that daily life and involvement should be meaningful. Activities are meaningful when they reflect a person's interests and lifestyle are enjoyable to the person, help the person to feel useful, and provide a sense of belonging. Maintaining contact and interaction with the community is an important aspect of a person's well-being and facilitates feelings of connectedness and self-esteem. Involvement in community includes interactions such as assisting the resident to maintain his/her ability to independently shop, attend the community theater, local concerts, library, and participate in community groups.

All residents have a need for engagement in meaningful activities. For residents with dementia, the lack of engaging activities can cause boredom, loneliness, and frustration, resulting in distress and agitation. Activities must be individualized and customized based on the resident's previous lifestyle (occupation, family, hobbies), preferences, and comforts.

The surveyors will be checking to make sure appropriate activities are provides for a resident who exhibits unusual amounts of energy or walking without purpose, engages in behaviors not conducive with a therapeutic home-like environment, exhibits behavior that require a less stimulating environment to discontinue behaviors not welcomed by others sharing their social space, goes through others' belongings, has withdrawn from previous activity interests or customary routines and isolates self in his/her room or bed most of the day, excessively seeks attention from staff and/or peers, who lacks awareness of personal safety, or has delusional and hallucinatory behavior that is stressful to her/him.

The stated goal of the survey process for this tag is to "*Use the Activities Critical Element pathway and the guidance above to investigate concerns related to activities which are based on the resident's comprehensive assessment and care plan, and meet the resident's interests and preferences, and support his or her physical, mental, and psychosocial well-being.*"

F680 Qualifications of Activity Professional

The activities program must be directed by a qualified professional who is a qualified therapeutic recreation specialist or an activities professional who (i) Is licensed or registered, if applicable, by the State in which practicing: and (ii) Is (A) Eligible for certification as a therapeutic recreation specialist or as an activities professional by a recognized accrediting body on or after October 1, 1990: or (B) Has 2 years of experience in a social or recreational program within the last 5 years, one of which was full-time in a therapeutic activities program: or (C) Is a qualified occupational therapist or occupational therapy assistant: or (D) Has completed a training course approved by the State.

This tag outlines the types of credentials required of any person who is employed as the Activity Director.

483.25 Quality of Care

This section outlines requirements for the quality of care that must be provided to residents. Each of these tags may be cited for substandard quality of care. Activities and Social Services are mentioned explicitly in two of the tags. Other tags specify that conditions, such as incontinence, pain management, or the need for tube feeding, should be handled in a way that does not impact the residents' ability to participate in activities of their choice.

***Tag F684 Quality of Care**

Quality of care is a fundamental principle that applies to all treatment and care provided to facility residents. Based on the comprehensive assessment of a resident, the facility must ensure that residents receive treatment and care in accordance with professional standards of practice, the comprehensive person-centered care plan, and the resident's choices.

This tag states that the resident must receive the types and quality of care indicated as needed by the assessment and outlined in the care plan. Activities and psychosocial needs are addressed specifically:

Activities/Psychosocial Needs — Care plan interventions for activities must be based on the resident's assessment and include the resident's choices, personal beliefs, interests, ethnic/cultural practices and spiritual values, as appropriate. In addition, the resident's assessment may identify psychosocial needs, such as fear, loneliness, anxiety, or depression. Interventions to address the needs must be included in the plan of care. (For concerns related to the provision of activities, refer to Tag F679. For concerns regarding medically related social services, refer to Tag F745.)

***Tag F689 Free of Accident Hazards/Supervision/Devices**

This tag sets the expectation that the environment will be free of accident hazards and that each resident will receive adequate supervision and assistance to be able to avoid accidental injury.

483.3 Physician Services

Tags F710-F715 refer to physician's services.

483.35 Nursing Services

Tags F725-F732 refer to nursing services.

483.40 Behavioral Health Services

The section on Behavioral Health Services is very important for social service and activity professionals. Tags F742-F745 have potential for substandard quality of care.

Tag F740 Behavioral Health Services

Each resident must receive and the facility must provide the necessary behavioral health care and services to attain or maintain the highest practicable physical, mental, and psychosocial well-being, in accordance with the comprehensive assessment and plan of care. Behavioral health encompasses a resident's whole emotional and mental well-being, which includes, but is not limited to the prevention and treatment of mental and substance use disorders.

The facility must provide necessary behavioral health care and services which include:

- *Ensuring that the necessary care and services are person-centered and reflect the resident's goals for care, while maximizing the resident's dignity, autonomy, privacy, socialization, independence, choice, and safety;*
- *Ensuring that direct care staff interact and communicate in a manner that promotes mental and psychosocial well-being.*
- *Providing meaningful activities which promote engagement, and positive meaningful relationships between residents and staff, families, other residents and the community. Meaningful activities are those that address the resident's customary routines, interests, preferences, etc. and enhance the resident's well-being;*
- *Providing an environment and atmosphere that is conducive to mental and psychosocial well-being;*
- *Ensuring that pharmacological interventions are only used when non-pharmacological interventions are ineffective or when clinically indicated.*

Tag F741 Sufficient/Competent Staff — Behavioral Health Needs

The facility must have sufficient staff who provide direct services to residents with the appropriate competencies and skills sets to provide nursing and related services to assure resident safety and attain or maintain the highest practicable physical, mental and psychosocial well-being of each resident, as determined by resident assessments and individual plans of care and considering the number, acuity, and diagnoses of the facility's resident population in accordance with 483.70 (e). These competencies and skills sets include but are not limited to, knowledge of and appropriate training and supervision for: Caring for residents with mental and psychosocial disorders as well as residents with a history of trauma and/or post-traumatic stress disorder, that have been identified in the facility assessment.

***Tag F742 Treatment Services for Mental/Psychosocial Concerns**

Based on the comprehensive assessment of a resident, the facility must ensure that a resident who displays or is diagnosed with mental disorder or psychosocial adjustment difficulty, or who has a history of trauma and/or post-traumatic stress disorder, receives appropriate treatment and services to correct the assessed problem or to attain the highest practicable mental and psychosocial well-being.

Appropriate treatment for trauma and PTSD are covered by this tag.

***Tag F743 No Pattern of Behavioral Difficulties Unless Unavoidable**

A resident whose assessment did not reveal or who does not have a diagnosis of a mental or psychosocial adjustment difficulty or a documented history of trauma and/or post-traumatic stress disorder does not display a pattern of decreased social interaction and/or increased withdrawn, angry, or depressive behaviors, unless the resident's clinical condition demonstrates that development of such as pattern was unavoidable.

***Tag F744 Treatment/Services for Dementia**

A resident who displays or is diagnosed with dementia receives the appropriate treatment and services to attain or maintain his or her highest practicable physical, mental, and psychosocial well-being.

***Tag F745 Provision of Medically Related Social Services**

The facility must provide medically related social services to attain or maintain the highest practicable physical, mental, and psychosocial well-being of each resident.

This tag outlines the scope of social services to be provided by the facility, as described earlier in this book.

483.45 Pharmacy Services

This section looks at pharmacy services. The only tag that is relevant for activities or social services deals with the use of psychoactive drugs. Citations of this tag may indicate substandard quality of care.

***Tag F758 Free from Unnecessary Psychotropic Meds/PRN Use**

A psychotropic drug is any drug that affects brain activities associated with mental processes and behavior. These drugs include, but are not limited to, drugs in the following categories: anti-psychotic, anti-depressant, anti-anxiety, and hypnotic.

The intent of this requirement is that:

- *each resident's entire drug/medication regimen is managed and monitored to promote or maintain the resident's highest practicable mental, physical, and psychosocial well-being;*
- *the facility implements gradual dose reductions (GDR) and non-pharmacological interventions, unless contraindicated, prior to initiating or instead of continuing psychotropic medication; and*
- *PRN orders for psychotropic medications are only used when the medication is necessary and PRN use is limited.*

Appropriate activities are one of the ways the facility may reduce the need for psychoactive medications.

483.50 Laboratory, Radiology, and Other Diagnostic Services

Tags F770-F779 refer to Laboratory, Radiology, and Other Diagnostic Services

483.55 Dental Services

Tags F790-F791 refer to dental services.

483.60 Food and Nutrition

The facility must provide each resident with a nourishing, palatable, well-balanced diet that meets his or her daily nutritional and special dietary needs, taking into consideration the preferences of each resident.

One tag mentions activities.

Tag F811 Feeding Assistant — Training/Supervision/Resident

Paid feeding assistants may assist eligible residents to eat and drink at meal times, snack times, or during activities or social events as needed, whenever the facility can provide the necessary supervision.

The feeding assistants are supervised by an RN or LPN. Activity professionals can act as feeding assistants only after they have completed a state-approved training course for paid feeding assistants

483.65 Specialized Rehabilitative Services

Recreational therapy services are evaluated using these tags/

Tag F825 Provide/Obtain Specialized Rehab Services

If specialized rehabilitative services such as but not limited to physical therapy, speech-language pathology, occupational therapy, respiratory therapy, and rehabilitative services for mental illness and intellectual disability or services of a lesser intensity as set forth as 483.120, are required in the resident's comprehensive plan of care, the facility must provide the required services or obtain the required services from an outside resource that is a provider of specialized rehabilitative services.

Tag F826 Rehab Services — Physician Order/Qualified Person

Specialized rehabilitative services must be provided under the written order of a physician by qualified personnel.

483.70 Administration

Tags F835-F851 discuss administration. One tag is relevant for social services. Another tag is relevant for all staff.

Tag F842 Resident Records — Identifiable Information

The medical record shall reflect a resident's progress toward achieving their person-centered plan of care objectives and goals and the improvement and maintenance of their clinical, functional, mental, and psychosocial status. Staff must document a resident's medical and non-medical status when any positive or negative condition change occurs, at a periodic reassessment, and during the annual comprehensive assessment. The medical record must also reflect the resident's condition and the care and services provided across all disciplines to ensure information is available to facilitate communication among the interdisciplinary team.

The medical record must contain an accurate representation of the actual experiences of the resident and include enough information to provide a picture of the resident's progress, including his/her response to treatments and/or services, and changes in his/her condition, plan of care goals, objectives, and/or interventions.

Except for the annual comprehensive assessment, periodic reassessments when a significant change in status occurs, and quarterly monitoring assessments, regulations do not define the documentation frequency of a resident's progress. Professional standards of practice however suggests documentation include a resident's care plan implementation progress.

All health care providers are required to keep resident records confidential.

How often should the professional write in the progress notes? The questions surveyors are instructed to ask themselves include: Is there enough recorded documentation for staff to conduct a care program and to revise the program as necessary to respond to the changing status of the resident as a result of interventions? How is the clinical record used in managing the resident's progress in maintaining or improving functional abilities and psychosocial status?

*Tag F850 Qualifications of Social Worker

Any facility with more than 120 beds must employ a qualified social worker on a full-time basis. A qualified social worker is an individual with a minimum of a bachelor's degree in social work or a bachelor's degree in a human service field including, but not limited to, sociology, gerontology, special education, rehabilitation counseling, and psychology and one year of supervised social work experience in a health care setting working directly with individuals.

483.75 Quality Assurance and Performance Improvement

The facility must have a functioning quality assurance committee, which meets at least quarterly and develops and implements appropriate plans of action to correct quality deficiencies.

Tags F865-F868 describe the requirements for the quality assurance and performance improvement program. These requirements were discussed in Chapter 17.

483.80 Infection Control

Tags F880-F883 describe infection control issues. These requirements were discussed in Chapter 17.

483.85 Compliance and Ethics Program

Tag F895 describes the compliance and ethics program which becomes part of the survey process in 2018.

483.90 Physical Environment

Tags F906-F926 describe the requirements for the physical environment of the facility.

Tag F907 Space and Equipment

Provide sufficient space and equipment in dining, health services, recreation, and program areas to enable staff to provide residents with needed services as required by these standards and as identified in each resident's assessment and plan of care

See Tag F920

Tag F920 Requirements for Dining and Activity Rooms

The facility must provide one or more rooms designated for resident dining and activities. These rooms must be well lighted, well ventilated, adequately furnished and have sufficient space to accommodate all activities.

Carole B. Lewis in her book *Improving Mobility in Older Persons* (Aspen Publications, 1989) states: "The lens of the eye becomes thicker with age and the person needs more light to see correctly. Treatment suggestion: use a lot of light (200 watts) especially in functional areas (e.g., reading spots, kitchens, and bathrooms.)" (p. 95). The facility must have adequate ventilation and, if a room is a non-smoking area, the signage indicating such must meet state requirements. The facility's rooms must be adequately furnished. Furnishings are structurally sound and functional (e.g., chairs of varying sizes to meet varying needs of residents, wheelchairs can fit under the dining room table). The activity room must have sufficient space to accommodate all activities. Space should be adaptable to a variety of uses and resident needs. Residents and staff have maximum flexibility in arranging furniture to accommodate residents who use walkers, wheelchairs, and other mobility aids. No crowding evident. Space does not limit resident access.

483.95 Training Requirements

Tags F940-F949 describe training requirements. Three training requirements are part of Phase 2 implementation. Seven more requirements are part of Phase 3.

Surveys

Each of the settings providing treatment services and health care to elderly, psychiatric, and MR/DD clients are governed by federal and state regulations.

CMS (Centers for Medicare and Medicaid Services) is responsible for issuing the Federal Register (federal regulations). Each state then reviews these federal guidelines and interprets them for state regulations, which will be in compliance with the federal government standards. In some cases the state may add regulations. It may not remove regulations.

In order to be a participant in the Medicare/Medicaid program, long-term care facilities and other agencies are reviewed and certified. Also, to receive a license by the state to operate as a business, the facilities need to be reviewed and re-licensed annually.

Every aspect of the facility is reviewed for compliance with both federal and state regulations. Because activities are required and extremely important to the well-being of the resident, they are reviewed yearly in this process. The department head needs to be very clear on what the requirements are for the department. Documentation needs to be presented to the surveyors upon request. You will also have the opportunity to share with them the special programs that you have implemented. The table above outlines some important considerations that will help you do well in the survey process.

Compliance with Regulations

Compliance with health care regulations is required. The goal of the federal government is for every health care facility to be in **substantial compliance** with all regulations. Substantial compliance means that the facility is providing a reasonable quality of care to its residents. There can be no deficiencies (services or equipment that do not meet standards) that cause actual harm to any resident and no more than the potential for minimal harm.

Prior to the implementation of the OBRA Final Rule in July 1995, there were instances of facilities not caring if one or two tags were out. For repeated minor deficiencies, there were no

Things to Remember about Survey

1. Know your regulations.
2. Be friendly and welcome conversation about what you do. Surveyors play an important role in assuring quality of care and quality of life.
3. Have records of participation, calendars from the past three months, bedside logs, resident council information (member list and minutes of meetings), and PR available for review. Present a packet of information (approved by your administrator) to the surveyors when they first get to the facility.
4. Have your office and supplies neatly organized and labeled.
5. Be responsible for your department but do not involve yourself in issues related to other departments. They are better trained to do these themselves, just as you are for the service your department provides.
6. Discussion and clarity are important in communicating what and why you do something. If your treatments follow from your assessments and you have made sure that the treatments are carried out according to the resident care plans, there should be no problem during survey.
7. Be yourself.

penalties. The facilities knew that they could implement a plan of correction and stay in business. If they were out of compliance again by the next survey, there was still no penalty.

The OBRA Final Rule changed that. Now there are required penalties for every facility that is out of substantial compliance. The intent of the new process is to have facilities stay in compliance year round and not experience the previous "yo-yo" compliance at survey time.

When deciding on the penalties, the surveyors look at the severity and scope for deficiencies found in **Quality of Care**, **Quality of Life**, or **Resident Behavior and Facility Practices**. Severity measures the level of harm being caused by the deficiency as shown in Table 2. Scope refers to the number of residents who are affected by the deficiency. See Table 3.

The surveyors look at the cause of the deficiency as well as the number of deficiencies to determine the scope. If the deficiencies are because the facility does not have a policy or system, the deficiency will probably be widespread. If the deficiency results from inadequate implementation, there will probably be a pattern of deficiency. If only one or a very limited number of residents are affected, the scope is isolated.

If the deficiencies are serious enough or widespread enough, the surveyors will find that the facility is providing a Substandard Quality of Care. This is an official term that means a certain level of deficiency is found during survey. Any Immediate Jeopardy is Substandard Quality of Care. Any pattern of Actual Harm or widespread Actual Harm (Level 3) or Potential for More Than Minimal Harm (Level 2) that is widespread is also considered Substandard Quality of Care. In Table 4 the white areas are areas of Substantial Compliance, the light gray areas are out of Substantial Compliance, but not considered Substandard Care. The dark gray areas are Substandard Care. The boldface letters in the bottom of each box are used by CMS to label the boxes in the chart. Refer to them if you are given a letter to describe the results of a survey. The chart also shows the level of penalty required for facilities that are out of substantial compliance.

The penalties in the chart above increase depending on the category of penalties.

Table 2: Level of harm

Level 1: No actual harm with potential for minimal harm	Nothing has happened to a resident and the worst that can happen is a minor negative impact.
Level 2: No actual harm with potential for more than minimal harm that is not immediate jeopardy.	The resident has been impacted in a minor negative way and/or there is a potential for significant harm that has not actually happened yet.
Level 3: Actual harm that is not immediate jeopardy	The resident has been significantly harmed by some practice at the facility and has been prevented from reaching his/her highest practicable level of well-being.
Level 4: Immediate jeopardy	Immediate jeopardy is a situation where immediate corrective action is necessary because what the facility is doing either has caused or may cause serious injury, serious harm, or death to a resident in the facility.

Table 3: Scope of deficiencies

Isolated	One or a very limited number of residents, staff, or locations are involved.
Pattern	More than a limited number of residents, staff, or locations are involved or the same resident has been affected by the deficiency on repeated occasions.
Widespread	The problems causing the deficiency exist throughout the facility and large portions of the residents have been affected or might be affected.

Table 4: Penalties for deficiencies

		SCOPE		
		Isolated	**Pattern**	**Widespread**
SEVERITY	**Level 4.** Immediate jeopardy to resident health/safety	Plan of Correction Required: Cat. 3 Optional: Cat. 2 Optional: Cat. 1 **J**	Plan of Correction Required: Cat 3 Optional: Cat 2 Optional: Cat 1 **K**	Plan of Correction Required: Cat 3 Optional: Cat 2 Optional: Cat 1 **L**
	Level 3. Actual harm that is not Immediate Jeopardy	Plan of Correction Required*: Cat. 2 Optional: Cat. 1 **G**	Plan of Correction Required*: Cat. 2 Optional: Cat. 1 **H**	Plan of Correction Required*: Cat 2 Optional: Temporary Management. Optional: Cat. 1 **I**
	Level 2. No actual harm with potential for more than minimal harm that is not immediate jeopardy	Plan of Correction Required*: Cat. 1 Optional: Cat. 2 **D**	Plan of Correction Required*: Cat. 1 Optional: Cat. 2 **E**	Plan of Correction Required*: Cat. 2 Optional: Cat. 1 **F**
	Level 1. No actual harm with potential for minimal harm	No remedies No Plan of Correction Commitment to correct **A**	Plan of Correction **B**	Plan of Correction **C**

* It is possible to terminate the operation of the facility instead of imposing these penalties. If termination is not chosen, these penalties are required.

Category 1 penalties include:

- Directed plan of correction;
- State monitor and/or
- Directed in-service training

Category 2 penalties include:

- Denial of payment for new admissions;
- Denial of payment for all residents and/or
- Civil penalties of $50 to $3,000 per day

Category 3 penalties include:

- Temporary management
- Termination
- Optional civil monetary penalties of $3,050 to $10,000 per day

There are two more conditions for compliance in addition to these penalties. They state that:

- Denial of payment for new admissions must be imposed when a facility is not in substantial compliance within three months after being found out of compliance.
- Denial of payment and state monitoring must be imposed when a facility has been found to have provided substandard quality of care on three consecutive standard surveys.

The new penalty structure makes it more important than ever for a facility to be in compliance with regulations. One of the best ways for professionals to do their part is to participate in the quality assurance process at their facility and to regularly check the compliance of their department using the Survey Checklist forms at the end of this section.

Professionals will be asked to give input to the plan of corrections. This is the plan that the facility creates to "fix" the identified problem. It is a response to the CMS form known as the *Statement of Deficiencies* or #2567 form.

The plan of corrections must include the following areas of information:

- How the corrective action will be accomplished for residents found to have been affected by the deficient practice.
- How the facility will identify other residents having the potential to be affected by the same deficient practice.
- What measures will be put into place or systemic changes made to ensure that the deficient practice will not recur.
- How the facility will monitor its corrective actions to ensure that the deficient practice is being corrected and will not recur. (This will be the Quality Assurance and Performance Improvement program that the facility is mandated to have in place.)

Surveyor Protocols

This section describes the survey process and what the surveyors are looking for under the new regulations. Surveys consist of observation, interviews, and record reviews.

During the observation phase surveyors observe staff over all shifts to determine if the activity portions of the comprehensive care plan are being implemented. Questions they ask include: is the resident transported, notified of activities of preference, and helped with in-room supplies?

The interview phase includes discussions with residents and families. The surveyors will also interview the activity staff, social services, CNAs, and charge nurses. The surveyors are looking for understanding of person-centered programs from all members of the staff and whether the staff knows the appropriate information about each resident to run programs that are in compliance with regulations.

The record review covers:

- Assessments, including having knowledge of longstanding interests, customary routine, and personal preferences
- Care plan records, which should show that: the resident has participated in activities, life roles are considered, adaptations have been made, new hobbies or skills have been developed, existing interests have been encouraged, and community events are available for interested residents. All disciplines that are responsible for the activities should have their roles clearly identified.
- Care plan revision, where the surveyors ask if changes are made when goals are not met and when the resident refuses to participate. They also check to see if new activities are added, as appropriate.

The facility will most likely be in compliance with the activity portion of the survey if they:

- Recognized and assessed preferences, choices, and specific conditions
- Implemented activities in accordance with the care plan
- Monitored and evaluated responses
- Revised approaches as appropriate
- Documented that all of these steps were taken

Deficiencies are most likely to have psychosocial outcomes and surveyors are instructed to use the Psychosocial Outcome Severity Guide to determine level of severity. This can be found in the State Operators Manual. Ask your administrator for a copy to review.

CMS Quality Indicator Survey

The Quality Indicator Survey (QIS) is a new computer-assisted, long-term care survey process used by selected State Survey Agencies and CMS to determine if Medicare and Medicaid certified nursing homes meet federal requirements. It is important to note that federal regulations and interpretive guidelines have not changed — only the survey process itself.

This new survey was designed to improve consistency and accuracy of quality of care and quality of life problems. The surveyors will review all triggered regulatory areas and, with the help of the computerized program, be able to more clearly and accurately focus on those facilities with the largest numbers of quality concerns.

CMS selected a company to conduct the initial QIS training and the subsequent training of a state's designated QIS trainers. Surveyors who successfully complete all QIS training components will be entered in the CMS Learning Management System as a Registered QIS Surveyor.

The QIS Survey is a two-stage process:

1. Surveyors look at regulatory areas
2. Surveyors objectively investigate any regulatory areas that are triggered.

Table 5 shows the QIS Process as it goes from the off-site survey preparation to conducting the exit conference. It is important for all staff to understand the process from beginning to end so that they are comfortable with the design of this new survey process.

Table 6 shows the differences between the traditional survey and the QIS survey. This will be helpful to review before your community's survey window.

Table 5: Overview of the QIS Process

	Offsite Survey Preparation	
	Onsite Survey Preparation	
Entrance Conference	Reconcile Stage I Sample	Facility Tour
	Initial Team Meeting	
	Stage I Preliminary Investigation	
Census and Admission Sample Reviews	Mandatory Facility-Level Tasks (non-staged)	Stage I Team Meeting
	Transition from Stage I to Stage II Draw Stage II Sample	
	Stage II Investigation	
Care Area Investigations	Triggered Facility-Level Tasks Continue Mandatory Facility-Level Tasks	Stage II Team Meeting
	Stage II Analysis and Decision Making: Integration of Information Decisions to Cite or Not to Cite	
	Conduct the Exit Conference	

Table 6: Differences between the Traditional Survey and the QIS

Traditional Survey	QIS
Automation	
• Survey team collects data and records findings on paper. • The computer is only used to prepare the deficiencies recorded on the CMS-2567.	• Each survey team member uses a tablet PC throughout the survey process to record findings that are synthesized and organized by the QIS software.
Offsite	
• Review OSCAR 3 and 4 report. • Survey team uses QM/QI's report offsite to identify preliminary sample of residents (about 20% of facility census) and areas of concern.	• Review the OSCAR 3 Report and current complaints. • Download the MDS data to tablet PC. • DCT selects a random sample of residents for Stage I.
Entrance Information	
• Review of Roster Sample Matrix Form (CMS 802).	• Obtain alphabetical resident census with room numbers and units. • List of new admissions over last 30 days.
Tour	
• Gather information about pre-selected residents and new concerns. • Determine whether pre-selected residents are still appropriate.	• No sample selection. • Initial overview of facility.
Sample Selection	

• Sample size determined by facility census.
• Residents selected based on QM/QI percentiles and issues identified offsite and on tour.
	• The DCT provides a random selected sample of residents for the following:
	  ◦ Admission sample is a review of 30 current or discharged resident records.
	  ◦ Census sample includes 40 current residents for observation, interview, and record review.

Survey Structure	

• Resident sample is about 20% of facility census for resident observations, interviews, and record reviews
  ◦ Phase I: Focused and comprehensive reviews based on QM/QI report and issues identified from offsite information and facility tour.
  ◦ Phase II: Focused record reviews.
  ◦ Facility and environmental tasks completed during the survey.
	• Stage I: Preliminary investigation of regulatory areas in the admission and census samples and mandatory facility-level tasks started.
	• Stage II: Completion of in-depth investigation of triggered care areas and/or facility-level tasks based on Stage I findings.

Group Interview	
• Meet with Resident Group/Council. • Includes Resident Council minutes review to identify concerns.	• Interview with Resident Council President or Representative.

The survey process is tailored to the newest changes and implementation of phases 1-3 and is a combination of the traditional and the QIS survey process. Be sure to acquaint yourself with both of these in order to feel comfortable during the survey process.

Critical Element Pathways

The survey process, which combines elements of the traditional survey and the QIS survey, includes a long list of Critical Element Pathways to help surveyors. Pathways include:

- SNF Beneficiary Protection Notification Review
- Dining Observation
- Infection Prevention, Control & Immunizations
- Kitchen Observation
- Medication Administration Observation
- Resident Council Interview
- Quality Assessment and Assurance (QAA) and Quality Assurance and Performance Improvement (QAPI) Plan Review
- Abuse Critical Element Pathway
- Environmental Observations
- Sufficient and Competent Nurse Staffing Review
- Personal Funds Review
- Activities Critical Element Pathway
- Activities of Daily Living (ADL) Critical Element Pathway
- Behavioral and Emotional Status Critical Element Pathway
- Urinary Catheter or Urinary Tract Infection Critical Element Pathway
- Communication and Sensory Problems (Includes Hearing and Vision) Critical Element Pathway
- Dental Status and Services Critical Element Pathway
- Dialysis Critical Element Pathway
- General Critical Element Pathway
- Hospice and End of Life Care and Services Critical Element Pathway
- Death Critical Element Pathway
- Nutrition Critical Element Pathway
- Pain Recognition and Management Critical Element Pathway
- Physical Restraints Critical Element Pathway
- Pressure Ulcer/Injury Critical Element Pathway
- Specialized Rehabilitative or Restorative Services Critical Element Pathway
- Respiratory Care Critical Element Pathway
- Unnecessary Medications, Psychotropic Medications, and Medication Regimen Review Critical Element Pathway
- Medication Storage and Labeling
- Preadmission Screening and Resident Review Critical Element Pathway
- Extended Survey
- Hydration Critical Element Pathway
- Tube Feeding Status Critical Element Pathway
- Positioning, Mobility & Range of Motion (ROM) Critical Element Pathway
- Hospitalization Critical Element Pathway
- Bladder or Bowel Incontinence Critical Element Pathway
- Accidents Critical Element Pathway
- Neglect Critical Element Pathway
- Resident Assessment Critical Element Pathway
- Discharge Critical Element Pathway
- Dementia Care Critical Element Pathway

You can download these at www.cmscompliancegroup.com/2017/08/29/ltc-survey-pathways-entrance-form/. You can review the Resident Council Interview Pathway form on page 313

CMS Focused Surveys

In addition to the normal survey process, there are also CMS Focused Surveys. These surveys are specialized surveys with a focus on MDS and Staffing, Dementia, Medication Related Events, and Infection Control.

MDS 2014 was the first focused MDS survey. It started with 25 facilities and will be expanded.

Dementia 2014 was also the first focused survey on dementia. It was piloted in five states and expanded in 2015. It included more focus on non-pharmacological interventions for residents living with dementia.

Medication-Related Events was implemented in 2014.

Infection Control is a three-year pilot project. During this time all surveys will be educational only (no citations). More surveys will be completed in 2017.

Survey Groups

There are several different survey groups that may be responsible for looking at your facility. The major ones are in the following list:

CMS

Centers for Medicare and Medicaid Services: Responsible for ensuring that minimum federal standards are met. Required of all long-term care facilities. Usually sub-contract with state to do their surveys.

State Department of Health, Licensing, and Certification Division

State surveys are required at least every twelve months unless the state requests an extension. The surveyors may also survey specific state regulations concerning long-term care services.

JCAHO

Joint Commission on Accreditation of Healthcare Organizations: This is a private credentialing body that conducts voluntary surveys. Standards are usually more stringent with a different focus than state and federal regulations. The intent of this survey process is to acknowledge a higher level of standards above federal, state, and corporate standards. There is a charge to the facility for this survey process. More and more nursing facilities are requesting this accreditation because the services being provided in many facilities are more specialized and resident based.

CARF: The Rehabilitation Accreditation Commission

CARF: The Rehabilitation Accreditation Commission: This is a private credentialing body that conducts voluntary surveys. CARF Standards apply to rehab services. There is a charge for this survey.

Peer Review

The peer review survey process is a voluntary process requested by the facility. The team may be comprised of management staff from the corporation that owns the facility, a peer review team of a sister facility, or a survey team comprised of staff members from a professional long-term care organization or community group. There are usually no fees associated with this process, as it is an assurance review process in preparation for any of the above reviews.

Federal Regulations

The federal regulations are standard to all states. In 1987 the Omnibus Budget Reconciliation Act (discussed earlier in the chapter) was enacted. All nursing facilities or "long-term care facilities" participating in Medicare and Medicaid are subject to the Act. The regulations serve as the basis for survey activities for the purpose of determining whether a facility meets the requirements for participation in Medicare and Medicaid.

State Regulations

Each state also has regulations for licensing and certification of long-term care facilities. These regulations may be stricter than the federal regulations but not more lenient. They will be used in addition to the federal regulations for survey purposes. It is not possible in the scope of this book to review each state's requirements. A copy of the state regulations should be available in the facility. If not, a copy can be reviewed at the county law library.

Corporate or Facility Policy

Many corporations standardize policies and procedures in all of their facilities across the United States. Others allow facilities to adopt their own policies and procedures. Independently owned facilities adopt standardized procedures or create their own. Again, these policies and procedures can be stricter than federal and state law but may not be more lenient. A copy should be available in the facility and in the activity department.

If a policy is no longer applicable or needs to be revised, this should be brought to the attention of the administrator. Facility polices and procedures must be followed, just as state and federal laws must be followed. It is in the best interest of the professional to follow all laws, regulations, and policies. They serve as a protection and provide a rationale for any action that may be taken in the care and treatment of the people we serve.

Survey Checklists

You should use the survey checklists on the following pages to see if your program will pass survey.

OBRA '87
Quality of Life Review Form

Facility:________________________________ Date:____________

F675 A–Quality of Life
"A facility must care for its residents in a manner and in an environment that promotes maintenance or enhancement of each resident's quality of life."

Requirement	Interpretation	+ = Met - = Not Met
F557 Dignity	Focus on a resident as an individual Respect for space and property Treating residents respectfully as adults Promoting independence and dignity in dining	

Self-Determination and Participation. The resident has the right to —		
F679 Choose activities, schedules, and health care consistent with his or her interests, assessment, and plans of care	Accommodating individual schedules and needs according to resident's requests and previous lifestyle and interests	
F586 Interact with members of the community both inside and outside the facility	Facilitating involvement in community groups and matters that were important to resident before admission	
F555 Make choices about aspects of his or her life in the facility *that are significant to the resident*	Providing smoking areas for residents who smoke Working around the resident's schedule (including television programs)	

F565 Participation in resident and family groups in the facility	Provide a private space for family and resident groups upon request	
F585 Facility must provide a designated staff person responsible for providing assistance and responding to written requests that result from group meetings	This staff person listens, records, and assists administration with following through with grievances and recommendations	
F558 Accommodation of Needs (1) adaptations of the facility's physical environment and staff behaviors to assist residents in maintaining independent functioning, dignity, well-being, and self-determination.	Accommodation of Needs pertains to how well the team is enhancing and maintaining independence vs. dependence on staff and environment including: telephone access, personal property, married couples, activities, social services, psychosocial functioning, homelike environment, activities of daily living, and accidents and prevention-assistive devices	
F559...Receive notice before the resident's room or roommate in the facility changes	Resident must have a say in who his/her roommate is and the timing of any change	

OBRA '87
Environment Review Form

Facility: ____________________________ Date: _____________

F584 — Environment
"The facility must provide a safe, clean, comfortable, and homelike environment, allowing the resident to use his or her personal belongings to the extent possible."

Be sure to review the *Environmental Assessment Form* to begin problem solving.

Requirements	Interpretation	+ = Met - = Not Met
De-emphasize institutional character	Encourage personal belongings.	
Cleanliness	How clean is the facility? Are there odors detected in any of the rooms and halls?	
Individuality	Do you get to know who this person is and what his/her past interests were by observing his/her room and personal things and style?	
Clutter	Are day rooms and private rooms cluttered? Is there space for wheelchair and equipment accessibility?	
Housekeeping and Maintenance Services	Assuring cleanliness and an infection-free environment for resident's equipment and supplies: toothbrush, dentures, denture cups, bedpans, urinals, feeding tubes, leg bags, catheter bags, pads, and positioning devices.	
Clean bed and bath linens that are in good condition	Are there adequate linens available? Are they in good condition and without stains?	
Private closet space in each room	Closets must be provided with ample space and accessible shelves for resident use.	
Adequate lighting	Lighting suitable to tasks that residents choose to perform or facility staff must perform. Minimal glare and comfortable to the visually impaired. Is lighting accessible to the resident?	
Comfortable and safe temperature levels	Ambient temperature levels to decrease likelihood of temperature changes that could affect well-being of residents. Are there any rooms that are noticeably too cold or too warm?	
Comfortable sound levels	Is conversation easy or do you have to raise your voice to be heard? Are there many distractions during group events? Are TVs and radios on too loud and too early or late at night?	

OBRA '87
Activities Potential Review Form

F679 Activities
"To create opportunities for each resident to have a meaningful life by supporting his/her domains of wellness (security, autonomy, growth, connectedness, identity, joy, and meaning)."

+ = Met
- = Not Met

Requirements	Interpretation	
All activities which are not Activities of Daily Living	These would be activity/leisure involvement that a resident pursues for a sense of well-being.	
Self-esteem	Focus on the individual. Meaningful activities that highlight the abilities and uniqueness of each resident.	
Health education	Nutrition related activities, wellness, leisure education, relaxation, understanding medical conditions and treatment plans.	
Pleasurable experiences	These can be social activities that encourage passive or active participation. What brings the pleasure is feeling safe, familiar surroundings, rekindling past interests.	
Opportunities for creative expression	Art, creative writing, oral histories, poetry, music, drama, gardening, cooking.	
Opportunities for achieving success	Can be incorporated in all activities at any level. Activities must be adapted and segmented into tasks for success at each level.	
Opportunities for achieving financial independence	Money management. Involvement in previous interests such as the stock market, investments, and banking.	
Opportunities for achieving emotional independence	Problem solving activities and situations. Creative and expressive outlets. Activities that promote self-respect and individuality. Life review. Activities that assist others so that the resident has the chance to continue giving to others.	

Medications in the Elderly

In the United States, the use of medications by the elderly is far too common. They consume over 30% of all prescription drugs and 40% of all non-prescription drugs. Those who are living in long-term care facilities average more than six drugs per resident. All medications cause a change in the body. Because of the normal changes in how the body functions as one ages, the additional changes caused by medications may have a significant effect on the person's overall well-being. The chart below outlines some of the typical changes related to age that help increase the impact of medications.

Adverse Drug Reactions

All drugs have the potential to cause a side effect or adverse reaction. The elderly are more likely to experience an adverse effect and are more likely to be hospitalized as a result.

Adverse drug reactions fall into three categories:

- They are a result of an allergic reaction to the medication.
- They are a result of a non-allergic reaction to a medication.
- They are considered to be an unusual or idiosyncratic reaction to a medication.

There are six general risk factors considered to increase the risk of an adverse drug reaction. Generally, individuals who are elderly have many of these risk factors, which increase the likelihood of experiencing a side effect to a medication. The risk factors are

Common Body Changes Associated with Aging

Cardiovascular Function: Congestive Heart Failure	• Decreased organ perfusion: as the heart weakens, it is less able to supply blood to the various vital organs. • Decreased metabolism: decreased blood flow to the liver or to the kidneys may result in decreased drug metabolism and excretion and, in turn, greater drug activity.
Central Nervous System: Degenerative Changes	• Over time, the central nervous system (CNS) may exhibit degeneration and also the tissues in the CNS often have an enhanced response to medications.
Kidney and Liver Function	• Decreased functional ability: may be a result of decreases in blood perfusion or a long-term disease process such as diabetes mellitus or high blood pressure. • Decreases in metabolism and excretion.
Body Composition Changes	• Decreased lean body mass: decreases in muscle mass and protein stores may influence the response to a medication. • Contributes to changes in drug activity.
Sensitivity to Drugs	• The tissues in the body and various receptor sites where medications exert their pharmaceutical activity may show increased sensitivity resulting in a greater response to a particular drug. This may result in an increased number of side effects.

- Age
- Number of drugs
- Duration of treatment
- Gender (female)
- Dosage
- Underlying condition

Medications are frequently grouped together by types because they are prescribed for similar disorders, they change the body in similar ways, and they frequently share common side effects. The chart on the next page shows some of the medication types that are most frequently prescribed for those who are older and common side effects.

Psychoactive or psychotropic medications are prescribed in order to modify behaviors, mood, or thought patterns. There are four types of psychoactive/psychotropic medications: anti-psychotics, anti-depressants, anti-anxiety, and sedatives. Because these medications alter mood and behavior, they need to be closely monitored for potential side effects. They are also considered chemical restraints in the OBRA '87 regulations and are to be used in the least restrictive way and only after all other interventions are unsuccessful. Activities are considered to be non-pharmacological interventions for disturbing behaviors, so they must be tried before medications are prescribed.

Psychoactive/psychotropic medications can have significant side effects. One of these is postural hypotension. This is a decrease in blood pressure upon standing or changing position, which causes lightheadedness and dizziness, placing a resident at higher risk for falls. Another side effect is tardive dyskinesia. This is a movement disorder caused by damage to the central nervous system. Some characteristics may be lip-smacking, spasms, chewing motions of mouth, and body swaying. Due to the potential for side effects, psychoactive or psychotropic medications need to be part of the care plan, so all staff are aware of these issue. Yet another significant side effect is metabolic problems: weight gain, elevated cholesterol, and elevated blood sugar.

An excellent resource that is always up to date for psychotropic medication is the chart *Quick Reference to Psychotropic Medication* by John Preston, Psy.D. This reference sheet can be downloaded for free at www.PsyD-fx.com.

Frequently Prescribed Medications and Their Side Effects		
Type	**Medication examples**	**Potential Side Effects**
Cardiovascular Medications	Digoxin Verapamil	Dizziness, weakness, syncope due to low blood pressure. Abnormal heart rhythm Confusion, depression
Diuretics	Lasix Hydrochlorothiazide	Dehydration Headache Weakness, fatigue Nausea, vomiting
Potassium Products		Stomach distress
Pain Medications	Tylenol with Codeine Vicodin Oxycontin	Stomach: bleeding, nausea, pain Dizziness, drowsiness, confusion, depression Narcotics: physical and psychological dependence
Antidiabetic Agents	Insulin Micronase	Low blood sugar (Hypoglycemia) Chills Nausea Nervousness Confusion Hunger Rapid, shallow breathing Fast heartbeat Fatigue
Stomach-Intestinal Medications	Tagamet Reglan Lomotil	Diarrhea Confusion Dizziness Depression
Psychoactive Medications: Antipsychotic Medications	Haldol Mellaril Thorazine Navane Risperdal Zyprexa	Drowsiness Low blood pressure Tremors, shaking Inability to sit still (akathesia) Tardive dyskinesia — irreversible abnormal movements of the mouth and tongue
Psychoactive Medications: Antidepressants	Elavil Desyrel Imipramine	Low blood pressure Fast heart rate Dry mouth, blurred vision, constipation Lethargy
Psychoactive Medications: Antidepressants	Prozac Paxil Zoloft	Insomnia Anxiety, nervousness Tremors
Psychoactive Medications: Anti-Anxiety and Sleeping Medications	Valium, BuSpar Ativan, Librium Xanax Klonopin Restoril Dalmane	Lethargy, tiredness Clumsiness, drunken walk Confusion Depression

19. Summary

The responsibilities and challenges of activity, recreational therapy, and social services professionals keep growing in direct proportion to the increased needs of the people we serve.

Increased emphasis has been placed on quality of care — regardless of where it is received. The type of staff performance once expected only in hospitals has now worked its way into standards of nursing homes, assisted living, and adult day centers. Federal regulations and voluntary accreditation standards have changed the face of long-term care forever. These changes have added to the work responsibilities for all staff members. The beauty of the change is that the focus is on the individual and how we, as a team, can assist each one in meeting goals and projecting outcomes. The medical model focused on the diagnosis and now our functional/holistic model focuses on how a person heals, what gives him/her the resilience to meet new challenges, how the environment either enhances or negatively impacts his/her ability to improve and have a high quality of life.

As you have seen in the flow of information in this book, the authors have attempted to bring you full circle with why the services are important, who the people we serve might be, what the environment offers, and how we, as staff, make a profound difference in individual lives — regardless of cognitive and functional abilities and/or limitations.

The impact of quality programming and teamwork are inspirational and do make a difference in both our lives and the lives of the individuals who find themselves in need of our services.

Many things change but, as Socrates observed far back in history, much remains the same:

> I consider the old who have gone before us along a road which we must all travel in our turn and it is good we should ask them of the nature of that road.

The work that you put your spirit and soul into will not only make an impact on the people we serve living today in long-term care settings, but create increasingly higher standards for the generations in the future.

A. Abbreviations

$\bar{c}$	with
$\bar{s}$	without
AC	Activity Coordinator
ADL	activities of daily living
AKA	above the knee amputation; also known as
AM	morning
amt	amount
ASHD	arteriosclerotic heart disease
B&C	board and care
bid	2x daily
bp	blood pressure
CAA	Care Area Assessment
CAT	Care Area Trigger
c/o	complain of
CHF	congestive heart failure
COPD	chronic obstructive pulmonary disease
CPR	cardiopulmonary resuscitation
CTRS	Certified Therapeutic Recreation Specialist
CVA	cerebral vascular accident
d/c	discontinue
DD	developmentally disabled
DME	durable medical equipment
DON	Director of Nursing
dx	diagnosis
ETOH	alcohol
fx	fracture
GI	gastrointestinal
gm	gram
H&P	history and physical
HBV	Hepatitis B Virus
HIPAA	Health Information Portability and Accountability Act
HIV	Human Immunodeficiency Virus
HOH	hard of hearing
I	independent
IDT	interdisciplinary team
IM	intramuscular
IV	intravenous
L	left
lb	pound
LE	lower extremity
MDS	Minimum Data Set
mg	milligram
MI	mentally ill; myocardial infarction
MS	multiple sclerosis
noc	night
NPO	nothing by mouth
∅	no/none
OBRA	Omnibus Budget Reconciliation Act
OOB	out of bed
OT	Occupational Therapy
PHI	personal health information
PM	afternoon, evening
PO	by mouth
PoC	Plan of Correction
PPS	Prospective Payment System
prn	as necessary
Pt	patient
PT	Physical Therapy
q	every
qd	every day
qh	every hour
R	right
r/t	related to
RA	rheumatoid arthritis; restorative aide
RAI	Resident Assessment Instrument
RAP	Resident Assessment Protocol
rehab	rehabilitation
res.	resident
ROM	range of motion
RT	Respiratory Therapist; Recreational Therapist
RUG	Resident Utilization Group
Rx	prescription
/s	without

s/p status post (after)
SNF skilled nursing facility
SOB shortness of breath
SP/ST Speech Pathologist, Therapist
SSC/SSD Social Services Coordinator/Director
stat immediately
T-22 Title 22 (California)
THR total hip replacement
TIA transient ischemic attack
tid 3x daily
tx treatment; therapy
UE upper extremity
URI upper respiratory infection
UTI urinary tract infection
w/c wheel chair
WFL within functional limits
wk week
WNL within normal limits
wt weight
X times

B. Minimum Data Set and the Resident Assessment System

Facilities in the United States that receive Medicare funds are required to use a specific, standardized assessment on every resident admitted to the facility. This standardized assessment, called the Minimum Data Set (MDS), is an interdisciplinary assessment. Each member of the interdisciplinary team is required to conduct his/her own assessment of the resident, analyze the resident's status, and then summarize that information on the MDS form within 14 days of the resident's admission to the facility.

The MDS provides health care workers in long-term care settings with two advantages: 1. it standardizes medical vocabulary across the nation and 2. it provides the mechanism for the collection of information: demographic information, mortality and morbidity statistics, and treatment outcomes. The MDS has been used long enough for us to be able to recognize when a "score" on the MDS indicates health or when it indicates the need to provide some kind of treatment. A book that is used with the MDS, called *Resident Assessment System for Long-term Care*, outlines which scores or combination of scores point up the need for specific interventions.

The MDS 3.0 report form is shown in this appendix.

Resident ________ Identifier ________ Date ________

MINIMUM DATA SET (MDS) - Version 3.0
RESIDENT ASSESSMENT AND CARE SCREENING
Nursing Home Comprehensive (NC) Item Set

Section A	**Identification Information**
A0050. Type of Record	
Enter Code ☐	1. **Add new record** → Continue to A0100, Facility Provider Numbers 2. **Modify existing record** → Continue to A0100, Facility Provider Numbers 3. **Inactivate existing record** → Skip to X0150, Type of Provider
A0100. Facility Provider Numbers	
	A. National Provider Identifier (NPI): ☐☐☐☐☐☐☐☐☐☐ **B. CMS Certification Number (CCN):** ☐☐☐☐☐☐☐☐☐☐☐☐ **C. State Provider Number:** ☐☐☐☐☐☐☐☐☐☐☐☐☐☐☐
A0200. Type of Provider	
Enter Code ☐	**Type of provider** 1. **Nursing home (SNF/NF)** 2. **Swing Bed**
A0310. Type of Assessment	
Enter Code ☐☐	**A. Federal OBRA Reason for Assessment** 01. **Admission** assessment (required by day 14) 02. **Quarterly** review assessment 03. **Annual** assessment 04. **Significant change in status** assessment 05. **Significant correction** to **prior comprehensive** assessment 06. **Significant correction** to **prior quarterly** assessment 99. **None of the above**
Enter Code ☐☐	**B. PPS Assessment** **PPS Scheduled Assessments for a Medicare Part A Stay** 01. **5-day** scheduled assessment 02. **14-day** scheduled assessment 03. **30-day** scheduled assessment 04. **60-day** scheduled assessment 05. **90-day** scheduled assessment **PPS Unscheduled Assessments for a Medicare Part A Stay** 07. **Unscheduled assessment used for PPS** (OMRA, significant or clinical change, or significant correction assessment) **Not PPS Assessment** 99. **None of the above**
Enter Code ☐	**C. PPS Other Medicare Required Assessment - OMRA** 0. **No** 1. **Start of therapy** assessment 2. **End of therapy** assessment 3. **Both Start and End of therapy** assessment 4. **Change of therapy** assessment
Enter Code ☐	**D. Is this a Swing Bed clinical change assessment?** Complete only if A0200 = 2 0. **No** 1. **Yes**
Enter Code ☐	**E. Is this assessment the first assessment** (OBRA, Scheduled PPS, or Discharge) **since the most recent admission/entry or reentry?** 0. **No** 1. **Yes**

A0310 continued on next page

Resident ______________________ Identifier ______________________ Date ______________

Section A — Identification Information

A0310. Type of Assessment - Continued

Enter Code [ ][ ]

F. Entry/discharge reporting
01. **Entry** tracking record
10. **Discharge** assessment-**return not anticipated**
11. **Discharge** assessment-**return anticipated**
12. **Death in facility** tracking record
99. **None of the above**

Enter Code [ ]

G. Type of discharge - Complete only if A0310F = 10 or 11
1. **Planned**
2. **Unplanned**

Enter Code [ ]

H. Is this a SNF Part A PPS Discharge Assessment?
0. **No**
1. **Yes**

A0410. Unit Certification or Licensure Designation

Enter Code [ ]

1. **Unit is neither Medicare nor Medicaid certified and MDS data is not required by the State**
2. **Unit is neither Medicare nor Medicaid certified but MDS data is required by the State**
3. **Unit is Medicare and/or Medicaid certified**

A0500. Legal Name of Resident

A. First name: [ ][ ][ ][ ][ ][ ][ ][ ][ ][ ][ ][ ]

B. Middle initial: [ ]

C. Last name: [ ][ ][ ][ ][ ][ ][ ][ ][ ][ ][ ][ ][ ][ ][ ][ ][ ][ ]

D. Suffix: [ ][ ][ ]

A0600. Social Security and Medicare Numbers

A. Social Security Number: [ ][ ][ ] – [ ][ ] – [ ][ ][ ][ ]

B. Medicare number (or comparable railroad insurance number): [ ][ ][ ][ ][ ][ ][ ][ ][ ][ ][ ][ ]

A0700. Medicaid Number - Enter "+" if pending, "N" if not a Medicaid recipient

[ ][ ][ ][ ][ ][ ][ ][ ][ ][ ][ ][ ][ ][ ]

A0800. Gender

Enter Code [ ]

1. **Male**
2. **Female**

A0900. Birth Date

[ ][ ] – [ ][ ] – [ ][ ][ ][ ]
Month Day Year

A1000. Race/Ethnicity

↓ Check all that apply

- [ ] **A. American Indian or Alaska Native**
- [ ] **B. Asian**
- [ ] **C. Black or African American**
- [ ] **D. Hispanic or Latino**
- [ ] **E. Native Hawaiian or Other Pacific Islander**
- [ ] **F. White**

Resident ______________________ Identifier ______________ Date __________

Section A — Identification Information

A1100. Language

Enter Code [ ]

A. Does the resident need or want an interpreter to communicate with a doctor or health care staff?

0. **No** → Skip to A1200, Marital Status
1. **Yes** → Specify in A1100B, Preferred language
9. **Unable to determine** → Skip to A1200, Marital Status

B. Preferred language:

A1200. Marital Status

Enter Code [ ]

1. **Never married**
2. **Married**
3. **Widowed**
4. **Separated**
5. **Divorced**

A1300. Optional Resident Items

A. Medical record number:

B. Room number:

C. Name by which resident prefers to be addressed:

D. Lifetime occupation(s) - put "/" between two occupations:

A1500. Preadmission Screening and Resident Review (PASRR)

Complete only if A0310A = 01, 03, 04, or 05

Enter Code [ ]

Is the resident currently considered by the state level II PASRR process to have serious mental illness and/or intellectual disability ("mental retardation" in federal regulation) or a related condition?

0. **No** → Skip to A1550, Conditions Related to ID/DD Status
1. **Yes** → Continue to A1510, Level II Preadmission Screening and Resident Review (PASRR) Conditions
9. **Not a Medicaid-certified unit** → Skip to A1550, Conditions Related to ID/DD Status

A1510. Level II Preadmission Screening and Resident Review (PASRR) Conditions

Complete only if A0310A = 01, 03, 04, or 05

↓ **Check all that apply**

- [ ] **A. Serious mental illness**
- [ ] **B. Intellectual Disability ("mental retardation" in federal regulation)**
- [ ] **C. Other related conditions**

Resident ____________ Identifier ____________ Date ____________

Section A — Identification Information

A1550. Conditions Related to ID/DD Status
If the resident is 22 years of age or older, complete only if A0310A = 01
If the resident is 21 years of age or younger, complete only if A0310A = 01, 03, 04, or 05

↓ **Check all conditions that are related to ID/DD status** that were manifested before age 22, and are likely to continue indefinitely

	ID/DD With Organic Condition
☐	**A. Down syndrome**
☐	**B. Autism**
☐	**C. Epilepsy**
☐	**D. Other organic condition related to ID/DD**
	ID/DD Without Organic Condition
☐	**E. ID/DD with no organic condition**
	No ID/DD
☐	**Z. None of the above**

Most Recent Admission/Entry or Reentry into this Facility

A1600. Entry Date

☐☐ – ☐☐ – ☐☐☐☐
Month Day Year

A1700. Type of Entry

Enter Code ☐
1. **Admission**
2. **Reentry**

A1800. Entered From

Enter Code ☐☐
01. **Community** (private home/apt., board/care, assisted living, group home)
02. **Another nursing home or swing bed**
03. **Acute hospital**
04. **Psychiatric hospital**
05. **Inpatient rehabilitation facility**
06. **ID/DD facility**
07. **Hospice**
09. **Long Term Care Hospital** (LTCH)
99. **Other**

A1900. Admission Date (Date this episode of care in this facility began)

☐☐ – ☐☐ – ☐☐☐☐
Month Day Year

A2000. Discharge Date
Complete only if A0310F = 10, 11, or 12

☐☐ – ☐☐ – ☐☐☐☐
Month Day Year

Resident ______ Identifier ______ Date ______

Section A — Identification Information

A2100. Discharge Status
Complete only if A0310F = 10, 11, or 12

Enter Code

01. **Community** (private home/apt., board/care, assisted living, group home)
02. **Another nursing home or swing bed**
03. **Acute hospital**
04. **Psychiatric hospital**
05. **Inpatient rehabilitation facility**
06. **ID/DD facility**
07. **Hospice**
08. **Deceased**
09. **Long Term Care Hospital** (LTCH)
99. **Other**

A2200. Previous Assessment Reference Date for Significant Correction
Complete only if A0310A = 05 or 06

Month – Day – Year

A2300. Assessment Reference Date

Observation end date:

Month – Day – Year

A2400. Medicare Stay

Enter Code

A. Has the resident had a Medicare-covered stay since the most recent entry?

0. **No** → Skip to B0100, Comatose
1. **Yes** → Continue to A2400B, Start date of most recent Medicare stay

B. Start date of most recent Medicare stay:

Month – Day – Year

C. End date of most recent Medicare stay - Enter dashes if stay is ongoing:

Month – Day – Year

Resident ______________________ Identifier ______________ Date __________

Look back period for all items is 7 days unless another time frame is indicated

Section B — Hearing, Speech, and Vision

B0100. Comatose

Enter Code	**Persistent vegetative state/no discernible consciousness** 0. **No** → Continue to B0200, Hearing 1. **Yes** → Skip to G0110, Activities of Daily Living (ADL) Assistance

B0200. Hearing

Enter Code	**Ability to hear** (with hearing aid or hearing appliances if normally used) 0. **Adequate** - no difficulty in normal conversation, social interaction, listening to TV 1. **Minimal difficulty** - difficulty in some environments (e.g., when person speaks softly or setting is noisy) 2. **Moderate difficulty** - speaker has to increase volume and speak distinctly 3. **Highly impaired** - absence of useful hearing

B0300. Hearing Aid

Enter Code	**Hearing aid or other hearing appliance used** in completing B0200, Hearing 0. **No** 1. **Yes**

B0600. Speech Clarity

Enter Code	**Select best description of speech pattern** 0. **Clear speech** - distinct intelligible words 1. **Unclear speech** - slurred or mumbled words 2. **No speech** - absence of spoken words

B0700. Makes Self Understood

Enter Code	**Ability to express ideas and wants,** consider both verbal and non-verbal expression 0. **Understood** 1. **Usually understood** - difficulty communicating some words or finishing thoughts **but** is able if prompted or given time 2. **Sometimes understood** - ability is limited to making concrete requests 3. **Rarely/never understood**

B0800. Ability To Understand Others

Enter Code	**Understanding verbal content, however able** (with hearing aid or device if used) 0. **Understands** - clear comprehension 1. **Usually understands** - misses some part/intent of message **but** comprehends most conversation 2. **Sometimes understands** - responds adequately to simple, direct communication only 3. **Rarely/never understands**

B1000. Vision

Enter Code	**Ability to see in adequate light** (with glasses or other visual appliances) 0. **Adequate** - sees fine detail, such as regular print in newspapers/books 1. **Impaired** - sees large print, but not regular print in newspapers/books 2. **Moderately impaired** - limited vision; not able to see newspaper headlines but can identify objects 3. **Highly impaired** - object identification in question, but eyes appear to follow objects 4. **Severely impaired** - no vision or sees only light, colors or shapes; eyes do not appear to follow objects

B1200. Corrective Lenses

Enter Code	**Corrective lenses (contacts, glasses, or magnifying glass) used** in completing B1000, Vision 0. **No** 1. **Yes**

Resident ______________________ Identifier ______________ Date ______________

Section C — Cognitive Patterns

C0100. Should Brief Interview for Mental Status (C0200-C0500) be Conducted?
Attempt to conduct interview with all residents

Enter Code [ ]
0. **No** (resident is rarely/never understood) → Skip to and complete C0700-C1000, Staff Assessment for Mental Status
1. **Yes** → Continue to C0200, Repetition of Three Words

Brief Interview for Mental Status (BIMS)

C0200. Repetition of Three Words

Enter Code [ ]

Ask resident: *"I am going to say three words for you to remember. Please repeat the words after I have said all three. The words are:* ***sock, blue, and bed.*** *Now tell me the three words."*

Number of words repeated after first attempt
0. **None**
1. **One**
2. **Two**
3. **Three**

After the resident's first attempt, repeat the words using cues ("*sock, something to wear; blue, a color; bed, a piece of furniture*"). You may repeat the words up to two more times.

C0300. Temporal Orientation (orientation to year, month, and day)

Enter Code [ ]

Ask resident: "*Please tell me what year it is right now.*"
A. Able to report correct year
0. **Missed by > 5 years** or no answer
1. **Missed by 2-5 years**
2. **Missed by 1 year**
3. **Correct**

Enter Code [ ]

Ask resident: "*What month are we in right now?*"
B. Able to report correct month
0. **Missed by > 1 month** or no answer
1. **Missed by 6 days to 1 month**
2. **Accurate within 5 days**

Enter Code [ ]

Ask resident: "*What day of the week is today?*"
C. Able to report correct day of the week
0. **Incorrect** or no answer
1. **Correct**

C0400. Recall

Ask resident: "*Let's go back to an earlier question. What were those three words that I asked you to repeat?*"
If unable to remember a word, give cue (something to wear; a color; a piece of furniture) for that word.

Enter Code [ ]

A. Able to recall "sock"
0. **No** - could not recall
1. **Yes, after cueing** ("something to wear")
2. **Yes, no cue required**

Enter Code [ ]

B. Able to recall "blue"
0. **No** - could not recall
1. **Yes, after cueing** ("a color")
2. **Yes, no cue required**

Enter Code [ ]

C. Able to recall "bed"
0. **No** - could not recall
1. **Yes, after cueing** ("a piece of furniture")
2. **Yes, no cue required**

C0500. BIMS Summary Score

Enter Score [ ][ ]

Add scores for questions C0200-C0400 and fill in total score (00-15)
Enter 99 if the resident was unable to complete the interview

Resident ______________________ Identifier ______________ Date ________

Section C | Cognitive Patterns

C0600. Should the Staff Assessment for Mental Status (C0700 - C1000) be Conducted?

Enter Code [ ]
0. **No** (resident was able to complete Brief Interview for Mental Status) → Skip to C1310, Signs and Symptoms of Delirium
1. **Yes** (resident was unable to complete Brief Interview for Mental Status) → Continue to C0700, Short-term Memory OK

Staff Assessment for Mental Status

Do not conduct if Brief Interview for Mental Status (C0200-C0500) was completed

C0700. Short-term Memory OK

Enter Code [ ] **Seems or appears to recall after 5 minutes**
0. **Memory OK**
1. **Memory problem**

C0800. Long-term Memory OK

Enter Code [ ] **Seems or appears to recall long past**
0. **Memory OK**
1. **Memory problem**

C0900. Memory/Recall Ability

↓ **Check all that the resident was normally able to recall**

- [ ] **A. Current season**
- [ ] **B. Location of own room**
- [ ] **C. Staff names and faces**
- [ ] **D. That he or she is in a nursing home/hospital swing bed**
- [ ] **Z. None of the above** were recalled

C1000. Cognitive Skills for Daily Decision Making

Enter Code [ ] **Made decisions regarding tasks of daily life**
0. **Independent** - decisions consistent/reasonable
1. **Modified independence** - some difficulty in new situations only
2. **Moderately impaired** - decisions poor; cues/supervision required
3. **Severely impaired** - never/rarely made decisions

Delirium

C1310. Signs and Symptoms of Delirium (from CAM©)

Code **after completing** Brief Interview for Mental Status or Staff Assessment, and reviewing medical record

A. Acute Onset Mental Status Change

Enter Code [ ] **Is there evidence of an acute change in mental status** from the resident's baseline?
0. **No**
1. **Yes**

Coding:
0. **Behavior not present**
1. **Behavior continuously present, does not fluctuate**
2. **Behavior present, fluctuates** (comes and goes, changes in severity)

↓ **Enter Codes in Boxes**

[ ] **B. Inattention** - Did the resident have difficulty focusing attention, for example being easily distractible, or having difficulty keeping track of what was being said?

[ ] **C. Disorganized thinking** - Was the resident's thinking disorganized or incoherent (rambling or irrelevant conversation, unclear or illogical flow of ideas, or unpredictable switching from subject to subject)?

[ ] **D. Altered level of consciousness** - Did the resident have altered level of consciousness as indicated by any of the following criteria?
- **vigilant** - startled easily to any sound or touch
- **lethargic** - repeatedly dozed off when being asked questions, but responded to voice or touch
- **stuporous** - very difficult to arouse and keep aroused for the interview
- **comatose** - could not be aroused

Resident ______ Identifier ______ Date ______

Section D — Mood

D0100. Should Resident Mood Interview be Conducted? - Attempt to conduct interview with all residents

Enter Code [ ]

0. **No** (resident is rarely/never understood) → Skip to and complete D0500-D0600, Staff Assessment of Resident Mood (PHQ-9-OV)
1. **Yes** → Continue to D0200, Resident Mood Interview (PHQ-9©)

D0200. Resident Mood Interview (PHQ-9©)

Say to resident: *"Over the last 2 weeks, have you been bothered by any of the following problems?"*

If symptom is present, enter 1 (yes) in column 1, Symptom Presence.
If yes in column 1, then ask the resident: "*About **how often** have you been bothered by this?*"
Read and show the resident a card with the symptom frequency choices. Indicate response in column 2, Symptom Frequency.

1. Symptom Presence
0. **No** (enter 0 in column 2)
1. **Yes** (enter 0-3 in column 2)
9. **No response** (leave column 2 blank)

2. Symptom Frequency
0. **Never or 1 day**
1. **2-6 days** (several days)
2. **7-11 days** (half or more of the days)
3. **12-14 days** (nearly every day)

	1. Symptom Presence	2. Symptom Frequency
	↓ Enter Scores in Boxes	↓
A. *Little interest or pleasure in doing things*	[ ]	[ ]
B. *Feeling down, depressed, or hopeless*	[ ]	[ ]
C. *Trouble falling or staying asleep, or sleeping too much*	[ ]	[ ]
D. *Feeling tired or having little energy*	[ ]	[ ]
E. *Poor appetite or overeating*	[ ]	[ ]
F. *Feeling bad about yourself - or that you are a failure or have let yourself or your family down*	[ ]	[ ]
G. *Trouble concentrating on things, such as reading the newspaper or watching television*	[ ]	[ ]
H. *Moving or speaking so slowly that other people could have noticed. Or the opposite - being so fidgety or restless that you have been moving around a lot more than usual*	[ ]	[ ]
I. *Thoughts that you would be better off dead, or of hurting yourself in some way*	[ ]	[ ]

D0300. Total Severity Score

Enter Score [ ][ ]

Add scores for all frequency responses in Column 2, Symptom Frequency. Total score must be between 00 and 27.
Enter 99 if unable to complete interview (i.e., Symptom Frequency is blank for 3 or more items).

D0350. Safety Notification - Complete only if D0200I1 = 1 indicating possibility of resident self harm

Enter Code [ ]

Was responsible staff or provider informed that there is a potential for resident self harm?
0. **No**
1. **Yes**

Resident ________________ Identifier ________________ Date ________________

Section D	Mood

D0500. Staff Assessment of Resident Mood (PHQ-9-OV*)
Do not conduct if Resident Mood Interview (D0200-D0300) was completed

Over the last 2 weeks, did the resident have any of the following problems or behaviors?

If symptom is present, enter 1 (yes) in column 1, Symptom Presence.
Then move to column 2, Symptom Frequency, and indicate symptom frequency.

1. Symptom Presence
0. **No** (enter 0 in column 2)
1. **Yes** (enter 0-3 in column 2)

2. Symptom Frequency
0. **Never or 1 day**
1. **2-6 days** (several days)
2. **7-11 days** (half or more of the days)
3. **12-14 days** (nearly every day)

	1. Symptom Presence	2. Symptom Frequency
	↓ Enter Scores in Boxes ↓	
A. Little interest or pleasure in doing things	☐	☐
B. Feeling or appearing down, depressed, or hopeless	☐	☐
C. Trouble falling or staying asleep, or sleeping too much	☐	☐
D. Feeling tired or having little energy	☐	☐
E. Poor appetite or overeating	☐	☐
F. Indicating that s/he feels bad about self, is a failure, or has let self or family down	☐	☐
G. Trouble concentrating on things, such as reading the newspaper or watching television	☐	☐
H. Moving or speaking so slowly that other people have noticed. Or the opposite - being so fidgety or restless that s/he has been moving around a lot more than usual	☐	☐
I. States that life isn't worth living, wishes for death, or attempts to harm self	☐	☐
J. Being short-tempered, easily annoyed	☐	☐

D0600. Total Severity Score

Enter Score	
☐☐	**Add scores for all frequency responses in Column 2**, Symptom Frequency. Total score must be between 00 and 30.

D0650. Safety Notification - Complete only if D0500I1 = 1 indicating possibility of resident self harm

Enter Code	
☐	**Was responsible staff or provider informed that there is a potential for resident self harm?** 0. **No** 1. **Yes**

Resident ____________ Identifier ____________ Date ____________

Section E Behavior

E0100. Potential Indicators of Psychosis

↓ Check all that apply

- ☐ **A. Hallucinations** (perceptual experiences in the absence of real external sensory stimuli)
- ☐ **B. Delusions** (misconceptions or beliefs that are firmly held, contrary to reality)
- ☐ **Z. None of the above**

Behavioral Symptoms

E0200. Behavioral Symptom - Presence & Frequency

Note presence of symptoms and their frequency

Coding:	↓ Enter Codes in Boxes	
Coding: 0. **Behavior not exhibited** 1. **Behavior of this type occurred 1 to 3 days** 2. **Behavior of this type occurred 4 to 6 days,** but less than daily 3. **Behavior of this type occurred daily**	☐	**A. Physical behavioral symptoms directed toward others** (e.g., hitting, kicking, pushing, scratching, grabbing, abusing others sexually)
	☐	**B. Verbal behavioral symptoms directed toward others** (e.g., threatening others, screaming at others, cursing at others)
	☐	**C. Other behavioral symptoms not directed toward others** (e.g., physical symptoms such as hitting or scratching self, pacing, rummaging, public sexual acts, disrobing in public, throwing or smearing food or bodily wastes, or verbal/vocal symptoms like screaming, disruptive sounds)

E0300. Overall Presence of Behavioral Symptoms

Enter Code ☐ **Were any behavioral symptoms in questions E0200 coded 1, 2, or 3?**
0. **No** → Skip to E0800, Rejection of Care
1. **Yes** → Considering all of E0200, Behavioral Symptoms, answer E0500 and E0600 below

E0500. Impact on Resident

Did any of the identified symptom(s):

Enter Code ☐ **A. Put the resident at significant risk for physical illness or injury?**
0. **No**
1. **Yes**

Enter Code ☐ **B. Significantly interfere with the resident's care?**
0. **No**
1. **Yes**

Enter Code ☐ **C. Significantly interfere with the resident's participation in activities or social interactions?**
0. **No**
1. **Yes**

E0600. Impact on Others

Did any of the identified symptom(s):

Enter Code ☐ **A. Put others at significant risk for physical injury?**
0. **No**
1. **Yes**

Enter Code ☐ **B. Significantly intrude on the privacy or activity of others?**
0. **No**
1. **Yes**

Enter Code ☐ **C. Significantly disrupt care or living environment?**
0. **No**
1. **Yes**

E0800. Rejection of Care - Presence & Frequency

Enter Code ☐ **Did the resident reject evaluation or care** (e.g., bloodwork, taking medications, ADL assistance) **that is necessary to achieve the resident's goals for health and well-being?** Do not include behaviors that have already been addressed (e.g., by discussion or care planning with the resident or family), and determined to be consistent with resident values, preferences, or goals.
0. **Behavior not exhibited**
1. **Behavior of this type occurred 1 to 3 days**
2. **Behavior of this type occurred 4 to 6 days,** but less than daily
3. **Behavior of this type occurred daily**

Resident ______________ Identifier ______________ Date ______________

Section E	**Behavior**
E0900. Wandering - Presence & Frequency	
Enter Code ☐	**Has the resident wandered?** 0. **Behavior not exhibited** → Skip to E1100, Change in Behavioral or Other Symptoms 1. **Behavior of this type occurred 1 to 3 days** 2. **Behavior of this type occurred 4 to 6 days**, but less than daily 3. **Behavior of this type occurred daily**
E1000. Wandering - Impact	
Enter Code ☐	**A. Does the wandering place the resident at significant risk of getting to a potentially dangerous place** (e.g., stairs, outside of the facility)? 0. **No** 1. **Yes**
Enter Code ☐	**B. Does the wandering significantly intrude on the privacy or activities of others?** 0. **No** 1. **Yes**
E1100. Change in Behavior or Other Symptoms Consider all of the symptoms assessed in items E0100 through E1000	
Enter Code ☐	How does resident's current behavior status, care rejection, or wandering **compare to prior assessment (OBRA or Scheduled PPS)?** 0. **Same** 1. **Improved** 2. **Worse** 3. **N/A** because no prior MDS assessment

Resident ______ Identifier ______ Date ______

Section F — Preferences for Customary Routine and Activities

F0300. Should Interview for Daily and Activity Preferences be Conducted? - Attempt to interview all residents able to communicate. If resident is unable to complete, attempt to complete interview with family member or significant other

Enter Code ☐

0. **No** (resident is rarely/never understood and family/significant other not available) → Skip to and complete F0800, Staff Assessment of Daily and Activity Preferences
1. **Yes** → Continue to F0400, Interview for Daily Preferences

F0400. Interview for Daily Preferences

Show resident the response options and say: **"*While you are in this facility...*"**

	↓ Enter Codes in Boxes	
Coding: 1. **Very important** 2. **Somewhat important** 3. **Not very important** 4. **Not important at all** 5. **Important, but can't do or no choice** 9. **No response or non-responsive**	☐	**A.** *how important is it to you to **choose what clothes to wear?***
	☐	**B.** *how important is it to you to **take care of your personal belongings or things?***
	☐	**C.** *how important is it to you to **choose between a tub bath, shower, bed bath, or sponge bath?***
	☐	**D.** *how important is it to you to **have snacks available between meals?***
	☐	**E.** *how important is it to you to **choose your own bedtime?***
	☐	**F.** *how important is it to you to **have your family or a close friend involved in discussions about your care?***
	☐	**G.** *how important is it to you to **be able to use the phone in private?***
	☐	**H.** *how important is it to you to **have a place to lock your things to keep them safe?***

F0500. Interview for Activity Preferences

Show resident the response options and say: **"*While you are in this facility...*"**

	↓ Enter Codes in Boxes	
Coding: 1. **Very important** 2. **Somewhat important** 3. **Not very important** 4. **Not important at all** 5. **Important, but can't do or no choice** 9. **No response or non-responsive**	☐	**A.** *how important is it to you to **have books, newspapers, and magazines to read?***
	☐	**B.** *how important is it to you to **listen to music you like?***
	☐	**C.** *how important is it to you to **be around animals such as pets?***
	☐	**D.** *how important is it to you to **keep up with the news?***
	☐	**E.** *how important is it to you to **do things with groups of people?***
	☐	**F.** *how important is it to you to **do your favorite activities?***
	☐	**G.** *how important is it to you to **go outside to get fresh air when the weather is good?***
	☐	**H.** *how important is it to you to **participate in religious services or practices?***

F0600. Daily and Activity Preferences Primary Respondent

Enter Code ☐

Indicate primary respondent for Daily and Activity Preferences (F0400 and F0500)

1. **Resident**
2. **Family or significant other** (close friend or other representative)
9. **Interview could not be completed** by resident or family/significant other ("No response" to 3 or more items")

Resident ______________________ Identifier ______________ Date ____________

Section F	Preferences for Customary Routine and Activities

F0700. Should the Staff Assessment of Daily and Activity Preferences be Conducted?

Enter Code	
☐	0. **No** (because Interview for Daily and Activity Preferences (F0400 and F0500) was completed by resident or family/significant other) → Skip to and complete G0110, Activities of Daily Living (ADL) Assistance 1. **Yes** (because 3 or more items in Interview for Daily and Activity Preferences (F0400 and F0500) were not completed by resident or family/significant other) → Continue to F0800, Staff Assessment of Daily and Activity Preferences

F0800. Staff Assessment of Daily and Activity Preferences

Do not conduct if Interview for Daily and Activity Preferences (F0400-F0500) was completed

Resident Prefers:

↓ Check all that apply	
☐	**A. Choosing clothes to wear**
☐	**B. Caring for personal belongings**
☐	**C. Receiving tub bath**
☐	**D. Receiving shower**
☐	**E. Receiving bed bath**
☐	**F. Receiving sponge bath**
☐	**G. Snacks between meals**
☐	**H. Staying up past 8:00 p.m.**
☐	**I. Family or significant other involvement in care discussions**
☐	**J. Use of phone in private**
☐	**K. Place to lock personal belongings**
☐	**L. Reading books, newspapers, or magazines**
☐	**M. Listening to music**
☐	**N. Being around animals such as pets**
☐	**O. Keeping up with the news**
☐	**P. Doing things with groups of people**
☐	**Q. Participating in favorite activities**
☐	**R. Spending time away from the nursing home**
☐	**S. Spending time outdoors**
☐	**T. Participating in religious activities or practices**
☐	**Z. None of the above**

Resident ______ Identifier ______ Date ______

Section G Functional Status

G0110. Activities of Daily Living (ADL) Assistance
Refer to the ADL flow chart in the RAI manual to facilitate accurate coding

Instructions for Rule of 3

- When an activity occurs three times at any one given level, code that level.
- When an activity occurs three times at multiple levels, code the most dependent, exceptions are total dependence (4), activity must require full assist every time, and activity did not occur (8), activity must not have occurred at all. Example, three times extensive assistance (3) and three times limited assistance (2), code extensive assistance (3).
- When an activity occurs at various levels, but not three times at any given level, apply the following:
  - When there is a combination of full staff performance, and extensive assistance, code extensive assistance.
  - When there is a combination of full staff performance, weight bearing assistance and/or non-weight bearing assistance code limited assistance (2).

If none of the above are met, code supervision.

1. ADL Self-Performance
Code for **resident's performance** over all shifts - not including setup. If the ADL activity occurred 3 or more times at various levels of assistance, code the most dependent - except for total dependence, which requires full staff performance every time

Coding:

Activity Occurred 3 or More Times

0. **Independent** - no help or staff oversight at any time
1. **Supervision** - oversight, encouragement or cueing
2. **Limited assistance** - resident highly involved in activity; staff provide guided maneuvering of limbs or other non-weight-bearing assistance
3. **Extensive assistance** - resident involved in activity, staff provide weight-bearing support
4. **Total dependence** - full staff performance every time during entire 7-day period

Activity Occurred 2 or Fewer Times

7. **Activity occurred only once or twice** - activity did occur but only once or twice
8. **Activity did not occur** - activity did not occur or family and/or non-facility staff provided care 100% of the time for that activity over the entire 7-day period

2. ADL Support Provided
Code for **most support provided** over all shifts; code regardless of resident's self-performance classification

Coding:

0. **No** setup or physical help from staff
1. **Setup** help only
2. **One** person physical assist
3. **Two+** persons physical assist
8. ADL activity itself **did not occur** or family and/or non-facility staff provided care 100% of the time for that activity over the entire 7-day period

	1. Self-Performance	2. Support
	↓ Enter Codes in Boxes ↓	
A. Bed mobility - how resident moves to and from lying position, turns side to side, and positions body while in bed or alternate sleep furniture	☐	☐
B. Transfer - how resident moves between surfaces including to or from: bed, chair, wheelchair, standing position (**excludes** to/from bath/toilet)	☐	☐
C. Walk in room - how resident walks between locations in his/her room	☐	☐
D. Walk in corridor - how resident walks in corridor on unit	☐	☐
E. Locomotion on unit - how resident moves between locations in his/her room and adjacent corridor on same floor. If in wheelchair, self-sufficiency once in chair	☐	☐
F. Locomotion off unit - how resident moves to and returns from off-unit locations (e.g., areas set aside for dining, activities or treatments). **If facility has only one floor**, how resident moves to and from distant areas on the floor. If in wheelchair, self-sufficiency once in chair	☐	☐
G. Dressing - how resident puts on, fastens and takes off all items of clothing, including donning/removing a prosthesis or TED hose. Dressing includes putting on and changing pajamas and housedresses	☐	☐
H. Eating - how resident eats and drinks, regardless of skill. Do not include eating/drinking during medication pass. Includes intake of nourishment by other means (e.g., tube feeding, total parenteral nutrition, IV fluids administered for nutrition or hydration)	☐	☐
I. Toilet use - how resident uses the toilet room, commode, bedpan, or urinal; transfers on/off toilet; cleanses self after elimination; changes pad; manages ostomy or catheter; and adjusts clothes. Do not include emptying of bedpan, urinal, bedside commode, catheter bag or ostomy bag	☐	☐
J. Personal hygiene - how resident maintains personal hygiene, including combing hair, brushing teeth, shaving, applying makeup, washing/drying face and hands (**excludes** baths and showers)	☐	☐

Resident ______ Identifier ______ Date ______

Section G — Functional Status

G0120. Bathing

How resident takes full-body bath/shower, sponge bath, and transfers in/out of tub/shower (**excludes** washing of back and hair). Code for **most dependent** in self-performance and support

Enter Code ☐ **A. Self-performance**
0. **Independent** - no help provided
1. **Supervision** - oversight help only
2. **Physical help limited to transfer only**
3. **Physical help in part of bathing activity**
4. **Total dependence**
8. **Activity itself did not occur** or family and/or non-facility staff provided care 100% of the time for that activity over the entire 7-day period

Enter Code ☐ **B. Support provided**
(Bathing support codes are as defined in item **G0110 column 2, ADL Support Provided**, above)

G0300. Balance During Transitions and Walking

After observing the resident, **code the following walking and transition items for most dependent**

Coding:
0. **Steady at all times**
1. **Not steady, but able to stabilize without staff assistance**
2. **Not steady, only able to stabilize with staff assistance**
8. **Activity did not occur**

↓ **Enter Codes in Boxes**

☐	**A. Moving from seated to standing position**
☐	**B. Walking** (with assistive device if used)
☐	**C. Turning around** and facing the opposite direction while walking
☐	**D. Moving on and off toilet**
☐	**E. Surface-to-surface transfer** (transfer between bed and chair or wheelchair)

G0400. Functional Limitation in Range of Motion

Code for limitation that interfered with daily functions or placed resident at risk of injury

Coding:
0. **No impairment**
1. **Impairment on one side**
2. **Impairment on both sides**

↓ **Enter Codes in Boxes**

☐	**A. Upper extremity** (shoulder, elbow, wrist, hand)
☐	**B. Lower extremity** (hip, knee, ankle, foot)

G0600. Mobility Devices

↓ **Check all that were normally used**

☐	**A. Cane/crutch**
☐	**B. Walker**
☐	**C. Wheelchair** (manual or electric)
☐	**D. Limb prosthesis**
☐	**Z. None of the above** were used

G0900. Functional Rehabilitation Potential

Complete only if A0310A = 01

Enter Code ☐ **A. Resident believes he or she is capable of increased independence** in at least some ADLs
0. **No**
1. **Yes**
9. **Unable to determine**

Enter Code ☐ **B. Direct care staff believe resident is capable of increased independence** in at least some ADLs
0. **No**
1. **Yes**

Resident ______________________ Identifier ______________ Date __________

Section GG — Functional Abilities and Goals - Admission (Start of SNF PPS Stay)

GG0130. Self-Care (Assessment period is days 1 through 3 of the SNF PPS Stay starting with A2400B)
Complete only if A0310B = 01

Code the resident's usual performance at the start of the SNF PPS stay (admission) for each activity using the 6-point scale. If activity was not attempted at the start of the SNF PPS stay (admission), code the reason. Code the resident's end of SNF PPS stay (discharge) goal(s) using the 6-point scale. Do not use codes 07, 09, or 88 to code end of SNF PPS stay (discharge) goals.

Coding:

Safety and **Quality of Performance -** If helper assistance is required because resident's performance is unsafe or of poor quality, score according to amount of assistance provided.

Activities may be completed with or without assistive devices.

06. **Independent** - Resident completes the activity by him/herself with no assistance from a helper.
05. **Setup or clean-up assistance** - Helper SETS UP or CLEANS UP; resident completes activity. Helper assists only prior to or following the activity.
04. **Supervision or touching assistance** - Helper provides VERBAL CUES or TOUCHING/STEADYING assistance as resident completes activity. Assistance may be provided throughout the activity or intermittently.
03. **Partial/moderate assistance** - Helper does LESS THAN HALF the effort. Helper lifts, holds, or supports trunk or limbs, but provides less than half the effort.
02. **Substantial/maximal assistance** - Helper does MORE THAN HALF the effort. Helper lifts or holds trunk or limbs and provides more than half the effort.
01. **Dependent** - Helper does ALL of the effort. Resident does none of the effort to complete the activity. Or, the assistance of 2 or more helpers is required for the resident to complete the activity.

If activity was not attempted, code reason:

07. **Resident refused.**
09. **Not applicable.**
88. Not attempted due to **medical condition or safety concerns.**

1. Admission Performance	2. Discharge Goal	
↓ Enter Codes in Boxes ↓		
☐☐	☐☐	**A. Eating:** The ability to use suitable utensils to bring food to the mouth and swallow food once the meal is presented on a table/tray. Includes modified food consistency.
☐☐	☐☐	**B. Oral hygiene:** The ability to use suitable items to clean teeth. [Dentures (if applicable): The ability to remove and replace dentures from and to the mouth, and manage equipment for soaking and rinsing them.]
☐☐	☐☐	**C. Toileting hygiene:** The ability to maintain perineal hygiene, adjust clothes before and after using the toilet, commode, bedpan, or urinal. If managing an ostomy, include wiping the opening but not managing equipment.

Resident ______ Identifier ______ Date ______

Section GG — Functional Abilities and Goals - Admission (Start of SNF PPS Stay)

GG0170. Mobility (Assessment period is days 1 through 3 of the SNF PPS Stay starting with A2400B)
Complete only if A0310B = 01

Code the resident's usual performance at the start of the SNF PPS stay (admission) for each activity using the 6-point scale. If activity was not attempted at the start of the SNF PPS stay (admission), code the reason. Code the resident's end of SNF PPS stay (discharge) goal(s) using the 6-point scale. Do not use codes 07, 09, or 88 to code end of SNF PPS stay (discharge) goals.

Coding:

Safety and **Quality of Performance** - If helper assistance is required because resident's performance is unsafe or of poor quality, score according to amount of assistance provided.

Activities may be completed with or without assistive devices.

- 06. **Independent** - Resident completes the activity by him/herself with no assistance from a helper.
- 05. **Setup or clean-up assistance** - Helper SETS UP or CLEANS UP; resident completes activity. Helper assists only prior to or following the activity.
- 04. **Supervision or touching assistance** - Helper provides VERBAL CUES or TOUCHING/STEADYING assistance as resident completes activity. Assistance may be provided throughout the activity or intermittently.
- 03. **Partial/moderate assistance** - Helper does LESS THAN HALF the effort. Helper lifts, holds, or supports trunk or limbs, but provides less than half the effort.
- 02. **Substantial/maximal assistance** - Helper does MORE THAN HALF the effort. Helper lifts or holds trunk or limbs and provides more than half the effort.
- 01. **Dependent** - Helper does ALL of the effort. Resident does none of the effort to complete the activity. Or, the assistance of 2 or more helpers is required for the resident to complete the activity.

If activity was not attempted, code reason:

- 07. **Resident refused.**
- 09. **Not applicable.**
- 88. Not attempted due to **medical condition or safety concerns.**

1. Admission Performance	2. Discharge Goal	
↓ Enter Codes in Boxes ↓		
☐☐	☐☐	**B. Sit to lying:** The ability to move from sitting on side of bed to lying flat on the bed.
☐☐	☐☐	**C. Lying to sitting on side of bed:** The ability to safely move from lying on the back to sitting on the side of the bed with feet flat on the floor, and with no back support.
☐☐	☐☐	**D. Sit to stand:** The ability to safely come to a standing position from sitting in a chair or on the side of the bed.
☐☐	☐☐	**E. Chair/bed-to-chair transfer:** The ability to safely transfer to and from a bed to a chair (or wheelchair).
☐☐	☐☐	**F. Toilet transfer:** The ability to safely get on and off a toilet or commode.
	☐	**H1. Does the resident walk?** 0. **No**, and walking goal is not clinically indicated → Skip to GG0170Q1, Does the resident use a wheelchair/scooter? 1. **No**, and walking goal is clinically indicated → Code the resident's discharge goal(s) for items GG0170J and GG0170K 2. **Yes** → Continue to GG0170J, Walk 50 feet with two turns
☐☐	☐☐	**J. Walk 50 feet with two turns:** Once standing, the ability to walk at least 50 feet and make two turns.
☐☐	☐☐	**K. Walk 150 feet:** Once standing, the ability to walk at least 150 feet in a corridor or similar space.
	☐	**Q1. Does the resident use a wheelchair/scooter?** 0. **No** → Skip to GG0130, Self Care (Discharge) 1. **Yes** → Continue to GG0170R, Wheel 50 feet with two turns
☐☐	☐☐	**R. Wheel 50 feet with two turns:** Once seated in wheelchair/scooter, can wheel at least 50 feet and make two turns.
	☐	**RR1. Indicate the type of wheelchair/scooter used.** 1. **Manual** 2. **Motorized**
☐☐	☐☐	**S. Wheel 150 feet:** Once seated in wheelchair/scooter, can wheel at least 150 feet in a corridor or similar space.
	☐	**SS1. Indicate the type of wheelchair/scooter used.** 1. **Manual** 2. **Motorized**

Resident ______ Identifier ______ Date ______

Section GG	Functional Abilities and Goals - Discharge (End of SNF PPS Stay)

GG0130. Self-Care (Assessment period is the last 3 days of the SNF PPS Stay ending on A2400C)
Complete only if A0310G is not = 2 **and** A0310H = 1 **and** A2400C minus A2400B is greater than 2 **and** A2100 is not = 03

Code the resident's usual performance at the end of the SNF PPS stay for each activity using the 6-point scale. If an activity was not attempted at the end of the SNF PPS stay, code the reason.

Coding:

Safety and **Quality of Performance -** If helper assistance is required because resident's performance is unsafe or of poor quality, score according to amount of assistance provided.

Activities may be completed with or without assistive devices.

06. **Independent** - Resident completes the activity by him/herself with no assistance from a helper.
05. **Setup or clean-up assistance** - Helper SETS UP or CLEANS UP; resident completes activity. Helper assists only prior to or following the activity.
04. **Supervision or touching assistance** - Helper provides VERBAL CUES or TOUCHING/STEADYING assistance as resident completes activity. Assistance may be provided throughout the activity or intermittently.
03. **Partial/moderate assistance** - Helper does LESS THAN HALF the effort. Helper lifts, holds, or supports trunk or limbs, but provides less than half the effort.
02. **Substantial/maximal assistance** - Helper does MORE THAN HALF the effort. Helper lifts or holds trunk or limbs and provides more than half the effort.
01. **Dependent** - Helper does ALL of the effort. Resident does none of the effort to complete the activity. Or, the assistance of 2 or more helpers is required for the resident to complete the activity.

If activity was not attempted, code reason:

07. **Resident refused.**
09. **Not applicable.**
88. Not attempted due to **medical condition or safety concerns.**

3. Discharge Performance	
Enter Code	**A. Eating:** The ability to use suitable utensils to bring food to the mouth and swallow food once the meal is presented on a table/tray. Includes modified food consistency.
Enter Code	**B. Oral hygiene:** The ability to use suitable items to clean teeth. [Dentures (if applicable): The ability to remove and replace dentures from and to the mouth, and manage equipment for soaking and rinsing them.]
Enter Code	**C. Toileting hygiene:** The ability to maintain perineal hygiene, adjust clothes before and after using the toilet, commode, bedpan, or urinal. If managing an ostomy, include wiping the opening but not managing equipment.

Resident ______________________ Identifier ______________ Date ____________

Section GG — Functional Abilities and Goals - Discharge (End of SNF PPS Stay)

GG0170. Mobility (Assessment period is the last 3 days of the SNF PPS Stay ending on A2400C)
Complete only if A0310G is not = 2 **and** A0310H = 1 **and** A2400C minus A2400B is greater than 2 **and** A2100 is not = 03

Code the resident's usual performance at the end of the SNF PPS stay for each activity using the 6-point scale. If an activity was not attempted at the end of the SNF PPS stay, code the reason.

Coding:

Safety and **Quality of Performance** - If helper assistance is required because resident's performance is unsafe or of poor quality, score according to amount of assistance provided.

Activities may be completed with or without assistive devices.

- 06. **Independent** - Resident completes the activity by him/herself with no assistance from a helper.
- 05. **Setup or clean-up assistance** - Helper SETS UP or CLEANS UP; resident completes activity. Helper assists only prior to or following the activity.
- 04. **Supervision or touching assistance** - Helper provides VERBAL CUES or TOUCHING/STEADYING assistance as resident completes activity. Assistance may be provided throughout the activity or intermittently.
- 03. **Partial/moderate assistance** - Helper does LESS THAN HALF the effort. Helper lifts, holds, or supports trunk or limbs, but provides less than half the effort.
- 02. **Substantial/maximal assistance** - Helper does MORE THAN HALF the effort. Helper lifts or holds trunk or limbs and provides more than half the effort.
- 01. **Dependent** - Helper does ALL of the effort. Resident does none of the effort to complete the activity. Or, the assistance of 2 or more helpers is required for the resident to complete the activity.

If activity was not attempted, code reason:

- 07. **Resident refused.**
- 09. **Not applicable.**
- 88. Not attempted due to **medical condition or safety concerns.**

3. Discharge Performance (Enter Codes in Boxes)	
☐☐	**B. Sit to lying:** The ability to move from sitting on side of bed to lying flat on the bed.
☐☐	**C. Lying to sitting on side of bed:** The ability to safely move from lying on the back to sitting on the side of the bed with feet flat on the floor, and with no back support.
☐☐	**D. Sit to stand:** The ability to safely come to a standing position from sitting in a chair or on the side of the bed.
☐☐	**E. Chair/bed-to-chair transfer:** The ability to safely transfer to and from a bed to a chair (or wheelchair).
☐☐	**F. Toilet transfer:** The ability to safely get on and off a toilet or commode.
☐	**H3. Does the resident walk?** 0. **No** → Skip to GG0170Q3, Does the resident use a wheelchair/scooter? 2. **Yes** → Continue to GG0170J, Walk 50 feet with two turns
☐☐	**J. Walk 50 feet with two turns:** Once standing, the ability to walk at least 50 feet and make two turns.
☐☐	**K. Walk 150 feet:** Once standing, the ability to walk at least 150 feet in a corridor or similar space.
☐	**Q3. Does the resident use a wheelchair/scooter?** 0. **No** → Skip to H0100, Appliances 1. **Yes** → Continue to GG0170R, Wheel 50 feet with two turns
☐☐	**R. Wheel 50 feet with two turns:** Once seated in wheelchair/scooter, can wheel at least 50 feet and make two turns.
☐	**RR3. Indicate the type of wheelchair/scooter used.** 1. **Manual** 2. **Motorized**
☐☐	**S. Wheel 150 feet:** Once seated in wheelchair/scooter, can wheel at least 150 feet in a corridor or similar space.
☐	**SS3. Indicate the type of wheelchair/scooter used.** 1. **Manual** 2. **Motorized**

Resident ______________ Identifier ______________ Date ______________

Section H	Bladder and Bowel

H0100. Appliances

↓ Check all that apply	
☐	**A. Indwelling catheter** (including suprapubic catheter and nephrostomy tube)
☐	**B. External catheter**
☐	**C. Ostomy** (including urostomy, ileostomy, and colostomy)
☐	**D. Intermittent catheterization**
☐	**Z. None of the above**

H0200. Urinary Toileting Program

Enter Code ☐	**A. Has a trial of a toileting program (e.g., scheduled toileting, prompted voiding, or bladder training)** been attempted on admission/entry or reentry or since urinary incontinence was noted in this facility? 0. **No** → Skip to H0300, Urinary Continence 1. **Yes** → Continue to H0200B, Response 9. **Unable to determine** → Skip to H0200C, Current toileting program or trial
Enter Code ☐	**B. Response -** What was the resident's response to the trial program? 0. **No improvement** 1. **Decreased wetness** 2. **Completely dry** (continent) 9. **Unable to determine** or trial in progress
Enter Code ☐	**C. Current toileting program or trial** - Is a toileting program (e.g., scheduled toileting, prompted voiding, or bladder training) currently being used to manage the resident's urinary continence? 0. **No** 1. **Yes**

H0300. Urinary Continence

Enter Code ☐	**Urinary continence -** Select the one category that best describes the resident 0. **Always continent** 1. **Occasionally incontinent** (less than 7 episodes of incontinence) 2. **Frequently incontinent** (7 or more episodes of urinary incontinence, but at least one episode of continent voiding) 3. **Always incontinent** (no episodes of continent voiding) 9. **Not rated,** resident had a catheter (indwelling, condom), urinary ostomy, or no urine output for the entire 7 days

H0400. Bowel Continence

Enter Code ☐	**Bowel continence -** Select the one category that best describes the resident 0. **Always continent** 1. **Occasionally incontinent** (one episode of bowel incontinence) 2. **Frequently incontinent** (2 or more episodes of bowel incontinence, but at least one continent bowel movement) 3. **Always incontinent** (no episodes of continent bowel movements) 9. **Not rated,** resident had an ostomy or did not have a bowel movement for the entire 7 days

H0500. Bowel Toileting Program

Enter Code ☐	**Is a toileting program currently being used to manage the resident's bowel continence?** 0. **No** 1. **Yes**

H0600. Bowel Patterns

Enter Code ☐	**Constipation present?** 0. **No** 1. **Yes**

Resident ______________________ Identifier ______________ Date ____________

Section I — Active Diagnoses

Active Diagnoses in the last 7 days - Check all that apply
Diagnoses listed in parentheses are provided as examples and should not be considered as all-inclusive lists

Cancer

- ☐ **I0100. Cancer** (with or without metastasis)

Heart/Circulation

- ☐ **I0200. Anemia** (e.g., aplastic, iron deficiency, pernicious, and sickle cell)
- ☐ **I0300. Atrial Fibrillation or Other Dysrhythmias** (e.g., bradycardias and tachycardias)
- ☐ **I0400. Coronary Artery Disease (CAD)** (e.g., angina, myocardial infarction, and atherosclerotic heart disease (ASHD))
- ☐ **I0500. Deep Venous Thrombosis (DVT), Pulmonary Embolus (PE), or Pulmonary Thrombo-Embolism (PTE)**
- ☐ **I0600. Heart Failure** (e.g., congestive heart failure (CHF) and pulmonary edema)
- ☐ **I0700. Hypertension**
- ☐ **I0800. Orthostatic Hypotension**
- ☐ **I0900. Peripheral Vascular Disease (PVD) or Peripheral Arterial Disease (PAD)**

Gastrointestinal

- ☐ **I1100. Cirrhosis**
- ☐ **I1200. Gastroesophageal Reflux Disease (GERD) or Ulcer** (e.g., esophageal, gastric, and peptic ulcers)
- ☐ **I1300. Ulcerative Colitis, Crohn's Disease, or Inflammatory Bowel Disease**

Genitourinary

- ☐ **I1400. Benign Prostatic Hyperplasia (BPH)**
- ☐ **I1500. Renal Insufficiency, Renal Failure, or End-Stage Renal Disease (ESRD)**
- ☐ **I1550. Neurogenic Bladder**
- ☐ **I1650. Obstructive Uropathy**

Infections

- ☐ **I1700. Multidrug-Resistant Organism (MDRO)**
- ☐ **I2000. Pneumonia**
- ☐ **I2100. Septicemia**
- ☐ **I2200. Tuberculosis**
- ☐ **I2300. Urinary Tract Infection (UTI) (LAST 30 DAYS)**
- ☐ **I2400. Viral Hepatitis** (e.g., Hepatitis A, B, C, D, and E)
- ☐ **I2500. Wound Infection** (other than foot)

Metabolic

- ☐ **I2900. Diabetes Mellitus (DM)** (e.g., diabetic retinopathy, nephropathy, and neuropathy)
- ☐ **I3100. Hyponatremia**
- ☐ **I3200. Hyperkalemia**
- ☐ **I3300. Hyperlipidemia** (e.g., hypercholesterolemia)
- ☐ **I3400. Thyroid Disorder** (e.g., hypothyroidism, hyperthyroidism, and Hashimoto's thyroiditis)

Musculoskeletal

- ☐ **I3700. Arthritis** (e.g., degenerative joint disease (DJD), osteoarthritis, and rheumatoid arthritis (RA))
- ☐ **I3800. Osteoporosis**
- ☐ **I3900. Hip Fracture** - any hip fracture that has a relationship to current status, treatments, monitoring (e.g., sub-capital fractures, and fractures of the trochanter and femoral neck)
- ☐ **I4000. Other Fracture**

Neurological

- ☐ **I4200. Alzheimer's Disease**
- ☐ **I4300. Aphasia**
- ☐ **I4400. Cerebral Palsy**
- ☐ **I4500. Cerebrovascular Accident (CVA), Transient Ischemic Attack (TIA), or Stroke**
- ☐ **I4800. Non-Alzheimer's Dementia** (e.g. Lewy body dementia, vascular or multi-infarct dementia; mixed dementia; frontotemporal dementia such as Pick's disease; and dementia related to stroke, Parkinson's or Creutzfeldt-Jakob diseases)

Neurological Diagnoses continued on next page

Resident ______ Identifier ______ Date ______

Section I — Active Diagnoses

Active Diagnoses in the last 7 days - Check all that apply
Diagnoses listed in parentheses are provided as examples and should not be considered as all-inclusive lists

Neurological - Continued

- ☐ **I4900. Hemiplegia or Hemiparesis**
- ☐ **I5000. Paraplegia**
- ☐ **I5100. Quadriplegia**
- ☐ **I5200. Multiple Sclerosis (MS)**
- ☐ **I5250. Huntington's Disease**
- ☐ **I5300. Parkinson's Disease**
- ☐ **I5350. Tourette's Syndrome**
- ☐ **I5400. Seizure Disorder or Epilepsy**
- ☐ **I5500. Traumatic Brain Injury (TBI)**

Nutritional

- ☐ **I5600. Malnutrition** (protein or calorie) or at risk for malnutrition

Psychiatric/Mood Disorder

- ☐ **I5700. Anxiety Disorder**
- ☐ **I5800. Depression** (other than bipolar)
- ☐ **I5900. Manic Depression** (bipolar disease)
- ☐ **I5950. Psychotic Disorder** (other than schizophrenia)
- ☐ **I6000. Schizophrenia** (e.g., schizoaffective and schizophreniform disorders)
- ☐ **I6100. Post Traumatic Stress Disorder (PTSD)**

Pulmonary

- ☐ **I6200. Asthma, Chronic Obstructive Pulmonary Disease (COPD), or Chronic Lung Disease** (e.g., chronic bronchitis and restrictive lung diseases such as asbestosis)
- ☐ **I6300. Respiratory Failure**

Vision

- ☐ **I6500. Cataracts, Glaucoma, or Macular Degeneration**

None of Above

- ☐ **I7900. None of the above active diagnoses** within the last 7 days

Other

I8000. Additional active diagnoses
Enter diagnosis on line and ICD code in boxes. Include the decimal for the code in the appropriate box.

A. ______ ☐☐☐☐☐☐☐☐

B. ______ ☐☐☐☐☐☐☐☐

C. ______ ☐☐☐☐☐☐☐☐

D. ______ ☐☐☐☐☐☐☐☐

E. ______ ☐☐☐☐☐☐☐☐

F. ______ ☐☐☐☐☐☐☐☐

G. ______ ☐☐☐☐☐☐☐☐

H. ______ ☐☐☐☐☐☐☐☐

I. ______ ☐☐☐☐☐☐☐☐

J. ______ ☐☐☐☐☐☐☐☐

Resident ______ Identifier ______ Date ______

Section J Health Conditions

J0100. Pain Management - Complete for all residents, regardless of current pain level

At any time in the last **5** days, has the resident:

Enter Code	
☐	**A. Received scheduled pain medication regimen?** 0. **No** 1. **Yes**
☐	**B. Received PRN pain medications OR was offered and declined?** 0. **No** 1. **Yes**
☐	**C. Received non-medication intervention for pain?** 0. **No** 1. **Yes**

J0200. Should Pain Assessment Interview be Conducted?
Attempt to conduct interview with all residents. If resident is comatose, skip to J1100, Shortness of Breath (dyspnea)

Enter Code	
☐	0. **No** (resident is rarely/never understood) → Skip to and complete J0800, Indicators of Pain or Possible Pain 1. **Yes** → Continue to J0300, Pain Presence

Pain Assessment Interview

J0300. Pain Presence

Enter Code	
☐	Ask resident: "***Have you had pain or hurting at any time*** *in the last 5 days?*" 0. **No** → Skip to J1100, Shortness of Breath 1. **Yes** → Continue to J0400, Pain Frequency 9. **Unable to answer** → Skip to J0800, Indicators of Pain or Possible Pain

J0400. Pain Frequency

Enter Code	
☐	Ask resident: "***How much of the time have you experienced pain or hurting*** *over the last 5 days?*" 1. **Almost constantly** 2. **Frequently** 3. **Occasionally** 4. **Rarely** 9. **Unable to answer**

J0500. Pain Effect on Function

Enter Code	
☐	**A.** Ask resident: "*Over the past 5 days,* ***has pain made it hard for you to sleep at night?***" 0. **No** 1. **Yes** 9. **Unable to answer**
☐	**B.** Ask resident: "*Over the past 5 days,* ***have you limited your day-to-day activities because of pain?***" 0. **No** 1. **Yes** 9. **Unable to answer**

J0600. Pain Intensity - Administer **ONLY ONE** of the following pain intensity questions (A or B)

Enter Rating ☐☐	**A. Numeric Rating Scale (00-10)** Ask resident: "*Please rate your worst pain over the last 5 days on a zero to ten scale, with zero being no pain and ten as the worst pain you can imagine.*" (Show resident 00 -10 pain scale) **Enter two-digit response. Enter 99 if unable to answer.**
Enter Code ☐	**B. Verbal Descriptor Scale** Ask resident: "*Please rate the intensity of your worst pain over the last 5 days.*" (Show resident verbal scale) 1. **Mild** 2. **Moderate** 3. **Severe** 4. **Very severe, horrible** 9. **Unable to answer**

Resident ______________________ Identifier ______________ Date __________

Section J — Health Conditions

J0700. Should the Staff Assessment for Pain be Conducted?

Enter Code	
☐	0. **No** (J0400 = 1 thru 4) → Skip to J1100, Shortness of Breath (dyspnea) 1. **Yes** (J0400 = 9) → Continue to J0800, Indicators of Pain or Possible Pain

Staff Assessment for Pain

J0800. Indicators of Pain or Possible Pain in the last 5 days

↓ Check all that apply	
☐	**A. Non-verbal sounds** (e.g., crying, whining, gasping, moaning, or groaning)
☐	**B. Vocal complaints of pain** (e.g., that hurts, ouch, stop)
☐	**C. Facial expressions** (e.g., grimaces, winces, wrinkled forehead, furrowed brow, clenched teeth or jaw)
☐	**D. Protective body movements or postures** (e.g., bracing, guarding, rubbing or massaging a body part/area, clutching or holding a body part during movement)
☐	**Z. None of these signs observed or documented** → If checked, skip to J1100, Shortness of Breath (dyspnea)

J0850. Frequency of Indicator of Pain or Possible Pain in the last 5 days

Enter Code	
☐	Frequency with which resident complains or shows evidence of pain or possible pain 1. **Indicators of pain** or possible pain observed **1 to 2 days** 2. **Indicators of pain** or possible pain observed **3 to 4 days** 3. **Indicators of pain** or possible pain observed **daily**

Other Health Conditions

J1100. Shortness of Breath (dyspnea)

↓ Check all that apply	
☐	**A. Shortness of breath** or trouble breathing **with exertion** (e.g., walking, bathing, transferring)
☐	**B. Shortness of breath** or trouble breathing **when sitting at rest**
☐	**C. Shortness of breath** or trouble breathing **when lying flat**
☐	**Z. None of the above**

J1300. Current Tobacco Use

Enter Code	
☐	**Tobacco use** 0. **No** 1. **Yes**

J1400. Prognosis

Enter Code	
☐	Does the resident have a condition or chronic disease that may result in a **life expectancy of less than 6 months?** (Requires physician documentation) 0. **No** 1. **Yes**

J1550. Problem Conditions

↓ Check all that apply	
☐	**A. Fever**
☐	**B. Vomiting**
☐	**C. Dehydrated**
☐	**D. Internal bleeding**
☐	**Z. None of the above**

Resident ____________ Identifier ____________ Date ____________

Section J	Health Conditions

J1700. Fall History on Admission/Entry or Reentry
Complete only if A0310A = 01 or A0310E = 1

Enter Code ☐	**A.** Did the resident have a fall any time in the **last month** prior to admission/entry or reentry? 0. **No** 1. **Yes** 9. **Unable to determine**
Enter Code ☐	**B.** Did the resident have a fall any time in the **last 2-6 months** prior to admission/entry or reentry? 0. **No** 1. **Yes** 9. **Unable to determine**
Enter Code ☐	**C.** Did the resident have any **fracture related to a fall in the 6 months** prior to admission/entry or reentry? 0. **No** 1. **Yes** 9. **Unable to determine**

J1800. Any Falls Since Admission/Entry or Reentry or Prior Assessment (OBRA or Scheduled PPS), whichever is more recent

Enter Code ☐	Has the resident **had any falls since admission/entry or reentry or the prior assessment** (OBRA or Scheduled PPS), whichever is more recent? 0. **No** → Skip to K0100, Swallowing Disorder 1. **Yes** → Continue to J1900, Number of Falls Since Admission/Entry or Reentry or Prior Assessment (OBRA or Scheduled PPS)

J1900. Number of Falls Since Admission/Entry or Reentry or Prior Assessment (OBRA or Scheduled PPS), whichever is more recent

	↓ Enter Codes in Boxes	
Coding: 0. **None** 1. **One** 2. **Two or more**	☐	**A. No injury** - no evidence of any injury is noted on physical assessment by the nurse or primary care clinician; no complaints of pain or injury by the resident; no change in the resident's behavior is noted after the fall
	☐	**B. Injury (except major)** - skin tears, abrasions, lacerations, superficial bruises, hematomas and sprains; or any fall-related injury that causes the resident to complain of pain
	☐	**C. Major injury** - bone fractures, joint dislocations, closed head injuries with altered consciousness, subdural hematoma

Resident ______________ Identifier ______________ Date ______________

Section K Swallowing/Nutritional Status

K0100. Swallowing Disorder
Signs and symptoms of possible swallowing disorder

↓ Check all that apply	
☐	**A. Loss of liquids/solids from mouth when eating or drinking**
☐	**B. Holding food in mouth/cheeks or residual food in mouth after meals**
☐	**C. Coughing or choking during meals or when swallowing medications**
☐	**D. Complaints of difficulty or pain with swallowing**
☐	**Z. None of the above**

K0200. Height and Weight - While measuring, if the number is X.1 - X.4 round down; X.5 or greater round up

☐☐ inches	**A. Height** (in inches). Record most recent height measure since the most recent admission/entry or reentry
☐☐☐ pounds	**B. Weight** (in pounds). Base weight on most recent measure in last 30 days; measure weight consistently, according to standard facility practice (e.g., in a.m. after voiding, before meal, with shoes off, etc.)

K0300. Weight Loss

Enter Code ☐	**Loss of 5% or more in the last month or loss of 10% or more in last 6 months** 0. **No** or unknown 1. **Yes, on** physician-prescribed weight-loss regimen 2. **Yes, not on** physician-prescribed weight-loss regimen

K0310. Weight Gain

Enter Code ☐	**Gain of 5% or more in the last month or gain of 10% or more in last 6 months** 0. **No** or unknown 1. **Yes, on** physician-prescribed weight-gain regimen 2. **Yes, not on** physician-prescribed weight-gain regimen

K0510. Nutritional Approaches
Check all of the following nutritional approaches that were performed during the last **7 days**

1. **While NOT a Resident** Performed ***while NOT a resident*** of this facility and within the ***last 7 days***. Only check column 1 if resident entered (admission or reentry) IN THE LAST 7 DAYS. If resident last entered 7 or more days ago, leave column 1 blank 2. **While a Resident** Performed ***while a resident*** of this facility and within the ***last 7 days***	**1. While NOT a Resident**	**2. While a Resident**
	↓ **Check all that apply** ↓	
A. Parenteral/IV feeding	☐	☐
B. Feeding tube - nasogastric or abdominal (PEG)	☐	☐
C. Mechanically altered diet - require change in texture of food or liquids (e.g., pureed food, thickened liquids)	☐	☐
D. Therapeutic diet (e.g., low salt, diabetic, low cholesterol)	☐	☐
Z. None of the above	☐	☐

Resident ______ Identifier ______ Date ______

Section K | Swallowing/Nutritional Status

K0710. Percent Intake by Artificial Route - Complete K0710 only if Column 1 and/or Column 2 are checked for K0510A and/or K0510B

	1. While NOT a Resident	2. While a Resident	3. During Entire 7 Days
1. While NOT a Resident Performed ***while NOT a resident*** of this facility and within the ***last 7 days***. Only enter a code in column 1 if resident entered (admission or reentry) IN THE LAST 7 DAYS. If resident last entered 7 or more days ago, leave column 1 blank **2. While a Resident** Performed ***while a resident*** of this facility and within the ***last 7 days*** **3. During Entire 7 Days** Performed during the entire ***last 7 days***	↓	**Enter Codes**	↓
A. Proportion of total calories the resident received through parenteral or tube feeding 1. **25% or less** 2. **26-50%** 3. **51% or more**	☐	☐	☐
B. Average fluid intake per day by IV or tube feeding 1. **500 cc/day or less** 2. **501 cc/day or more**	☐	☐	☐

Section L | Oral/Dental Status

L0200. Dental

↓ Check all that apply	
☐	**A. Broken or loosely fitting full or partial denture** (chipped, cracked, uncleanable, or loose)
☐	**B. No natural teeth or tooth fragment(s)** (edentulous)
☐	**C. Abnormal mouth tissue** (ulcers, masses, oral lesions, including under denture or partial if one is worn)
☐	**D. Obvious or likely cavity or broken natural teeth**
☐	**E. Inflamed or bleeding gums or loose natural teeth**
☐	**F. Mouth or facial pain, discomfort or difficulty with chewing**
☐	**G. Unable to examine**
☐	**Z. None of the above were present**

Resident ______________________ Identifier ______________ Date ______________

Section M | Skin Conditions

Report based on highest stage of existing ulcer(s) at its worst; do not "reverse" stage

M0100. Determination of Pressure Ulcer Risk

↓ Check all that apply

- ☐ **A. Resident has a stage 1 or greater, a scar over bony prominence, or a non-removable dressing/device**
- ☐ **B. Formal assessment instrument/tool** (e.g., Braden, Norton, or other)
- ☐ **C. Clinical assessment**
- ☐ **Z. None of the above**

M0150. Risk of Pressure Ulcers

Enter Code ☐ **Is this resident at risk of developing pressure ulcers?**

0. **No**
1. **Yes**

M0210. Unhealed Pressure Ulcer(s)

Enter Code ☐ **Does this resident have one or more unhealed pressure ulcer(s) at Stage 1 or higher?**

0. **No** → Skip to M0900, Healed Pressure Ulcers
1. **Yes** → Continue to M0300, Current Number of Unhealed Pressure Ulcers at Each Stage

M0300. Current Number of Unhealed Pressure Ulcers at Each Stage

Enter Number ☐ **A. Number of Stage 1 pressure ulcers**
Stage 1: Intact skin with non-blanchable redness of a localized area usually over a bony prominence. Darkly pigmented skin may not have a visible blanching; in dark skin tones only it may appear with persistent blue or purple hues

B. Stage 2: Partial thickness loss of dermis presenting as a shallow open ulcer with a red or pink wound bed, without slough. May also present as an intact or open/ruptured blister

Enter Number ☐ 1. **Number of Stage 2 pressure ulcers -** If 0 → Skip to M0300C, Stage 3

Enter Number ☐ 2. **Number of these Stage 2 pressure ulcers that were present upon admission/entry or reentry** - enter how many were noted at the time of admission/entry or reentry

3. **Date of oldest Stage 2 pressure ulcer** - Enter dashes if date is unknown:

☐☐ – ☐☐ – ☐☐☐☐
Month Day Year

C. Stage 3: Full thickness tissue loss. Subcutaneous fat may be visible but bone, tendon or muscle is not exposed. Slough may be present but does not obscure the depth of tissue loss. May include undermining and tunneling

Enter Number ☐ 1. **Number of Stage 3 pressure ulcers** - If 0 → Skip to M0300D, Stage 4

Enter Number ☐ 2. **Number of these Stage 3 pressure ulcers that were present upon admission/entry or reentry** - enter how many were noted at the time of admission/entry or reentry

D. Stage 4: Full thickness tissue loss with exposed bone, tendon or muscle. Slough or eschar may be present on some parts of the wound bed. Often includes undermining and tunneling

Enter Number ☐ 1. **Number of Stage 4 pressure ulcers** - If 0 → Skip to M0300E, Unstageable - Non-removable dressing

Enter Number ☐ 2. **Number of these Stage 4 pressure ulcers that were present upon admission/entry or reentry** - enter how many were noted at the time of admission/entry or reentry

M0300 continued on next page

Resident ____________ Identifier ____________ Date ____________

Section M — Skin Conditions

M0300. Current Number of Unhealed Pressure Ulcers at Each Stage - Continued

E. Unstageable - Non-removable dressing: Known but not stageable due to non-removable dressing/device

Enter Number [ ] **1. Number of unstageable pressure ulcers due to non-removable dressing/device** - If 0 → Skip to M0300F, Unstageable - Slough and/or eschar

Enter Number [ ] **2. Number of these unstageable pressure ulcers that were present upon admission/entry or reentry** - enter how many were noted at the time of admission/entry or reentry

F. Unstageable - Slough and/or eschar: Known but not stageable due to coverage of wound bed by slough and/or eschar

Enter Number [ ] **1. Number of unstageable pressure ulcers due to coverage of wound bed by slough and/or eschar** - If 0 → Skip to M0300G, Unstageable - Deep tissue injury

Enter Number [ ] **2. Number of these unstageable pressure ulcers that were present upon admission/entry or reentry** - enter how many were noted at the time of admission/entry or reentry

G. Unstageable - Deep tissue injury: Suspected deep tissue injury in evolution

Enter Number [ ] **1. Number of unstageable pressure ulcers with suspected deep tissue injury in evolution** - If 0 → Skip to M0610, Dimension of Unhealed Stage 3 or 4 Pressure Ulcers or Eschar

Enter Number [ ] **2. Number of these unstageable pressure ulcers that were present upon admission/entry or reentry** - enter how many were noted at the time of admission/entry or reentry

M0610. Dimensions of Unhealed Stage 3 or 4 Pressure Ulcers or Eschar
Complete only if M0300C1, M0300D1 or M0300F1 is greater than 0

If the resident has one or more unhealed Stage 3 or 4 pressure ulcers or an unstageable pressure ulcer due to slough or eschar, identify the pressure ulcer with the largest surface area (length x width) and record in centimeters:

[ ][ ].[ ] cm **A. Pressure ulcer length:** Longest length from head to toe

[ ][ ].[ ] cm **B. Pressure ulcer width:** Widest width of the same pressure ulcer, side-to-side perpendicular (90-degree angle) to length

[ ][ ].[ ] cm **C. Pressure ulcer depth:** Depth of the same pressure ulcer from the visible surface to the deepest area (if depth is unknown, enter a dash in each box)

M0700. Most Severe Tissue Type for Any Pressure Ulcer

Enter Code [ ] Select the best description of the most severe type of tissue present in any pressure ulcer bed

1. **Epithelial tissue** - new skin growing in superficial ulcer. It can be light pink and shiny, even in persons with darkly pigmented skin
2. **Granulation tissue** - pink or red tissue with shiny, moist, granular appearance
3. **Slough** - yellow or white tissue that adheres to the ulcer bed in strings or thick clumps, or is mucinous
4. **Eschar** - black, brown, or tan tissue that adheres firmly to the wound bed or ulcer edges, may be softer or harder than surrounding skin
9. **None of the Above**

M0800. Worsening in Pressure Ulcer Status Since Prior Assessment (OBRA or Scheduled PPS) or Last Admission/Entry or Reentry
Complete only if A0310E = 0

Indicate the number of current pressure ulcers that were **not present or were at a lesser stage** on prior assessment (OBRA or scheduled PPS) or last entry. If no current pressure ulcer at a given stage, enter 0.

Enter Number [ ] **A. Stage 2**

Enter Number [ ] **B. Stage 3**

Enter Number [ ] **C. Stage 4**

Resident ______________________ Identifier ______________ Date ____________

Section M	Skin Conditions
M0900. Healed Pressure Ulcers Complete only if A0310E = 0	
Enter Code ☐	**A. Were pressure ulcers present on the prior assessment (OBRA or scheduled PPS)?** 0. **No** → Skip to M1030, Number of Venous and Arterial Ulcers 1. **Yes** → Continue to M0900B, Stage 2
	Indicate the number of pressure ulcers that were noted on the prior assessment (OBRA or scheduled PPS) that have completely closed (resurfaced with epithelium). If no healed pressure ulcer at a given stage since the prior assessment (OBRA or scheduled PPS), enter 0.
Enter Number ☐	**B. Stage 2**
Enter Number ☐	**C. Stage 3**
Enter Number ☐	**D. Stage 4**
M1030. Number of Venous and Arterial Ulcers	
Enter Number ☐	**Enter the total number of venous and arterial ulcers present**
M1040. Other Ulcers, Wounds and Skin Problems	
↓ Check all that apply	
	Foot Problems
☐	**A. Infection of the foot** (e.g., cellulitis, purulent drainage)
☐	**B. Diabetic foot ulcer(s)**
☐	**C. Other open lesion(s) on the foot**
	Other Problems
☐	**D. Open lesion(s) other than ulcers, rashes, cuts** (e.g., cancer lesion)
☐	**E. Surgical wound(s)**
☐	**F. Burn(s)** (second or third degree)
☐	**G. Skin tear(s)**
☐	**H. Moisture Associated Skin Damage (MASD)** (e.g., incontinence-associated dermatitis [IAD], perspiration, drainage)
	None of the Above
☐	**Z. None of the above** were present
M1200. Skin and Ulcer Treatments	
↓ Check all that apply	
☐	**A. Pressure reducing device for chair**
☐	**B. Pressure reducing device for bed**
☐	**C. Turning/repositioning program**
☐	**D. Nutrition or hydration intervention** to manage skin problems
☐	**E. Pressure ulcer care**
☐	**F. Surgical wound care**
☐	**G. Application of nonsurgical dressings** (with or without topical medications) other than to feet
☐	**H. Applications of ointments/medications** other than to feet
☐	**I. Application of dressings to feet** (with or without topical medications)
☐	**Z. None of the above** were provided

Resident ______________________ Identifier ______________ Date __________

Section N — Medications

N0300. Injections

Enter Days [ ]	**Record the number of days that injections of any type** were received during the last 7 days or since admission/entry or reentry if less than 7 days. If 0 → Skip to N0410, Medications Received

N0350. Insulin

Enter Days [ ]	**A. Insulin injections - Record the number of days that insulin injections** were received during the last 7 days or since admission/entry or reentry if less than 7 days
Enter Days [ ]	**B. Orders for insulin - Record the number of days the physician (or authorized assistant or practitioner) changed the resident's insulin orders** during the last 7 days or since admission/entry or reentry if less than 7 days

N0410. Medications Received

Indicate the number of DAYS the resident received the following medications by pharmacological classification, not how it is used, during the last 7 days or since admission/entry or reentry if less than 7 days. Enter "0" if medication was not received by the resident during the last 7 days

Enter Days [ ]	**A. Antipsychotic**
Enter Days [ ]	**B. Antianxiety**
Enter Days [ ]	**C. Antidepressant**
Enter Days [ ]	**D. Hypnotic**
Enter Days [ ]	**E. Anticoagulant** (e.g., warfarin, heparin, or low-molecular weight heparin)
Enter Days [ ]	**F. Antibiotic**
Enter Days [ ]	**G. Diuretic**
Enter Days [ ]	**H. Opioid**

N0450. Antipsychotic Medication Review

Enter Code [ ]	**A. Did the resident receive antipsychotic medications since admission/entry or reentry or the prior OBRA assessment, whichever is more recent?** 0. **No** - Antipsychotics were not received → Skip to O0100, Special Treatments, Procedures, and Programs 1. **Yes** - Antipsychotics were received on a routine basis only → Continue to N0450B, Has a GDR been attempted? 2. **Yes** - Antipsychotics were received on a PRN basis only → Continue to N0450B, Has a GDR been attempted? 3. **Yes** - Antipsychotics were received on a routine and PRN basis → Continue to N0450B, Has a GDR been attempted?
Enter Code [ ]	**B. Has a gradual dose reduction (GDR) been attempted?** 0. **No** → Skip to N0450D, Physician documented GDR as clinically contraindicated 1. **Yes** → Continue to N0450C, Date of last attempted GDR
	C. Date of last attempted GDR: [ ][ ] – [ ][ ] – [ ][ ][ ][ ] Month Day Year

N0450 continued on next page

Resident ____________ Identifier ____________ Date ____________

Section N	Medications

N0450. Antipsychotic Medication Review - Continued

Enter Code	
☐	**D. Physician documented GDR as clinically contraindicated** 0. **No** - GDR has not been documented by a physician as clinically contraindicated → Skip to O0100, Special Treatments, Procedures, and Programs 1. **Yes** - GDR has been documented by a physician as clinically contraindicated → Continue to N0450E, Date physician documented GDR as clinically contraindicated
	E. Date physician documented GDR as clinically contraindicated: ☐☐ - ☐☐ - ☐☐☐☐ Month Day Year

Resident ______________ Identifier ______________ Date ______________

Section O — Special Treatments, Procedures, and Programs

O0100. Special Treatments, Procedures, and Programs

Check all of the following treatments, procedures, and programs that were performed during the last **14 days**

1. **While NOT a Resident**
   Performed ***while NOT a resident*** of this facility and within the ***last 14 days***. Only check column 1 if resident entered (admission or reentry) IN THE LAST 14 DAYS. If resident last entered 14 or more days ago, leave column 1 blank
2. **While a Resident**
   Performed ***while a resident*** of this facility and within the ***last 14 days***

	1. While NOT a Resident	2. While a Resident
	↓ Check all that apply ↓	
Cancer Treatments		
A. Chemotherapy	☐	☐
B. Radiation	☐	☐
Respiratory Treatments		
C. Oxygen therapy	☐	☐
D. Suctioning	☐	☐
E. Tracheostomy care	☐	☐
F. Ventilator or respirator	☐	☐
G. BiPAP/CPAP	☐	☐
Other		
H. IV medications	☐	☐
I. Transfusions	☐	☐
J. Dialysis	☐	☐
K. Hospice care	☐	☐
L. Respite care		☐
M. Isolation or quarantine for active infectious disease (does not include standard body/fluid precautions)	☐	☐
None of the Above		
Z. None of the above	☐	☐

O0250. Influenza Vaccine - Refer to current version of RAI manual for current influenza vaccination season and reporting period

Enter Code ☐ **A.** Did the **resident receive the influenza vaccine *in this facility*** for this year's influenza vaccination season?
- 0. **No** → Skip to O0250C, If influenza vaccine not received, state reason
- 1. **Yes** → Continue to O0250B, Date influenza vaccine received

B. Date influenza vaccine received → Complete date and skip to O0300A, Is the resident's Pneumococcal vaccination up to date?

☐☐ – ☐☐ – ☐☐☐☐
Month Day Year

Enter Code ☐ **C. If influenza vaccine not received, state reason:**
1. **Resident not in this facility** during this year's influenza vaccination season
2. **Received outside of this facility**
3. **Not eligible** - medical contraindication
4. **Offered and declined**
5. **Not offered**
6. **Inability to obtain influenza vaccine** due to a declared shortage
9. **None of the above**

O0300. Pneumococcal Vaccine

Enter Code ☐ **A. Is the resident's Pneumococcal vaccination up to date?**
- 0. **No** → Continue to O0300B, If Pneumococcal vaccine not received, state reason
- 1. **Yes** → Skip to O0400, Therapies

Enter Code ☐ **B. If Pneumococcal vaccine not received, state reason:**
1. **Not eligible** - medical contraindication
2. **Offered and declined**
3. **Not offered**

Resident ______ Identifier ______ Date ______

Section O — Special Treatments, Procedures, and Programs

O0400. Therapies

A. Speech-Language Pathology and Audiology Services

Enter Number of Minutes [ ][ ][ ][ ]
1. **Individual minutes** - record the total number of minutes this therapy was administered to the resident **individually** in the last 7 days

Enter Number of Minutes [ ][ ][ ][ ]
2. **Concurrent minutes** - record the total number of minutes this therapy was administered to the resident **concurrently with one other resident** in the last 7 days

Enter Number of Minutes [ ][ ][ ][ ]
3. **Group minutes** - record the total number of minutes this therapy was administered to the resident as **part of a group of residents** in the last 7 days

If the sum of individual, concurrent, and group minutes is zero, → skip to O0400A5, Therapy start date

Enter Number of Minutes [ ][ ][ ][ ]
3A. **Co-treatment minutes** - record the total number of minutes this therapy was administered to the resident in **co-treatment sessions** in the last 7 days

Enter Number of Days [ ]
4. **Days** - record the **number of days** this therapy was administered for **at least 15 minutes** a day in the last 7 days

5. **Therapy start date** - record the date the most recent therapy regimen (since the most recent entry) started

[ ][ ] – [ ][ ] – [ ][ ][ ][ ]
Month Day Year

6. **Therapy end date** - record the date the most recent therapy regimen (since the most recent entry) ended - enter dashes if therapy is ongoing

[ ][ ] – [ ][ ] – [ ][ ][ ][ ]
Month Day Year

B. Occupational Therapy

Enter Number of Minutes [ ][ ][ ][ ]
1. **Individual minutes** - record the total number of minutes this therapy was administered to the resident **individually** in the last 7 days

Enter Number of Minutes [ ][ ][ ][ ]
2. **Concurrent minutes** - record the total number of minutes this therapy was administered to the resident **concurrently with one other resident** in the last 7 days

Enter Number of Minutes [ ][ ][ ][ ]
3. **Group minutes** - record the total number of minutes this therapy was administered to the resident as **part of a group of residents** in the last 7 days

If the sum of individual, concurrent, and group minutes is zero, → skip to O0400B5, Therapy start date

Enter Number of Minutes [ ][ ][ ][ ]
3A. **Co-treatment minutes** - record the total number of minutes this therapy was administered to the resident in **co-treatment sessions** in the last 7 days

Enter Number of Days [ ]
4. **Days** - record the **number of days** this therapy was administered for **at least 15 minutes** a day in the last 7 days

5. **Therapy start date** - record the date the most recent therapy regimen (since the most recent entry) started

[ ][ ] – [ ][ ] – [ ][ ][ ][ ]
Month Day Year

6. **Therapy end date** - record the date the most recent therapy regimen (since the most recent entry) ended - enter dashes if therapy is ongoing

[ ][ ] – [ ][ ] – [ ][ ][ ][ ]
Month Day Year

O0400 continued on next page

Resident ______ Identifier ______ Date ______

Section O — Special Treatments, Procedures, and Programs

O0400. Therapies - Continued

C. Physical Therapy

Enter Number of Minutes [ ][ ][ ][ ]
1. **Individual minutes** - record the total number of minutes this therapy was administered to the resident **individually** in the last 7 days

Enter Number of Minutes [ ][ ][ ][ ]
2. **Concurrent minutes** - record the total number of minutes this therapy was administered to the resident **concurrently with one other resident** in the last 7 days

Enter Number of Minutes [ ][ ][ ][ ]
3. **Group minutes** - record the total number of minutes this therapy was administered to the resident as **part of a group of residents** in the last 7 days

If the sum of individual, concurrent, and group minutes is zero, → skip to O0400C5, Therapy start date

Enter Number of Minutes [ ][ ][ ][ ]
3A. **Co-treatment minutes** - record the total number of minutes this therapy was administered to the resident in **co-treatment sessions** in the last 7 days

Enter Number of Days [ ]
4. **Days** - record the **number of days** this therapy was administered for **at least 15 minutes** a day in the last 7 days

5. **Therapy start date** - record the date the most recent therapy regimen (since the most recent entry) started

[ ][ ] - [ ][ ] - [ ][ ][ ][ ]
Month Day Year

6. **Therapy end date** - record the date the most recent therapy regimen (since the most recent entry) ended - enter dashes if therapy is ongoing

[ ][ ] - [ ][ ] - [ ][ ][ ][ ]
Month Day Year

D. Respiratory Therapy

Enter Number of Minutes [ ][ ][ ][ ]
1. **Total minutes** - record the total number of minutes this therapy was administered to the resident in the last 7 days
If zero, → skip to O0400E, Psychological Therapy

Enter Number of Days [ ]
2. **Days** - record the **number of days** this therapy was administered for **at least 15 minutes** a day in the last 7 days

E. Psychological Therapy (by any licensed mental health professional)

Enter Number of Minutes [ ][ ][ ][ ]
1. **Total minutes** - record the total number of minutes this therapy was administered to the resident in the last 7 days
If zero, → skip to O0400F, Recreational Therapy

Enter Number of Days [ ]
2. **Days** - record the **number of days** this therapy was administered for **at least 15 minutes** a day in the last 7 days

F. Recreational Therapy (includes recreational and music therapy)

Enter Number of Minutes [ ][ ][ ][ ]
1. **Total minutes** - record the total number of minutes this therapy was administered to the resident in the last 7 days
If zero, → skip to O0420, Distinct Calendar Days of Therapy

Enter Number of Days [ ]
2. **Days** - record the **number of days** this therapy was administered for **at least 15 minutes** a day in the last 7 days

O0420. Distinct Calendar Days of Therapy

Enter Number of Days [ ]
Record the number of calendar days that the resident received Speech-Language Pathology and Audiology Services, Occupational Therapy, or Physical Therapy for at least 15 minutes in the past 7 days.

O0450. Resumption of Therapy - Complete only if A0310C = 2 or 3 and A0310F = 99

Enter Code [ ]
A. **Has a previous rehabilitation therapy regimen (speech, occupational, and/or physical therapy) ended, as reported on this End of Therapy OMRA, and has this regimen now resumed at exactly the same level for each discipline?**
0. **No** → Skip to O0500, Restorative Nursing Programs
1. **Yes**

B. **Date on which therapy regimen resumed:**

[ ][ ] - [ ][ ] - [ ][ ][ ][ ]
Month Day Year

Resident ______ Identifier ______ Date ______

Section O	Special Treatments, Procedures, and Programs

O0500. Restorative Nursing Programs

Record the **number of days** each of the following restorative programs was performed (for at least 15 minutes a day) in the last 7 calendar days (enter 0 if none or less than 15 minutes daily)

Number of Days	Technique
☐	**A. Range of motion (passive)**
☐	**B. Range of motion (active)**
☐	**C. Splint or brace assistance**
Number of Days	**Training and Skill Practice In:**
☐	**D. Bed mobility**
☐	**E. Transfer**
☐	**F. Walking**
☐	**G. Dressing and/or grooming**
☐	**H. Eating and/or swallowing**
☐	**I. Amputation/prostheses care**
☐	**J. Communication**

O0600. Physician Examinations

Enter Days	
☐☐	Over the last 14 days, **on how many days did the physician (or authorized assistant or practitioner) examine the resident?**

O0700. Physician Orders

Enter Days	
☐☐	Over the last 14 days, **on how many days did the physician (or authorized assistant or practitioner) change the resident's orders?**

Resident ______________ Identifier ______________ Date ______________

Section P — Restraints and Alarms

P0100. Physical Restraints

Physical restraints are any manual method or physical or mechanical device, material or equipment attached or adjacent to the resident's body that the individual cannot remove easily which restricts freedom of movement or normal access to one's body

Coding	↓ Enter Codes in Boxes	
Coding: 0. **Not used** 1. **Used less than daily** 2. **Used daily**		**Used in Bed**
	☐	**A. Bed rail**
	☐	**B. Trunk restraint**
	☐	**C. Limb restraint**
	☐	**D. Other**
		Used in Chair or Out of Bed
	☐	**E. Trunk restraint**
	☐	**F. Limb restraint**
	☐	**G. Chair prevents rising**
	☐	**H. Other**

P0200. Alarms

An alarm is any physical or electronic device that monitors resident movement and alerts the staff when movement is detected

Coding	↓ Enter Codes in Boxes	
Coding: 0. **Not used** 1. **Used less than daily** 2. **Used daily**	☐	**A. Bed alarm**
	☐	**B. Chair alarm**
	☐	**C. Floor mat alarm**
	☐	**D. Motion sensor alarm**
	☐	**E. Wander/elopement alarm**
	☐	**F. Other alarm**

Resident ______________________ Identifier ______________ Date ______________

Section Q	Participation in Assessment and Goal Setting
Q0100. Participation in Assessment	
Enter Code ☐	**A. Resident participated in assessment** 0. **No** 1. **Yes**
Enter Code ☐	**B. Family or significant other participated in assessment** 0. **No** 1. **Yes** 9. **Resident has no family or significant other**
Enter Code ☐	**C. Guardian or legally authorized representative participated in assessment** 0. **No** 1. **Yes** 9. **Resident has no guardian or legally authorized representative**
Q0300. Resident's Overall Expectation Complete only if A0310E = 1	
Enter Code ☐	**A. Select one for resident's overall goal established during assessment process** 1. Expects to be **discharged to the community** 2. Expects to **remain in this facility** 3. Expects to be **discharged to another facility/institution** 9. **Unknown or uncertain**
Enter Code ☐	**B. Indicate information source for Q0300A** 1. **Resident** 2. If not resident, then **family or significant other** 3. If not resident, family, or significant other, then **guardian or legally authorized representative** 9. **Unknown or uncertain**
Q0400. Discharge Plan	
Enter Code ☐	**A. Is active discharge planning already occurring for the resident to return to the community?** 0. **No** 1. **Yes** → Skip to Q0600, Referral
Q0490. Resident's Preference to Avoid Being Asked Question Q0500B Complete only if A0310A = 02, 06, or 99	
Enter Code ☐	**Does the resident's clinical record document a request that this question be asked only on comprehensive assessments?** 0. **No** 1. **Yes** → Skip to Q0600, Referral
Q0500. Return to Community	
Enter Code ☐	**B. Ask the resident** (or family or significant other or guardian or legally authorized representative if resident is unable to understand or respond): **"Do you want to talk to someone about the possibility of leaving this facility and returning to live and receive services in the community?"** 0. **No** 1. **Yes** 9. **Unknown or uncertain**
Q0550. Resident's Preference to Avoid Being Asked Question Q0500B Again	
Enter Code ☐	**A. Does the resident** (or family or significant other or guardian or legally authorized representative if resident is unable to understand or respond) **want to be asked about returning to the community on all assessments?** (Rather than only on comprehensive assessments.) 0. **No** - then document in resident's clinical record and ask again only on the next comprehensive assessment 1. **Yes** 8. **Information not available**
Enter Code ☐	**B. Indicate information source for Q0550A** 1. **Resident** 2. If not resident, then **family or significant other** 3. If not resident, family or significant other, then **guardian or legally authorized representative** 9. **None of the above**

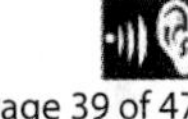

Resident ______________________ Identifier ______________ Date __________

Section Q	Participation in Assessment and Goal Setting
Q0600. Referral	
Enter Code ☐	**Has a referral been made to the Local Contact Agency?** (Document reasons in resident's clinical record) 0. **No** - referral not needed 1. **No** - referral is or may be needed (For more information see Appendix C, Care Area Assessment Resources #20) 2. **Yes** - referral made

Resident ______________________ Identifier ______________ Date ______

Section V — Care Area Assessment (CAA) Summary

V0100. Items From the Most Recent Prior OBRA or Scheduled PPS Assessment
Complete only if A0310E = 0 and if the following is true for the **prior assessment**: A0310A = 01- 06 or A0310B = 01- 05

Enter Code ☐☐	**A. Prior Assessment Federal OBRA Reason for Assessment** (A0310A value from prior assessment) 01. **Admission** assessment (required by day 14) 02. **Quarterly** review assessment 03. **Annual** assessment 04. **Significant change in status** assessment 05. **Significant correction** to **prior comprehensive** assessment 06. **Significant correction** to **prior quarterly** assessment 99. None of the above
Enter Code ☐☐	**B. Prior Assessment PPS Reason for Assessment** (A0310B value from prior assessment) 01. **5-day** scheduled assessment 02. **14-day** scheduled assessment 03. **30-day** scheduled assessment 04. **60-day** scheduled assessment 05. **90-day** scheduled assessment 07. **Unscheduled assessment used for PPS** (OMRA, significant or clinical change, or significant correction assessment) 99. None of the above
	C. Prior Assessment Reference Date (A2300 value from prior assessment) ☐☐ – ☐☐ – ☐☐☐☐ Month Day Year
Enter Score ☐☐	**D. Prior Assessment Brief Interview for Mental Status (BIMS) Summary Score** (C0500 value from prior assessment)
Enter Score ☐☐	**E. Prior Assessment Resident Mood Interview (PHQ-9©) Total Severity Score** (D0300 value from prior assessment)
Enter Score ☐☐	**F. Prior Assessment Staff Assessment of Resident Mood (PHQ-9-OV) Total Severity Score** (D0600 value from prior assessment)

Resident ______ Identifier ______ Date ______

Section V — Care Area Assessment (CAA) Summary

V0200. CAAs and Care Planning

1. Check column A if Care Area is triggered.
2. For each triggered Care Area, indicate whether a new care plan, care plan revision, or continuation of current care plan is necessary to address the problem(s) identified in your assessment of the care area. The Care Planning Decision column must be completed within 7 days of completing the RAI (MDS and CAA(s)). Check column B if the triggered care area is addressed in the care plan.
3. Indicate in the Location and Date of CAA Documentation column where information related to the CAA can be found. CAA documentation should include information on the complicating factors, risks, and any referrals for this resident for this care area.

A. CAA Results

Care Area	A. Care Area Triggered	B. Care Planning Decision	Location and Date of CAA documentation
	↓ Check all that apply ↓		
01. Delirium	☐	☐	
02. Cognitive Loss/Dementia	☐	☐	
03. Visual Function	☐	☐	
04. Communication	☐	☐	
05. ADL Functional/Rehabilitation Potential	☐	☐	
06. Urinary Incontinence and Indwelling Catheter	☐	☐	
07. Psychosocial Well-Being	☐	☐	
08. Mood State	☐	☐	
09. Behavioral Symptoms	☐	☐	
10. Activities	☐	☐	
11. Falls	☐	☐	
12. Nutritional Status	☐	☐	
13. Feeding Tube	☐	☐	
14. Dehydration/Fluid Maintenance	☐	☐	
15. Dental Care	☐	☐	
16. Pressure Ulcer	☐	☐	
17. Psychotropic Drug Use	☐	☐	
18. Physical Restraints	☐	☐	
19. Pain	☐	☐	
20. Return to Community Referral	☐	☐	

B. Signature of RN Coordinator for CAA Process and Date Signed

1. **Signature**

2. **Date** ☐☐ – ☐☐ – ☐☐☐☐ (Month, Day, Year)

C. Signature of Person Completing Care Plan Decision and Date Signed

1. **Signature**

2. **Date** ☐☐ – ☐☐ – ☐☐☐☐ (Month, Day, Year)

Resident ______ Identifier ______ Date ______

Section X — Correction Request

Complete Section X only if A0050 = 2 or 3

Identification of Record to be Modified/Inactivated - The following items identify the existing assessment record that is in error. In this section, reproduce the information EXACTLY as it appeared on the existing erroneous record, even if the information is incorrect. This information is necessary to locate the existing record in the National MDS Database.

X0150. Type of Provider (A0200 on existing record to be modified/inactivated)

Enter Code ☐

Type of provider
1. **Nursing home (SNF/NF)**
2. **Swing Bed**

X0200. Name of Resident (A0500 on existing record to be modified/inactivated)

A. **First name:** ☐☐☐☐☐☐☐☐☐☐☐☐

C. **Last name:** ☐☐☐☐☐☐☐☐☐☐☐☐☐☐☐☐☐☐

X0300. Gender (A0800 on existing record to be modified/inactivated)

Enter Code ☐

1. **Male**
2. **Female**

X0400. Birth Date (A0900 on existing record to be modified/inactivated)

☐☐ – ☐☐ – ☐☐☐☐
Month Day Year

X0500. Social Security Number (A0600A on existing record to be modified/inactivated)

☐☐☐ – ☐☐ – ☐☐☐☐

X0600. Type of Assessment (A0310 on existing record to be modified/inactivated)

Enter Code ☐☐

A. Federal OBRA Reason for Assessment
01. **Admission** assessment (required by day 14)
02. **Quarterly** review assessment
03. **Annual** assessment
04. **Significant change in status** assessment
05. **Significant correction** to **prior comprehensive** assessment
06. **Significant correction** to **prior quarterly** assessment
99. **None of the above**

Enter Code ☐☐

B. PPS Assessment
PPS Scheduled Assessments for a Medicare Part A Stay
01. **5-day** scheduled assessment
02. **14-day** scheduled assessment
03. **30-day** scheduled assessment
04. **60-day** scheduled assessment
05. **90-day** scheduled assessment

PPS Unscheduled Assessments for a Medicare Part A Stay
07. **Unscheduled assessment used for PPS** (OMRA, significant or clinical change, or significant correction assessment)

Not PPS Assessment
99. **None of the above**

Enter Code ☐

C. PPS Other Medicare Required Assessment - OMRA
0. **No**
1. **Start of therapy** assessment
2. **End of therapy** assessment
3. **Both Start and End of therapy** assessment
4. **Change of therapy** assessment

X0600 continued on next page

Resident ______ Identifier ______ Date ______

Section X — Correction Request

X0600. Type of Assessment - Continued

Enter Code	
☐	**D. Is this a Swing Bed clinical change assessment?** Complete only if X0150 = 2 0. **No** 1. **Yes**
☐☐	**F. Entry/discharge reporting** 01. **Entry** tracking record 10. **Discharge** assessment-**return not anticipated** 11. **Discharge** assessment-**return anticipated** 12. **Death in facility** tracking record 99. **None of the above**
☐	**H. Is this a SNF Part A PPS Discharge Assessment?** 0. **No** 1. **Yes**

X0700. Date on existing record to be modified/inactivated - **Complete one only**

	A. Assessment Reference Date (A2300 on existing record to be modified/inactivated) - Complete only if X0600F = 99 ☐☐ - ☐☐ - ☐☐☐☐ Month Day Year
	B. Discharge Date (A2000 on existing record to be modified/inactivated) - Complete only if X0600F = 10, 11, or 12 ☐☐ - ☐☐ - ☐☐☐☐ Month Day Year
	C. Entry Date (A1600 on existing record to be modified/inactivated) - Complete only if X0600F = 01 ☐☐ - ☐☐ - ☐☐☐☐ Month Day Year

Correction Attestation Section - Complete this section to explain and attest to the modification/inactivation request

X0800. Correction Number

Enter Number	
☐☐	**Enter the number of correction requests to modify/inactivate the existing record, including the present one**

X0900. Reasons for Modification - Complete only if Type of Record is to modify a record in error (A0050 = 2)

↓ **Check all that apply**

☐	**A. Transcription error**
☐	**B. Data entry error**
☐	**C. Software product error**
☐	**D. Item coding error**
☐	**E. End of Therapy - Resumption (EOT-R) date**
☐	**Z. Other error requiring modification** If "Other" checked, please specify: ______

X1050. Reasons for Inactivation - Complete only if Type of Record is to inactivate a record in error (A0050 = 3)

↓ **Check all that apply**

☐	**A. Event did not occur**
☐	**Z. Other error requiring inactivation** If "Other" checked, please specify: ______

Resident ______ Identifier ______ Date ______

Section X Correction Request

X1100. RN Assessment Coordinator Attestation of Completion

A. Attesting individual's first name:

☐☐☐☐☐☐☐☐☐☐☐☐

B. Attesting individual's last name:

☐☐☐☐☐☐☐☐☐☐☐☐☐☐☐☐☐☐

C. Attesting individual's title:

D. Signature

E. Attestation date

☐☐ – ☐☐ – ☐☐☐☐
Month Day Year

Resident ______________ Identifier ______________ Date ______________

Section Z	**Assessment Administration**

Z0100. Medicare Part A Billing

A. Medicare Part A HIPPS code (RUG group followed by assessment type indicator):

☐☐☐☐☐☐☐

B. RUG version code:

☐☐☐☐☐☐☐☐☐☐

Enter Code ☐ **C. Is this a Medicare Short Stay assessment?**
0. **No**
1. **Yes**

Z0150. Medicare Part A Non-Therapy Billing

A. Medicare Part A non-therapy HIPPS code (RUG group followed by assessment type indicator):

☐☐☐☐☐☐☐

B. RUG version code:

☐☐☐☐☐☐☐☐☐☐

Z0200. State Medicaid Billing (if required by the state)

A. RUG Case Mix group:

☐☐☐☐☐☐☐☐☐☐

B. RUG version code:

☐☐☐☐☐☐☐☐☐☐

Z0250. Alternate State Medicaid Billing (if required by the state)

A. RUG Case Mix group:

☐☐☐☐☐☐☐☐☐☐

B. RUG version code:

☐☐☐☐☐☐☐☐☐☐

Z0300. Insurance Billing

A. RUG billing code:

☐☐☐☐☐☐☐☐☐☐

B. RUG billing version:

☐☐☐☐☐☐☐☐☐☐

Resident ______________ Identifier ______________ Date ______________

Section Z — Assessment Administration

Z0400. Signature of Persons Completing the Assessment or Entry/Death Reporting

I certify that the accompanying information accurately reflects resident assessment information for this resident and that I collected or coordinated collection of this information on the dates specified. To the best of my knowledge, this information was collected in accordance with applicable Medicare and Medicaid requirements. I understand that this information is used as a basis for ensuring that residents receive appropriate and quality care, and as a basis for payment from federal funds. I further understand that payment of such federal funds and continued participation in the government-funded health care programs is conditioned on the accuracy and truthfulness of this information, and that I may be personally subject to or may subject my organization to substantial criminal, civil, and/or administrative penalties for submitting false information. I also certify that I am authorized to submit this information by this facility on its behalf.

Signature	Title	Sections	Date Section Completed
A.			
B.			
C.			
D.			
E.			
F.			
G.			
H.			
I.			
J.			
K.			
L.			

Z0500. Signature of RN Assessment Coordinator Verifying Assessment Completion

A. Signature:

B. Date RN Assessment Coordinator signed assessment as complete:

[ ][ ] – [ ][ ] – [ ][ ][ ][ ]
Month Day Year

C. Care Area Assessments

Care Area Assessments (CAAs) are the system of deciding which types of interventions will be needed. They are worked by scoring the MDS and reviewing the results in the book *Resident Assessment System for Long-term Care.* By reviewing the CAAs, each health care professional will be able to determine if there is a specific treatment required for the resident. The treatment interventions triggered by using CAAs indicate the basic, minimum standard of treatment for residents in long-term care facilities. Whether to implement a CAA treatment intervention is discussed in detail in Chapter 12.

There are 20 identified CAAs

- Delirium
- Cognitive Loss/Dementia
- Visual Function
- Communication
- Activities of Daily Living (ADLs) – Functional Status/Rehabilitation Potential
- Urinary Incontinence and Indwelling Catheter
- Psychosocial Well-Being
- Mood State
- Behavioral Symptoms
- Activities
- Fall(s)
- Nutritional Status
- Feeding Tube(s)
- Dehydration/Fluid Maintenance
- Dental Care
- Pressure Ulcer(s
- Psychotropic Medication Use
- Physical Restraints
- Pain
- Return to Community Referral

All professionals should be familiar with the MDS, the *Resident Assessment System for Long-term Care*, CAAs, and how to decide if a treatment intervention is indicated. *Chapter 12* provides an overview of many of the CAAs that may "trigger" the need for action by the professional. To help the reader develop a fuller understanding of the process, CAA examples have been included in this appendix. The CAAs in this book are from *Resident Assessment System for Long-term Care* published by the U.S. Department of Commerce, National Technical Information Service.

The next four pages show how the Activity CAA is worked for a man in, hopefully, a short-term stay while recovering from a fall. Following that are three Social Services CAAs: Psychosocial Well-Being, Mood State, and Behavioral Symptoms. The Social Services CAAs are based on the following case profile.

Mrs. R has been living at home with her husband as caregiver. Up until the last few months he was able to handle her care himself. She recently began leaving the home unattended, has been calling 911 for being held as a "prisoner," and has begun to be combative with her husband. She was admitted to the hospital after being found 2 miles from home in her nightgown and barefoot. She was subsequently transferred to the nursing home after it was deemed that her husband could no longer provide for her care. Her history: secretary at a real estate office, very concerned with her appearance, very involved with community services and church.

10. ACTIVITIES

Review of Indicators of Activities

✓	**Activity preferences prior to admission** (from interviews and clinical record)	**Supporting Documentation (Basis/reason for checking the item, including the location, date, and source (if applicable) of that information)**
☑	• Passive	Describes himself as happy in his routine. Reading, TV, and radio are his main interests. Family involved in care. Resident interview 10/5/2018
☐	• Active	
☐	• Outside the home	
☑	• Inside the home	
☐	• Centered almost entirely on family activities	
☐	• Centered almost entirely on non-family activities	
☐	• Group (F0500E) activities	
☑	• Solitary activities	
☐	• Involved in community service, volunteer activities	
☐	• Athletic	
☑	• Non-athletic	
✓	**Current activity pursuits** (from interviews and clinical record)	**Supporting Documentation**
☑	• Resident identifies leisure activities of interest	States interest in any food-related events, especially coffee and donuts. Resident interview 10/5/2018
☑	• Self-directed or done with others and/or planned by others	
☐	• Activities resident pursues when visitors are present	
☑	• Scheduled programs in which resident participates	
☐	• Activities of interest not currently available or offered to the resident	

✓	**Health issues** that result in reduced activity participation	**Supporting Documentation (Basis/reason for checking the item, including the location, date, and source (if applicable) of that information)**
☑	• Indicators of depression or anxiety (D0200, D0300, D0500, D0600)	Recent peptic ulcer and edema with stiffness in legs. Resolving but still weak. Uses 3-pt walker. Needs wheelchair for long distance mobility. Resident interview 10/5/2018 H&P 10/5/2018 PT Notes 10/5/2018
☐	• Use of psychoactive medications (N0410A-N0410D)	
☑	• Functional/mobility (G0110) or balance (G0300) problems; physical disability (G0300, G0400)	
☐	• Cognitive deficits (C0500, C0700-C1000), including stamina, ability to express self (B0700), understand others (B0800), make decisions (C1000)	
☑	• Unstable acute/chronic health problem (clinical record, O0100, J0100, J1100, J0700, J1400, J1550, I8000, M1040, M1200)	
☐	• Chronic health conditions, such as incontinence (H0300, H0400) or pain (J0300)	
☐	• Embarrassment or unease due to presence of equipment (O0100D, E, F), such as tubes, oxygen tank (O0100C), or colostomy bag (H0100) (observation, clinical record)	
☐	• Receives numerous treatments (O0100, O0400) that limit available time/energy (clinical record)	
☑	• Performs tasks slowly due to reduced energy reserves (observation, clinical record)	

✓	**Environmental or staffing issues** that hinder participation	**Supporting Documentation**
☐	• Physical barriers that prevent the resident from gaining access to the space where the activity is held (observation)	N/A
☐	• Need for additional staff responsible for social activities (observation)	
☐	• Lack of staff time to involve residents in current activity programs (observation)	
☐	• Resident's fragile nature results in feelings of intimidation by staff responsible for the activity (from observation, interviews, clinical record)	

✓	Unique skills or knowledge the resident has that he or she could pass on to others (from interviews and clinical record)	Supporting Documentation (Basis/reason for checking the item, including the location, date, and source (if applicable) of that information)
☐	• Games	N/A
☐	• Complex tasks such as knitting, or computer skills	
☐	• Topic that might interest others	
✓	**Issues** that result in reduced activity participation	**Supporting Documentation**
☐	• Resident is new to facility or has been in facility long enough to become bored with status quo (interview, clinical record)	Socialization was mainly at work, and with his wife and family. Interacts with others but not interested in making new friends. Wants to get out of his room and see "what is going on." Resident interview 10/5/2018
☐	• Psychosocial well-being issues, such as shyness, initiative, and social involvement	
☐	• Socially inappropriate behavior (E0200)	
☐	• Indicators of psychosis (E0100A-E0100C)	
☐	• Feelings of being unwelcome, due to issues such as those already involved in an activity drawing boundaries that are difficult to cross (observation, interview, clinical record)	
☐	• Limited opportunities for resident to get to know others through activities such as shared dining, afternoon refreshments, monthly birthday parties, reminiscence groups (observation, facility activity calendar)	
☐	• Available activities do not correspond to resident's values, attitudes, expectations (interview, clinical record) (F0500, F0800)	
☑	• Long history of unease in joining with others (interview, clinical record)	

Input from resident and/or family/representative regarding the care area. (Questions/Comments/Concerns/Preferences/Suggestions)
Family wants to encourage him to walk to activities of interest to increase strength. Also suggest he be introduced to men with similar interests and history

Analysis of Findings		Care Plan Considerations
Review indicators and supporting documentation, and draw conclusions. Document: • Description of the problem; • Causes and contributing factors; and • Risk factors related to the care area.	Care Plan Y/N	Document reason(s) care plan will/ will not be developed.
Mobility limited due to resolving health condition. Although content with in-room activities, there is the risk of spending too much time alone. This risk could impact condition and mood as well as pressure sores.	Y	Care plan will focus on supporting therapy goals to increase ambulation through involvement in related activities.

Referral(s) to another discipline(s) is warranted (to whom and why): No

Information regarding the CAA transferred to the CAA Summary (Section V of the MDS):
☑ Yes ☐ No

Signature/Title: E Martini Date: 10/08/18

7. PSYCHOSOCIAL WELL-BEING

Review of Indicators of Psychosocial Well-Being

✓	**Modifiable factors for relationship problems** (from resident, family, staff interviews and clinical record)	**Supporting Documentation (Basis/reason for checking the item, including the location, date, and source (if applicable) of that information)**
☑	• Resident says or indicates he or she feels lonely — Recent decline in social involvement and associated loneliness can be sign of acute health complications and depression	Social interaction has declined with onset of dementia. Husband does not think she is aware of this.
☐	• Resident indicates he or she feels distressed because of decline in social activities	
☑	• Over the past few years, resident has experienced absence of daily exchanges with relatives and friends	Very involved with community service & church in the past.
☐	• Resident is uneasy dealing with others	
☑	• Resident has conflicts with family, friends, roommate, other residents, or staff	Recently combative with husband & difficult to redirect.
☐	• Resident appears preoccupied with the past and unwilling to respond to needs of the present	
☐	• Resident seems unable or reluctant to begin to establish a social role in the facility; may be grieving lost status or roles	H&P 10/25/2018 husband interview
☐	• Recent change in family situation or social network, such as death of a close family member or friend	
✓	**Customary lifestyle** (from resident, family, staff interviews and clinical record) (Section F)	**Supporting Documentation**
☑	• Was lifestyle more satisfactory to the resident prior to admission to the nursing home?	See above.
☑	• Are current psychosocial/relationship problems consistent with resident's long-standing lifestyle or is this relatively new for the resident?	Undetermined at this time if her loss of former lifestyle is evident to her.
☐	• Has facility care plan to date been as consistent as possible with resident's prior lifestyle, preferences, and routines (F0400, F0600, F0800)?	

✓	**Diseases and conditions** that may impede ability to interact with others	**Supporting Documentation (Basis/reason for checking the item, including the location, date, and source (if applicable) of that information)**
☐	• Delirium (C1310, C1310A = 1, Delirium CAA)	Ongoing decline in recent year is the major contributory factor.
☐	• Intellectual disability /developmental disability (A1550)	
☐	• Alzheimer's disease (I4200)	
☐	• Aphasia (I4300)	
☑	• Other dementia (I4800)	
☐	• Depression (I5800)	
✓	**Health status factors** that may inhibit social involvement	**Supporting Documentation**
☑	• Decline in activities of daily living (G0110)	Declines are due to above, unlikely to resolve. Social interactions are primarily inhibited by her inability to recognize family and staff. family/staff interview 10/25/2018
☐	• Health problem, such as falls (J1700, J1800), pain (J0300, J0800), fatigue, etc.	
☑	• Mood (D0200A1, D0300, D0500A1, D0600) or behavior (E0200) problem that impacts interpersonal relationships or that arises because of social isolation (See Mood State and Behavioral Symptoms CAAs)	
☑	• Change in communication (B0700, B0800), vision (B1000), hearing (B0200), cognition (C0100, C0600)	
☑	• Medications with side effects that interfere with social interactions, such as incontinence, diarrhea, delirium, or sleepiness	
✓	**Environmental factors** that may inhibit social involvement	**Supporting Documentation**
☐	• Use of physical restraints (P0100)	Not related to her reduced social interaction. See above.
☑	• Change in residence leading to loss of autonomy and reduced self-esteem (A1700)	
☐	• Change in room assignment or dining location or table mates	
☐	• Living situation limits informal social interaction, such as isolation precautions (O0100M)	

CMS's RAI Version 3.0 Manual

Appendix C: CAA Resources
7. Psychosocial Well-Being

✓	**Strengths** to build upon (from resident, family, staff interviews and clinical record)	**Supporting Documentation (Basis/reason for checking the item, including the location, date, and source (if applicable) of that information)**
☐	• Activities in which resident appears especially at ease interacting with others	Was very proud of her accomplishments, took pride in her appearance. Very giving and concerned with others. Unsure if this can be built on with her decline in cognition and behavior. husband interview 11/25/2018
☐	• Certain situations appeal to resident more than others, such as small groups or 1:1 interactions rather than large groups	
☐	• Certain individuals who seem to bring out a more positive, optimistic side of the resident	
☑	• Positive traits that distinguished the resident as an individual prior to his or her illness	
☑	• What gave the resident a sense of satisfaction earlier in his or her life?	

October 2017 **Appendix C-31**

Input from resident and/or family/representative regarding the care area. (Questions/Comments/Concerns/Preferences/Suggestions)
Per husband: "Her appearance & behaviors just aren't who she was. I want her to be safe and cared for."

Analysis of Findings		**Care Plan Considerations**
Review indicators and supporting documentation, and draw conclusions. Document: • Description of the problem; • Causes and contributing factors; and • Risk factors related to the care area.	Care Plan Y/N	Document reason(s) care plan will/ will not be developed.
Mrs. R is no longer able to recognize her old friends or recall her previous lifestyle. She recognizes her husband but doesn't remember his visits. Not evident that she is distressed due to the above.	N	Decline in social involvement & conflicts with husband primarily due to her worsening dementia. No resolvable issues indentified. See Activity & Cognition CAA for intervention to maintain quality of life.

Referral(s) to another discipline(s) is warranted (to whom and why): No

Information regarding the CAA transferred to the CAA Summary (Section V of the MDS):
☑ Yes ☐ No

Signature/Title: M A Weeks, SSD Date: 11/28/18

8. MOOD STATE

Review of Indicators of Mood

✓	Psychosocial changes	Supporting Documentation (Basis/reason for checking the item, including the location, date, and source (if applicable) of that information)
☑	• Personal loss	Per husband & staff not evident that she is aware of changes. H&P 11/20/2018 interviews 11/20/2018
☑	• Recent move into or within the nursing home (A1700)	
☐	• Recent change in relationships, such as illness or loss of a relative or friend	
☐	• Recent change in health perception, such as perception of being seriously ill or too ill to return home (Q0300 - Q0600)	
☑	• Clinical or functional change that may affect the resident's dignity, such as new or worsening incontinence, communication, or decline	
✓	**Clinical issues** that can cause or contribute to a mood problem	**Supporting Documentation**
☐	• Relapse of an underlying mental health problem (I5700 – I6100)	Worsening dementia is the root cause of her poor appetite, restlessness, & poor concentration. Indicators present prior to admission & worsening per husband. interviews 11/20/2018 psych eval 10/30/2018
☐	• Psychiatric disorder (anxiety, depression, manic depression, schizophrenia, post-traumatic stress disorder) (I5700 – I6100)	
☐	• Alzheimer's disease (I4200)	
☐	• Delirium (C1310)	
☐	• Delusions (E0100B)	
☐	• Hallucinations (E0100A)	
☑	• Communication problems (B0700, B0800)	
☑	• Decline in Activities of Daily Living (ADLs) (G0110, clinical record)	
☐	• Infection (I1700 – I2500, clinical record)	
☐	• Pain (J0300 or J0800)	
☐	• Cardiac disease (I0200 – I0900)	
☐	• Thyroid abnormality (I3400)	
☐	• Dehydration (J1550C, clinical record)	
☐	• Metabolic disorder (I2900 – I3400)	
☐	• Neurological disease (I4200 – I5500)	
☐	• Recent cerebrovascular accident (I4500)	
☑	• Dementia, cognitive decline (I4800, clinical record)	
☐	• Cancer (I0100)	
☐	• Other (I8000)	

✓	**Medications** (from medication administration record and preadmission records if new admission)	**Supporting Documentation (Basis/reason for checking the item, including the location, date, and source (if applicable) of that information)**
☐	• Antibiotics (N0410F)	N/A
☐	• Anticholinergics	
☐	• Antihypertensives	
☐	• Anticonvulsants	
☐	• Antipsychotics (N0410A)	
☐	• Cardiac medications	
☐	• Cimetidine	
☐	• Clonidine	
☐	• Chemotherapeutic agents	
☐	• Digitalis	
☐	• Other	
☐	• Glaucoma medications	
☐	• Guanethidine	
☐	• Immuno-suppressive medications	
☐	• Methyldopa	
☐	• Narcotics	
☐	• Nitrates	
☐	• Propranolol	
☐	• Reserpine	
☐	• Steroids	
☐	• Stimulants	
✓	**Laboratory tests**	**Supporting Documentation**
☐	• Serum calcium	N/A
☐	• Thyroid function	
☐	• Blood glucose	
☐	• Potassium	
☐	• Porphyria	

Input from resident and/or family/representative regarding the care area. (Questions/Comments/Concerns/Preferences/Suggestions)
Per husband: She has always been an upbeat person. I don't think she's depressed now. She doesn't seem unhappy, just confused.

Analysis of Findings		**Care Plan Considerations**
Review indicators and supporting documentation, and draw conclusions. Document: • Description of the problem; • Causes and contributing factors; and • Risk factors related to the care area.	Care Plan Y/N	Document reason(s) care plan will/ will not be developed.
Mood indicators of poor appetite, restlessness, and poor sleep. Lack of interest related to her worsening dementia	N	Indicators not related to mood decline but due to her dementia & resulting behaviors. See Behavior CAA.

Referral(s) to another discipline(s) is warranted (to whom and why): N

Information regarding the CAA transferred to the CAA Summary (Section V of the MDS):
☑ Yes ☐ No

Signature/Title: M A Weeks, SSD Date: 11/28/18

9. BEHAVIORAL SYMPTOMS

Review of Indicators of Behavioral Symptoms

✓	Seriousness of the behavioral symptoms (E0300, E0800, E0900, E1100)	Supporting Documentation (Basis/reason for checking the item, including the location, date, and source (if applicable) of that information)
☐	• Resident is immediate threat to self – IMMEDIATE INTERVENTION REQUIRED (D0200I.1=1, D0500I.1=1, E1000 = 1)	Elopement/wandering no longer a danger in monitored environment.
☐	• Resident is immediate threat to others – IMMEDIATE INTERVENTION REQUIRED (E0600A)	
✓	**Nature of the behavioral disturbance** (resident interview, if possible; staff observations)	**Supporting Documentation**
☑	• Provoked or unprovoked	Hx of wandering & being combative with redirection. No pattern to resistance to care. She is often very sweet & accepting. Responds well to face to face instruction. staff/husband interview 11/22/18 H&P 11/10/18
☑	• Offensive or defensive	
☐	• Purposeful	
☐	• Occurs during specific activities, such as bath or transfers	
☑	• Pattern, such as certain times of the day, or varies over time	
☐	• Others in the vicinity are involved	
☐	• Reaction to a particular action, such as being physically moved	
☑	• Resident appears to startle easily	

✓	**Medication side effects** that can cause behavioral symptoms (from medication records)	**Supporting Documentation (Basis/reason for checking the item, including the location, date, and source (if applicable) of that information)**
☑	• New medication	Medications readjusted with recent hospitalization to address escalation of behaviors. Good response & more manageable behaviors. No s/e noted. Not contributing H&P 11/10/18
☑	• Change in dosage	
☐	• Antiparkinsonian drugs - may cause hypersexuality, socially inappropriate behavior	
☐	• Sedatives, centrally active antihypertensives, some cardiac drugs, anticholinergic agents can cause paranoid delusions, delirium	
☐	• Bronchodilators or other respiratory drugs, which can increase agitation and cause difficulty sleeping	
☐	• Caffeine	
☐	• Nicotine	
☐	• Medications that impair impulse control, such as benzodiazepines, sedatives, alcohol (or any product containing alcohol, such as some cough medicine)	
✓	**Illness or conditions** that can cause behavior problems	**Supporting Documentation**
☐	• Long-standing mental health problem associated with the behavioral disturbances, such as schizophrenia, bipolar disorder, depression, anxiety disorder, post-traumatic stress disorder (I5700 – I6100)	No change in physical condition N/A H&P 11/10/18
☐	• New or acute physical health problem or flare-up of a known chronic condition (I8000)	
☐	• Delusions (E0100B)	
☐	• Hallucinations (E0100A)	
☐	• Paranoia (from record)	
☐	• Constipation (H0600)	
☐	• Congestive heart failure (I0600)	
☐	• Infection (I1700 – I2500)	
☐	• Head injury (I5500, clinical record)	
☐	• Diabetes (I2900)	
☐	• Pain (J0300, J0800)	
☐	• Fever (J1550A, clinical record)	
☐	• Dehydration (J1550C, clinical record; see Dehydration CAA)	

✓	**Factors that can cause or exacerbate the behavior** (from observation, interview, record)	**Supporting Documentation (Basis/reason for checking the item, including the location, date, and source (if applicable) of that information)**
☐	• Frustration due to problem communicating discomfort or unmet need	Startles if approached quickly but not an exaggerated response. Fear not expressed verbally or facially. per husband: her behaviors are improved from those at home per staff: seems ill at ease in large groups interviews 11/20/18
☐	• Frustration, agitation due to need to urinate or have bowel movement	
☐	• Fear due to not recognizing caregiver	
☐	• Fear due to not recognizing the environment or misinterpreting the environment or actions of others	
☐	• Major unresolved sources of interpersonal conflict between the resident and family members, other residents, or staff (see Psychosocial Well-Being CAA)	
☑	• Recent change, such as new admission (A1700) or a new unit, assignment of new care staff, or withdrawal from a treatment program	
☐	• Departure from normal routines	
☐	• Sleep disturbance (D0500C = 1)	
☑	• Noisy, crowded area	
☐	• Dimly lit area	
☐	• Sensory impairment, such as hearing or vision problem (B0200, B1000)	
☐	• Restraints (P0100)	
☐	• Fatigue (D0500D = 1)	
☐	• Need for repositioning (M1200)	

✓	**Cognitive status problems** (also see Cognitive Loss CAT/CAA)	**Supporting Documentation**
☐	• Delirium (C1310), clinical record (Delirium CAT)	See previous notes. Dementia and cognition decline not reversible & and primary contributory factor to behaviors.
☑	• Dementia (I4800)	
☐	• Recent cognitive loss (clinical record, interviews with family, etc.)	
☐	• Alzheimer's disease (I4200)	
☐	• Effects of cerebrovascular accident (I4500)	

✓	Other Considerations	Supporting Documentation (Basis/reason for checking the item, including the location, date, and source (if applicable) of that information)
☐	• May be communicating discomfort, personal needs, preferences, fears, feeling ill	N/A
☐	• Persons exhibiting long-standing problem behaviors related to psychiatric conditions may place others in danger of physical assault, intimidation, or embarrassment and place themselves at increased risk of being stigmatized, isolated, abused, and neglected by loved ones or care givers	
☐	• The actions and responses of family members and caregivers can aggravate or even cause behavioral outbursts	

Input from resident and/or family/representative regarding the care area. (Questions/Comments/Concerns/Preferences/Suggestions)
She seems to be doing better here & with the medication changes. My goal is to have her safe and comfortable. I hope she remains able to walk and recognize me.

Analysis of Findings		**Care Plan Considerations**
Review indicators and supporting documentation, and draw conclusions. Document: • Description of the problem; • Causes and contributing factors; and • Risk factors related to the care area.	Care Plan Y/N	Document reason(s) care plan will/ will not be developed.
Decline in eating, ADL skills, sleeplessness, restlessness, cognition primarily due to unresolvable and worsening dementia. Risk factors include further cognitive decline, falls, incontinence, & decreased mobility.	Y	IDT will address risk factors & intervene to slow or minimize declines in areas itemized. IDT will seek pharmaceutical interventions to slow cognitive decline.

Referral(s) to another discipline(s) is warranted (to whom and why): PT/RTA to maintain amb & continence. MD for possible medication intervention. RD to avoid weight loss

Information regarding the CAA transferred to the CAA Summary (Section V of the MDS):
☑ Yes ☐ No

Signature/Title: M A Weeks, SSD Date: 11/28/18

References and Further Reading

Alzheimer's Association. (2017). Alzheimer's disease facts and figures. www.alz.org/facts.

American Health Care Association. (1996) Nursing facility subacute care: The quality and cost-effective alternative to hospital care. www.rai.to/subacute.htm

American Occupational Therapy Association. (1989). *Uniform terminology for reporting occupational therapy, 2nd ed.* Bethesda, MD.

American Psychiatric Association. (2013). *Diagnostic and statistical manual of mental disorders fifth edition.* Washington, DC.

Armstrong, Missy & Lauzen, Sarah. (1994). *Community integration program, 2nd edition.* Ravensdale, WA: Idyll Arbor, Inc.

Atkinson, R. C. & Shiffrin, R. M. (1971). The control of short-term memory and its control processes. *Scientific American, 225*, 82–90.

Ayres, A. Jean. (1971). *Sensory integration and learning disorders.* Los Angeles, CA: Western Psychological Services.

Best-Martini, E, (2006). "Let's get moving." *Creative Forecasting*, October, 2006.

Best-Martini, E. (2007). "Cognitive stimulation, cognitive retraining and mental wellness interventions: Implications for recreational therapy practice." *ATRA Newsletter*, *23*(2). Part One.

Best-Martini, E. & Botenhagen, K. 2003. *Exercise for frail elders*. Human Kinetics. Champaign, IL.

Blackman, J. A. (1990). *Medical aspects of developmental disabilities in children birth to three.* Gaithersburg, MD: Aspen Publications.

Bowlby, Carol. (1993). *Therapeutic activities with persons disabled by Alzheimer's disease and related disorders.* Gaithersburg, MD: Aspen Publishers.

Bradford, Leland P. (1976). *Making meetings work: A Guide for leaders and group members.* La Jolla, CA: University Associates.

Brasile, F., Skalko, T. K., & burlingame, j. (1998). *Perspectives in recreational therapy: Issues of a dynamic profession.* Ravensdale, WA: Idyll Arbor, Inc.

burlingame, j. (1999). Reprint from *Idyll Arbor's journal of recreational therapy practice.* www.IdyllArbor.com, April 1999.

burlingame, j. & Blaschko, T. M. (1991). *Therapy in intermediate care facilities for the mentally retarded.* Ravensdale, WA: Idyll Arbor, Inc.

burlingame, j. & Blaschko, T. M. (2010). *Assessment tools for recreational therapy and related fields, fourth edition.* Enumclaw, WA: Idyll Arbor, Inc.

Burnside, Irene Mortenson. (1978). *Working with the elderly: Group process and techniques*. Belmont, CA: Duxbury Press.

Buettner, L. & S. Fitzsimmons. (2003). *Dementia practice guidelines for recreational therapy: Treatment of disturbing behaviors.* ATRA. Alexandria: VA. p. 10

Campanelli, Linda & Leviton, Dan. (1989). "Intergenerational health promotion and rehabilitation: The adult health and development program model." *Topics in Geriatric Rehab, 4*(3) 61–69. Gaithersburg, MD: Aspen Publishing, Inc.

Campbell, Joseph with Moyer, Bill. (1988). *The power of myth.* New York, NY: Doubleday.

Capell, J., Dean, E., & Veenstra, G. (2008). The relationship between cultural competence and ethnocentrism of health care professionals. *Journal of Transcultural Nursing, 19*(2), 121–125. http://dx.doi.org/10.1177/1043659607312970

Caplan, Sandi. (1995). *Grief's courageous journey: A workbook.* Oakland, CA: New Harbinger.

Center for Medicare Services. (2010). *Resident assessment system for long-term care facilities.* Springfield, VA: U.S. Department of Commerce National Technical Information Service.

Colby, S. L. & Ortman, J. M. (2014). Projections of the size and composition of the U.S. population: 2014 to 2060, *Current Population Reports*, P25–1143, U.S. Census Bureau, Washington, DC.

Cross, T., Bazron, B., Dennis, K., & Isaacs, M. (1989). *Towards a culturally competent system of care.* Volume 2. Washington, DC: CASSP Technical Assistance Center, Center for Child Health and Mental Health Policy, Georgetown University Child Development Center.

Cunninghis, Richelle. (1995). *Reality activities: A how to manual for increasing orientation, second edition.* Ravensdale, WA: Idyll Arbor, Inc.

Cunninghis, R. N. & Best-Martini, E. (1996). *Quality assurance for activity programs, second edition.* Ravensdale, WA: Idyll Arbor, Inc.

D'Antonio-Nocera, Anne, DeBolt, Nancy, & Touhey, Nadine, Eds. (1996). *The professional activity manager and consultant.* Ravensdale, WA: Idyll Arbor, Inc.

de la Monte, Suzanne M. & Wands, Jack R. (2008). Alzheimer's disease is type 3 diabetes–evidence reviewed. *J Diabetes Sci Technol. 2008 Nov; 2*(6): 1101–1113.

Egede, L. (2006). Race, ethnicity, culture and disparities in health care. *Journal of General Intern Medicine, 21*(6):667–669.

Eliopoulos, Charlotte. (1993). *Gerontological nursing, third edition.* Philadelphia, PA: J. B. Lippincott Company.

Erikson, Erik H., Erikson, Joan M., & Kivnick, Helen Q. (1994). *Vital involvement in old age.* New York: W. W. Norton.

Feil, Naomi. (2012). *The validation breakthrough: Simple techniques for communicating with people with alzheimer's and other dementias, 3rd ed.* Baltimore: Health Professions Press.

Feldt, K. S. (2000). Checklist of nonverbal pain indicators. *Pain Management Nursing, 1*(1), 13–21.

Geriatric Video Productions. (1998). Treatment of pain in cognitively impaired compared with cognitively intact older patients with hip fractures. http://www.geriatricvideo.com/cfdocs/archives_titles.cfm?date=01-JAN-98&end_date=01-JAN-99.

Nolta, Michele M. (2010). *Care planning cookbook for activities and recreation.* San Diego, CA: Recreation Therapy Consultants.

Harris Lord, Janice. (1988). *Beyond sympathy: What to say and do for someone suffering an injury, illness or loss.* CA: Pathfinder Publishing.

Health Care Financing Administration. (1995). *State operations manual provider certification.* Springfield, VA: U.S. Department of Commerce National Technical Information Service.

Health Care Financing Administration. *RAI training manual.* Springfield, VA: U.S. Department of Commerce National Technical Information Service.

Hockenberry, M. J., Wilson, D, Winkelstein, M. L. (2005). *Wong's essentials of pediatric nursing, ed. 7*, St. Louis: Mosby.

Hoffner, Gloria, (2016). *Going places in Northern Europe: Armchair adventures and activities.* Enumclaw, WA: Idyll Arbor.

Hohman, M. (2013). Cultural humility: A lifelong practice (blog 9/10/13). www.Socialwork.sdsu.edu.

Hook, J. N., Davis, D. E., Owen, J., Worthington Jr., E. L., & Utsey, S. O. (2013). Cultural humility: Measuring openness to culturally diverse clients. *Journal of Counseling Psychology.* doi:10.1037/a0032595

Hopkins, H. L. & Smith, H. D. (1983). *Willard and Spackman's occupational therapy, sixth edition.* New York, NY: J. B. Lippincott Company.

Hospital Service. (1919, June 30). *The Red Cross Bulletin, 3*(27), 2–3. Referenced in James, A. "The conceptual development of recreational therapy" In Brasile, F., Skalko, T. K., & burlingame, j. (1998). *Perspectives in recreational therapy: issues of a dynamic profession.* Ravensdale, WA: Idyll Arbor.

Idyll Arbor's therapy dictionary (2001). Enumclaw, WA: Idyll Arbor, Inc.

Jones, N. A., & Bullock, J. (2012). The two or more races population: 2010. 2010 Census Briefs. http://www.census.gov/prod/cen2010/briefs/c2010br-13.pdf.

Jones, Rose. 2005. *Physical activity instruction of older adults.* Champaign, IL: Human Kinetics

Kaplan, H. I., Sadock, B. J., & Grebb, J. A. (1994). *Kaplan and Sadock's synopsis of psychiatry, seventh edition.* Baltimore: Williams and Wilkins.

Karam, C. (1989). *A practical guide to cardiac rehabilitation.* Gaithersburg, MD: Aspen Publications.

Katsinas, René, 1995, *Excess disability: Recognizing the hidden problem in long-term care,* presented at the American Therapeutic Recreation Association Conference, October, 1995.

Kemp, B., Brummel-Smith, K., & Ramsdell, J. W. (1990). *Geriatric rehabilitation.* Boston, MA: College Hill Publications.

Kisner, C. & Colby, L. A. (1990). *Therapeutic exercise: Foundations and techniques, second edition.* Philadelphia, PA: F. A. Davis.

Kosnik, W., Winslow, J., Kline, D., Rasinski, K., & Sekuler, R. (1988). Visual changes in daily life throughout adulthood. *Journal of Gerontology: Psychological Sciences, 43*:63-70.

Krames Communications. (1998). *Risk management: Your role in providing quality care.* Daly City, CA: Krames Communication.

Kübler-Ross, E. (2014). *On death and dying.* New York, NY: Macmillan Publishing Co., Inc.

Lewis, C. B. (1989). *Improving mobility in older persons: A manual for geriatric specialists.* Gaithersburg, MD: Aspen Publication.

Lewis, C. S. (2015). *A grief observed.* New York, NY: Bantam Books.

Lightner, Candy & Nancy Hathaway. (1990). *Giving Sorrow Words: How to cope with grief and get on with your life.* New York: Warner Books.

MacNeil, Richard D. & Teague, Michael L. (1987). *Aging and leisure vitality in later life.* Englewood Cliffs, NJ: Prentice Hall.

Manning, Doug. (1985). *Comforting those who grieve: A guide for helping others.* New York: Harper and Row.

McKay, M., Davis, M., & Fanning, P. (1983). *Messages: The communication skills book.* Oakland, CA: New Harbinger Publications.

Milner, C. (2010). *The Journal on Active Aging, 9*(1), 8. www.icaa.cc

National Center for Assisted Living. (2000). *Assisted living move-in/move out profiles.* May 28, 2000. http://www.ncal.org/about/resident.htm

National Center for Assisted Living. (2000). *Assisted living resident profile,* May 28,

2000 web site. http://www.ncal.org/about/resident.htm

National Therapeutic Recreation Society. (1998–1999). *NTRS Report 24*(1) p.17.

Newsfronts. *Contemporary Long-term Care 21*(5), 13.

Nolta, M. M. (2007). *Album for activity compliance.* San Diego, CA: Recreation Therapy Consultants.

Nolta, M. M. (2010). *MDS 3.0 care plan cookbook.* San Diego, CA: Recreation Therapy Consultants.

Nolta, M. M. (2010). *MDS 3.0 interview guidebook section f preference for customary routine and activities.* San Diego, CA: Recreation Therapy Consultants.

Office of Disease Prevention and Health Promotion, U.S. Department of Health & Human Services. (2014). Healthy people 2020. https://www.healthypeople.gov/2020/about/foundation-health-measures/Disparities.

Ortega, R. M., & Coulborn Faller, K. (2011). Training child welfare workers from an intersectional cultural humility perspective: A paradigm shift. *Child Welfare, 90*(5), 27–49.

Panati, C. (1989). *Extraordinary origins of everyday things.* New York: William Morrow

Parker, Sandra & Will, Carol. (1993). *Activities for the elderly volume 2, a guide to working with residents with significant physical and cognitive disabilities.* Ravensdale, WA: Idyll Arbor, Inc.

Peabody, Larry. (1982). *Deskbook on writing.* Olympia, WA: Writing Services.

Randall-David, E. (1989). *Strategies for working with culturally diverse communities and clients.* Bethesda, MD: Association for the Care of Children's Health.

Reber, A. S. (1985). *Dictionary of psychology.* New York, NY: Penguin Books.

Richardson-Brown, C. & Payton, G. (1993). *CompuPlan guide.* Indianapolis, IN: Med America Corporation.

Rodman, G. P., McEwen, C., & Wallace. S. L. (1973). *Primer on the rheumatic diseases.* Reprinted from *The Journal of the American Medical Association 224, no. 5* (April 30, 1973) (Supplement).

Romney, G. O. (1945). *Off the job living.* Washington, DC: McGrath Publishing Co. and National Recreation and Park Association. Referenced in James, A. The conceptual development of recreational therapy. In Brasile, F., Skalko, T. K., & burlingame, j. (1998). *Perspectives in Recreational therapy: Issues of a dynamic profession.* Ravensdale, WA: Idyll Arbor, Inc.

Rosenbloom, A. A. & Morgan, R. W. (1986). *Vision and aging.* NY: Fairchild Publishers.

Ross, Mildred & Burdick, Dona. (1981). *Sensory integration.* Thorofare, NJ: Slack, Inc.

Rowe, J. & Kahn, R. (1999). The future of aging. *Contemporary Long-Term Care, 22*(2), 38.

Schuldberg, J., Fox, N. S., Jones, C. A., Hunter, P., Mechard, M., & Stratton, M. (2012). Same, same but different: The development of cultural humility through an international volunteer experience. *International Journal of Humanities and Social Science, 2*(17), 17–30.

Seagull, B. (2007). *Mind your mind.* New Paltz, NY: Attainment Publications

Selden, Bernice. (1989). *The story of Walt Disney.* New York: Yearling Biography.

Selye, Hans. (1976). *The stress of life, revised edition.* New York: McGraw-Hill.

Simon, P. (1971). *Play and game theory in group work: A collection of papers by Neva Leona Boyd.* Referenced in James, A. The conceptual development of recreational therapy. In Brasile, F., Skalko, T. K., & burlingame, j. (1998). *Perspectives in recreational therapy: Issues of a dynamic profession.* Ravensdale, WA: Idyll Arbor, Inc.

Spirduso, W., Francis. K., & Macrae, P. (2005). *Physical dimensions of aging.* Champaign: IL: Human Kinetics

Staudacher, Carol. (1991). *Men and grief.* Oakland, CA: New Harbinger.

Sterns, A. K. (2010). *Living Through Personal Crisis.* Enumclaw, WA: Idyll Arbor.

Tariq, S. H., Tumosa, N., Chibnall, J. T., Perry III, H. M., & Morley, J. E. (2006). Comparison of the Saint Louis University mental status examination and the mini-mental state examination for detecting dementia and mild neurocognitive disorder: A pilot study. *Am J Geriatr Psychiatry, 14*(11):900-10.

Tervalon, M. & Murray-Garcia, J. (1998). Cultural humility versus cultural competence: A critical distinction in defining physician training outcomes in multicultural education. *Journal of Health Care for the Poor and Underserved, 9*(2), 117–125.

Toglia, J. P. (1992). Cognitive rehabilitation. In Zoltan. *Vision, Perception and Cognition, Third Edition.* Thorofare, NJ: Slack.

Uniack, Ann. (2012). *Documentation in a SNAP for activity programs, fourth edition.* Enumclaw, WA: Idyll Arbor.

Uniform Data System for Medical Rehabilitation. (1997). *Guide for the uniform data set for medical rehabilitation (including the FIM® instrument). Version 5.1.* Buffalo, NY: State University at Buffalo.

U.S. Administration on Aging. (2017). *Profile of older americans: 2015 report.* www.aoa.dhhs.gov/aoa/stats/profile/default.htm

U.S. Department of Health and Human Services. (1983). *CDC guidelines for isolation precautions in hospitals and cdc guidelines for infection control in hospital personnel.* Atlanta, GA: Centers for Disease Control.

Voelkl, J. E. (1988). *Risk management in therapeutic recreation: A component of quality assurance.* State College, PA: Venture Publishing.

Wallace, S., Levy-Storms, L, Kington, R., & Andersen, R. (1998). The persistence of race and ethnicity in the use of long-term care. *Journal of Gerontology: Social Sciences 53B*(2), S104-S112.

Weaver, G. R. (1986). Understanding and coping with cross-cultural adjustment stress. In R. M. Paige (Ed.), *Cross-cultural orientation, new conceptualizations and applications.* Lanham, MD: University Press of America.

Williams, J. M. (1987). *Cognitive stimulation in the home environment: The rehabilitation of cognitive disabilities.* New York, NY: Center for Applied Psychological Research, Memphis State University. Plenum Press.

Zoltan, Barbara. (1996). *Vision, perception and cognition: A manual for evaluation and treatment of the neurologically impaired adult, third edition.* Thorofare, NJ: Slack.

Zoltan, Barbara, Siev, Ellen, & Freishtat, Brenda. (1986). *The adult stroke patient: A manual for evaluation and treatment of perceptual and cognitive dysfunction.* Thorofare, NJ: Slack.

Index

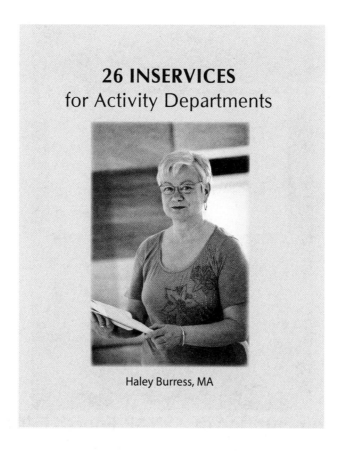

26 Inservices for Activity Departments

Haley Burress, 2016

Activity directors everywhere are searching for a way to get their staff, and the nursing staff, on board with activities. *26 Inservices for Activity Departments* will let you demonstrate your knowledge and credibility. It is your key to inspiring and empowering staff throughout your facility.

Without adding extra prep time to your already busy workload, *26 Inservices for Activity Departments* gives you the tools you need to make your staff meetings the most exciting part of your month.

The book includes 26 lesson plans for training sessions that last 30-60 minutes each. Many of the sessions are appropriate for more than your activities staff. They can be offered to nursing and other staff in your community to increase the cooperation between departments. Many suggest co-presentations with the heads of other departments.

The book includes:

- Easy to prepare inservice presentations for your staff
- Topics from safety on outings to federal regulations, appropriate for all levels of senior care.
- Sign in sheets and inservice descriptions that you can quickly file with human resources.
- Presentations that range from lecture and activities to scavenger hunts and observation tools.

Handouts or quizzes that the lesson plans require are included in the book for the Directors to copy and have them available for participants. *26 Inservices for Activity Departments* can be used by Directors in skilled nursing, assisted living, or independent living settings.

Item B710 Trade Paper, 120 pages $24.00 ISBN 9781611580426

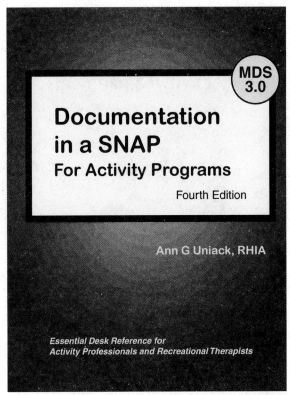

Documentation in a SNAP, Fourth Edition

Ann G. Uniack, 2012

This latest edition explains electronic records and security of health information for electronic records, faxes, and email. It also has everything you need to know about MDS 3.0 and recent changes to the survey process. Whether you are a new student or an experienced therapist who works in a nursing home, this book will help you improve your documentation and data security skills.

The purpose of this book is to create a system of documentation that supports the delivery of resident care. The clinical record may be either handwritten or electronic, but its purpose is to provide the activity professional with information to:

- assess each resident's needs
- develop a plan of care
- establish goals to be achieved and outcomes expected
- document interventions
- evaluate the success or need for revision of the care plan

Throughout this book you will find references specific to activity programs in nursing facilities and other situations that fall under OBRA guidelines. Federal regulations with interpretive guidelines and sections of the Resident Assessment Instrument (RAI) Version 3.0 Manual that describe documentation requirements are included. One can't play the game without knowing the rules.

Information is the key to meeting residents' needs. Health professionals turn to the clinical record for that information. Whether paper based or computerized, in order for the clinical record to be useful, accurate, and easy to find, documentation must be available for staff to make decisions for resident care.

In other words, DOCUMENTATION must be a SNAP! And this book shows you how.

Item B628 Trade Paper, 224 pages $42.00 ISBN 9781882883936

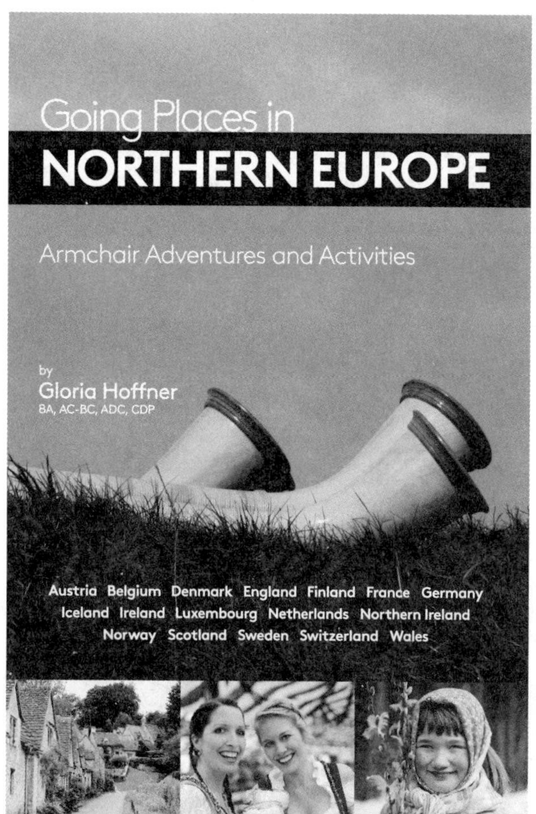

Going Places in Northern Europe: Armchair Adventures and Activities

Gloria Hoffner, 2016

Activity directors live and work in a multicultural world with residents, clients, and staff from many different places on the globe. A travel program allows activity staff to connect with the memories of residents who lived in other countries, have friends or relatives overseas, or who enjoyed traveling in their youth. It can even help improve connections between staff who may have been born in a foreign land and the residents they serve.

Each chapter in this book discusses one of 17 countries in Northern Europe. Each chapter covers the country's geography, language, national holidays, history, travel options, American roots, music and dance, food, and customs. Trivia questions for residents to answer are scattered throughout. DVD and online video suggestions for showing images and culture are included for each country.

This book is designed to be used for a travel activity lasting one hour, one day, or one week, and spread over daily, weekly, monthly, or annual sessions. It can provide new ways to celebrate special events, such as holidays including St. Patrick's Day and Bastille Day.

In addition, each chapter's Game section includes a fun and easy traditional game and a list of the cognitive and physical benefits of participation as outlined by the International Classification of Functioning, Disability, and Health (ICF) and by the guidelines of the International Classification of Health Interventions (ICHI).

Austria, Belgium, Denmark, England, Finland, France, Germany, Iceland, Ireland, Luxembourg, Netherlands, Northern Ireland, Norway, Scotland, Sweden, Switzerland, Wales.

Item B705 Trade Paper, 368 pages $24.00 ISBN 9781882883981

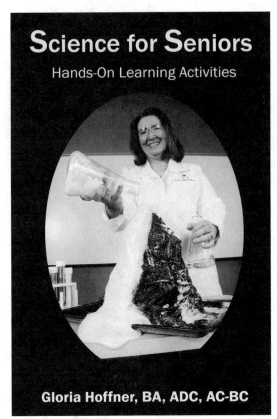

Science for Seniors: Hands-On Learning Activities

Gloria Hoffner, 2012

Science for Seniors shows activity leaders how to provide stimulating science activities that provide both entertainment and enlightenment as part of a life-long learning process.

Written in an informative and easy-to-follow style, *Science for Seniors* gives you basic science information and hands-on programs that any activity director or therapist can use with seniors of all intellectual and physical abilities.

Some of the topics covered in the book are volcanoes, oceans, global warming, rain forests, and outer space. With each subject, *Science for Seniors* provides step-by-step directions using ordinary household items such as eggs, water, baking soda, and salt. In addition to the hands-on activities, *Science for Seniors* provides with science trivia, questions to spark conversations, resource material, and opportunities for further study.

Gloria Hoffner is an award-winning and nationally certified activity consultant and a former journalist with the *Philadelphia Inquirer*, where she wrote frequently about science and seniors.

She is the founder of Guitar with Gloria and Science for Seniors, a national company that provides activity programs at communities in Pennsylvania, Delaware, and New Jersey.

The Science for Seniors program earned her a first place award in the 2010 National Certification Council of Activity Professionals' "Best Practice" award division. The award recognized Science for Seniors as the most outstanding new activity program design among retirement, assisted living, personal care, long-term care, and adult day center facilities.

Hoffner is also a frequent speaker at national and statewide conventions for professionals in the healthcare, activity, and certified therapeutic recreation fields.

Item B619 Trade Paper, 288 pages $28.00 ISBN 9781882883776

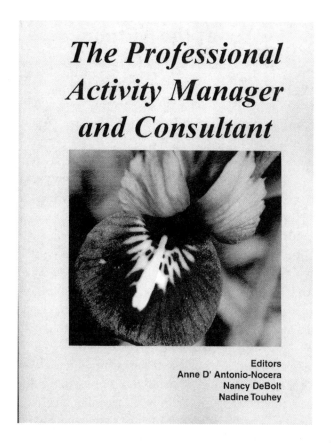

The Professional Activity Manager and Consultant

Edited by Anne D'Antonio-Nocera, Nancy DeBolt, and Nadine Touhey, 1996

This is the reference book that every manager or consultant needs to have! Whether you are a recreational therapist, activity professional, occupational therapist, or other type of therapist, this book provides you with hands-on instruction to excel at your job as a manager or consultant. The forty-two chapters are divided into ten sections: Introduction to Management and Consulting, Competency and Ethical Issues, Regulatory Issues, The Facility, Staffing, Adult Learning, Evaluation, Overview of Consulting, Consulting Techniques, and Managing a Consulting Business. The book contains many ready-made forms, checklists for quality assurance, and other quick reference sections.

Item B297 Trade Paper, Reproducible Forms, 452 pages $45.00 ISBN 9781882883240

About the Authors

Elizabeth (Betsy) Best-Martini

Elizabeth (Betsy) Best-Martini is a Recreational Therapist specializing in the field of gerontology. She has a Master of Science degree in Recreation Therapy / Administration. She is also a certified Caner Exercise Specialist.

Her consulting firm, *Recreation Consultation & Fit For Life* has provided recreational therapy consultation to over 200 retirement communities, skilled nursing settings, sub-acute settings, and residential/assisted care facilities in Northern California. Betsy has trained over 800 qualified activity professionals in Northern California.

In addition she provides one-to-one recreational therapy to clients needing assistance and assessment in the areas of physical activity. Betsy is a well-known presenter at national and state conferences for activity professionals and recreational therapists. She has been an academy faculty member of the American Therapeutic Recreation Association.

Her three publications are being used nationally and throughout Canada as training manuals for Activity Professionals and Recreational Therapists: *Long-Term Care 7th Edition, Exercise for Frail Elders,* and *Quality Assurance for Activity Programs.*

Betsy is a certified fitness instructor through the Senior Fitness Association. She writes a fitness column called "Let's Get Moving" for *Creative Forecasting*. She teaches two strength-training classes with older adults weekly in addition to teaching a certification class for students interested in becoming fitness instructors with frail elders and adults with special needs. She also provides training in Exercise for Frail Elders and Adults with Special Needs.

When enjoying her own leisure, she can be found gardening, hiking, exercising, and spending time with her husband, family, and many pets.

Mary Anne Weeks

Mary Anne Weeks has worked as a Social Worker (SSC) in nursing facilities since November of 1982. At that time, few facilities in California had yet realized a need for such a discipline so there were no "rules." Fortunately, Mary Anne had long ago, in 1965, worked as a summer intern in a prototype retirement home in Rochester, New York. Her past experience in this setting with various levels of care made the environment in nursing settings more familiar to her.

In the meantime, she had also received an undergraduate degree from the State University of New York, Genesee and pursued graduate work at University of California, Berkeley where she completed her Master Degree in Public Health.

Mary Anne lives in Sonoma, California, with her husband and two children. She is a Social Service Consultant in the specialty area of social services and is a lecturer at the community college level.

Priscilla Wirth

Priscilla Wirth is a Health Information Consultant for long-term care facilities. She is a Registered Health Information Administrator, receiving her degree from Seattle University. She has been in the health information profession since 1980.

Her Bachelor of Science degree and Master of Library Sciences were received from Northern Illinois University. Priscilla is currently practicing in Sonoma County, California, and is a member of the American Medical Record Association, the California Health Information Association, and the Network of Health Record Consultants. She is a lecturer at the community college level.